CLINICAL SLEEP MEDICINE

A Comprehensive Guide for Mental Health and Other Medical Professionals

Edited by

Emmanuel H. During, M.D.
Clete A. Kushida, M.D., Ph.D.

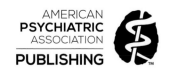

AMERICAN
PSYCHIATRIC
ASSOCIATION
PUBLISHING

If you wish to buy 50 or more copies of the same title, please go to www.appi.org/specialdiscounts for more information.

Copyright © 2021 American Psychiatric Association Publishing

ALL RIGHTS RESERVED

First Edition

Manufactured in the United States of America on acid-free paper
25 24 23 22 21   5 4 3 2 1

American Psychiatric Association Publishing
800 Maine Avenue SW, Suite 900
Washington, DC 20024-2812
www.appi.org

Library of Congress Cataloging-in-Publication Data
Names: During, Emmanuel H., 1976– editor. | Kushida, Clete Anthony, 1960– editor. | American Psychiatric Association Publishing, publisher.
Title: Clinical sleep medicine : a comprehensive guide for mental health and other medical professionals / edited by Emmanuel H. During, Clete A. Kushida.
Description: First edition. | Washington, DC : American Psychiatric Association Publishing, [2021] | Includes bibliographical references and index.
Identifiers: LCCN 2020023156 (print) | LCCN 2020023157 (ebook) | ISBN 9781615373000 (paperback ; alk. paper) | ISBN 9781615373161 (ebook)
Subjects: MESH: Sleep Wake Disorders | Mental Disorders | Mental Health Classification: LCC RC547 (print) | LCC RC547 (ebook) | NLM WL 108 | DDC 616.8/498—dc23
LC record available at https://lccn.loc.gov/2020023156
LC ebook record available at https://lccn.loc.gov/2020023157

British Library Cataloguing in Publication Data
A CIP record is available from the British Library.

CLINICAL SLEEP MEDICINE

A Comprehensive Guide for
Mental Health and
Other Medical Professionals

Contents

Contributors

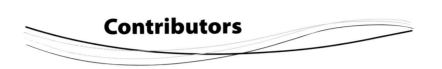

William Auyeung, M.D.
Stanford Center for Sleep Sciences and Medicine, Department of Psychiatry and Behavioral Sciences, Stanford University Medical Center, Palo Alto, California

Alon Y. Avidan, M.D., M.P.H.
Professor, Department of Neurology; Director, Sleep Disorders Center; and Chair, Faculty Executive Committee, David Geffen School of Medicine, University of California–Los Angeles, Los Angeles, California

Fiona Barwick, Ph.D., D.B.S.M.
Clinical Assistant Professor, Department of Psychiatry and Behavioral Sciences, Division of Sleep Medicine, Stanford University School of Medicine, Redwood City, California

Daniel Jin Blum, Ph.D.
Adjunct Clinical Instructor, Stanford University School of Medicine, Department of Psychiatry and Behavioral Sciences, Redwood City, California

Julia Buchfuhrer, D.O.
University of California–Irvine, Irvine, California

Mark Buchfuhrer, M.D.
Stanford University School of Medicine, Stanford, California

Michelle Cao, D.O.
Stanford Center for Sleep Sciences and Medicine, Department of Psychiatry and Behavioral Sciences, Stanford University Medical Center, Palo Alto, California

Joss Cohen, M.D.
Fellow, Department of Neurology, Cedars-Sinai Medical Center, Los Angeles, California

Emmanuel H. During, M.D.
Clinical Associate Professor, Department of Psychiatry and Behavioral Sciences–Division of Sleep Medicine and Department of Neurology and Neurological Sciences, Stanford University; Director, Stanford Parasomnia Clinic, Redwood City, California

Payal Kenia Gu, M.D.
Assistant Professor, Children's Hospital Los Angeles, Los Angeles, California

Christian Guilleminault, M.D.
Professor, Stanford Center for Sleep Sciences and Medicine, Department of Psychiatry and Behavioral Sciences, Stanford University Medical Center, Palo Alto, California

Birgit Högl, M.D.
Professor of Neurology and Sleep Medicine, Medical University of Innsbruck, Innsbruck, Austria

Michael J. Howell, M.D.
Associate Professor of Neurology, University of Minnesota, Minneapolis, Minnesota

Muna Irfan, M.D.
Assistant Professor of Neurology, University of Minnesota, Minneapolis Veterans Affair Medical Center, Minneapolis, Minnesota

Clete A. Kushida, M.D., Ph.D.
Division Chief and Medical Director, Stanford Sleep Medicine; Director, Stanford Center for Human Sleep Research; Professor, Department of Psychiatry and Behavioral Sciences, Stanford University Medical Center, Stanford University, California

Caroline Maness, M.D.
Neurology Resident, Emory Sleep Center and Department of Neurology, Emory University School of Medicine, Atlanta, Georgia

Mari Matsumura, M.P.H.
Sleep and Circadian Neurobiology Laboratory, Department of Psychiatry and Behavioral Sciences, Stanford University School of Medicine, Stanford, California

David N. Neubauer, M.D.
Associate Professor, Department of Psychiatry and Behavioral Sciences, Johns Hopkins University School of Medicine, Baltimore, Maryland

Seiji Nishino, M.D., Ph.D.
Sleep and Circadian Neurobiology Laboratory, Department of Psychiatry and Behavioral Sciences, Stanford University School of Medicine, Stanford, California

Taisuke Ono, M.D., Ph.D.
Sleep and Circadian Neurobiology Laboratory, Department of Psychiatry and Behavioral Sciences, Stanford University School of Medicine, Stanford, California

Daniella Palermo, M.D.
Clinical Instructor, Psychiatry and Human Behavior, Alpert Medical School of Brown University/Rhode Island Hospital, Providence, Rhode Island

Carlos H. Schenck, M.D.
Professor of Psychiatry, University of Minnesota, Minnesota Regional Sleep Disorders Center, Minneapolis, Minnesota

Logan Schneider, M.D.
Staff Neurologist, Stanford/VA Alzheimer's Research Center, VA Palo Alto Health Care System, Palo Alto; Clinical Assistant Professor (affiliated), Stanford Sleep Medicine Center, Redwood City, California

Katherine M. Sharkey, M.D., Ph.D., FAASM
Associate Professor, Medicine and Psychiatry and Human Behavior, Sleep for Science Research Laboratory, Alpert Medical School of Brown University/Rhode Island Hospital, Providence, Rhode Island

Gaurav Singh, M.D., M.P.H.
Staff Physician, Pulmonary, Critical Care, and Sleep Medicine Section, Veterans Affairs Palo Alto Health Care System, Palo Alto, California; Clinical Assistant Professor (affiliated), Division of Pulmonary, Allergy, and Critical Care Medicine, Stanford University, Palo Alto, California

Ambra Stefani, M.D.
Department of Neurology, Medical University of Innsbruck, Innsbruck, Austria

Lynn Marie Trotti, M.D., M.Sc.
Associate Professor of Neurology, Emory Sleep Center and Department of Neurology, Emory University School of Medicine, Atlanta, Georgia

Chester Wu, M.D.
The Menninger Clinic, Department of Psychiatry and Behavioral Sciences, Baylor College of Medicine, Houston, Texas

Jamie M. Zeitzer, Ph.D.
Associate Professor, Stanford University School of Medicine, Department of Psychiatry and Behavioral Sciences, Stanford Center for Sleep Sciences and Medicine, Palo Alto, California

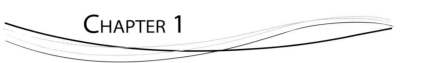

CHAPTER 1

Introduction

SLEEP DISORDERS AND MENTAL HEALTH

Emmanuel H. During, M.D.

The importance of sleep for well-being and general and mental health is increasingly being recognized. Sleep complaints are commonly associated with mental disorders and are even part of the diagnostic criteria for some, such as mood and anxiety disorders and PTSD. The relationship between sleep and psychiatric disorders is intertwined and, in some cases, bidirectional. Anxiety, psychosis, and depression often result in reduced sleep quality (sleep fragmentation, experience of unpleasant, unrefreshing sleep), quantity (increased or reduced), or pattern (changes in sleep schedule, loss of sleep consistency). Reciprocally, sleep disorders can contribute to the exacerbation of psychiatric symptoms and independently affect the prognosis. Finally, most psychotropic drugs have an effect on sleep and arousal and can aggravate a preexisting sleep abnormality.

This chapter aims to familiarize readers with current knowledge on the mutual effects of sleep and mental health and provide an integrated framework for students, clinicians, and researchers. It also serves as an introduction to this book, which covers throughout its 18 chapters the six main categories of sleep disorders: insomnia (Chapters 3–5), hypersomnia (Chapters 6–7), sleep-disordered breathing (Chapters 8–11), circadian disorders (Chapters 12–13), parasomnias (Chapters 14–16), and sleep-related movement disorders (Chapters 17–18).

Psychiatric Disorders and Sleep Disturbances

MAJOR DEPRESSIVE DISORDER

Sleep disturbances are associated with up to 90% cases of major depressive disorder (MDD) and can include insomnia and hypersomnia—two diagnostic criteria for MDD—as well as reduced sleep quality and nightmares (American Psychiatric Association 2013). Contrary to the depressive phase of bipolar disorder, often associated with hypersomnia, in MDD, insomnia is more common than hypersomnia. Conversely, patients with one of these complaints are about 10 times more likely to have MDD than are individuals who are satisfied with their sleep (Breslau et al. 1996; Ford and Kamerow 1989). Similarly, difficulty falling asleep and other symptoms of insomnia are associated with a two- to fivefold increased risk of developing depression at follow-up (Baglioni et al. 2011; Szklo-Coxe et al. 2010). Early morning insomnia is often considered a pathognomonic sign of depression, and the presence of insomnia during an episode of MDD is associated with a worse outcome (Minkel et al. 2017). Other sleep disorders, such as restless legs syndrome (RLS) or underlying obstructive sleep apnea (OSA) increase the risk of a mood disorder if left untreated (Earley and Silber 2010; Sharafkhaneh et al. 2005).

Polysomnographic studies consistently show changes in subjects with depression: increased sleep fragmentation, reduced slow-wave sleep (SWS) duration and delta power (14 Hz electroencephalographic activity), and increased REM sleep duration, with reduced sleep-to–REM onset latency, prolonged first REM sleep period, and increased eye movement density (number of rapid eye movements per minute of REM sleep). Among these changes, shortened REM latency and reduced SWS may be trait markers because they are present even between depressive episodes (Krystal 2012). REM sleep changes can also be found in asymptomatic subjects with a strong family history of depression and could therefore be an endophenotype for depressive disorder (Lauer et al. 1995).

Complaints of hypersomnia are often associated with so-called atypical depression, as well as with daytime fatigue and increased appetite. In MDD, hypersomnia appears to be more subjective than objective because it is usually not corroborated by objective findings of increased total sleep time (TST) on polysomnography or reduced sleep latency (time needed to fall asleep) on multiple sleep latency test (MSLT)—the gold-standard procedure for the evaluation of sleepiness (Nofzinger et al. 1991). The same is true of seasonal affective disorder. These differences distinguish complaints of hypersomnia associated with MDD from narcolepsy and "idiopathic hypersomnia" (see Chapters 6 and 7, respectively).

Complete sleep deprivation over only one night has dramatic antidepressant effects in most patients (Wirz-Justice and Van den Hoofdakker 1999). This effect may be mediated by brain-derived neurotrophic factor (Giese et al. 2014). Unfortunately, the therapeutic benefit of a single night of sleep deprivation abates as soon as sleep is restored, even if limited in duration (Wiegand et al. 1987). Attempts to artificially suppress REM sleep in the lab over several weeks, an effect observed with antidepressant drugs (due to their serotonergic, noradrenergic, and anticholinergic effects), have led to inconsistent results (Vogel et al. 1975). Bright light therapy proved to be useful in the treatment of seasonal affective disorder and may also have some utility in the treatment of MDD (Partonen and Lönnqvist 1998).

Approximately one-third of patients with MDD continue to experience sleep disturbances despite treatment of their depression (Krystal 2012). Such symptoms are associated with worse outcome, lower rate of remission, and slower recovery, with an increased risk of relapse in addition to the persistence of daytime symptoms of fatigue, excessive daytime sleepiness, and cognitive complaints (Dew et al. 1997; McCall et al. 2000; Reynolds et al. 1997). Sleep symptoms are also associated with increased suicidality and completed suicide, independent of MDD severity, based on several studies performed across age, ethnic, and cultural groups (Krystal 2012). As a proof of concept, most studies simultaneously treating mood symptoms and comorbid insomnia with pharmacotherapy or cognitive-behavioral therapy for insomnia have resulted in better outcomes in terms of not only sleep but also depression (Krystal 2012). The benefits on mood may be related to specific hypnotic drugs. For instance, eszopiclone may confer a benefit in terms of mood symptoms that has not been observed with extended-release zolpidem (Fava et al. 2011). Pharmacological and behavioral treatments of insomnia are topics covered in Chapters 4 and 5.

BIPOLAR DISORDER

Sleep is even more disturbed in bipolar disorder than in MDD. Reduced need for sleep is one of the diagnostic criteria for manic episodes; however, this symptom can be misinterpreted as insomnia (American Psychiatric Association 2013). If an individual has reduced sleep needs but spends the same amount of time in bed, he or she will spend less time sleeping and experience more sleep fragmentation (Wehr et al. 1987). The main difference from insomnia is that in mania, reduced sleep duration is not associated with reduced quality of life or daytime functioning. During the depressive phase of bipolar disorder, the complaint of hypersomnia is more common than that of insomnia, although both may alternate. However, as also seen in the case of MDD, this complaint is subjective—that is, not corroborated by polysomnography and MSLT (Nofzinger et al. 1991).

Sleep duration is reduced in mania; however, other changes during an acute episode are similar to those observed in MDD, including reduced SWS, reduced REM sleep latency, and increased eye movement density.

Manic episodes can be triggered by sleep deprivation in individuals with bipolar disorder (Wehr 1991). The mechanism remains unknown but could be related to the robust mood elevation observed after a single night of sleep deprivation in individuals with depression. The deleterious effect of sleep loss on mood stability and the natural observation that manic episodes contribute to sleep loss, which may in turn exacerbate mania, have practical implications. Lengthening sleep time can be used to treat and prevent mania.

In bipolar disorder, sleep disturbances are not limited to decompensation episodes. During periods of euthymia, as many as 70% of patients with bipolar disorder have sleep disturbance and 55% meet diagnostic criteria for insomnia (Harvey et al. 2005). Patients also report more daytime sleepiness on the Epworth Sleepiness Scale compared with control subjects (St-Amand et al. 2013). In some cases, these could presage a depressive relapse, because one study found that hypersomnia correlates with depressive symptoms at 6 months (Kaplan et al. 2011).

Sleep disturbances in bipolar disorder are not limited to insomnia and hypersomnia. Several studies have suggested that circadian disturbances may be a core mechanism triggering and perpetuating mood instability and cycling. Sleep disturbances may be prodromal symptoms of bipolar disorder in children (Anderson and Bradley 2013). Some actigraphy studies suggest patients with bipolar disorder have a tendency to experience delayed sleep phase (evening type) and greater variability in sleep patterns. This is, however, contradicted by findings of other possible circadian abnormalities (advanced sleep phase, irregular sleep-wake cycles) or only a few abnormalities on actigraphy-based studies (Anderson and Bradley 2013). Studies show patients with bipolar disorder have reduced melatonin secretion with reduced circadian amplitude, including reduced evening peaks of melatonin and increased sensitivity of melatonin levels to light (Nurnberger et al. 2000). This could be due to lower activity of N-acetylserotonin O-methyltransferase, an enzyme involved in melatonin synthesis (Etain et al. 2012). Supporting the hypothesis that reduced melatonin drive could contribute to mood instability, treatments with melatonin agonists such as ramelteon and agomelatine—a drug not available in the United States—have shown to be beneficial in patients with bipolar depression (Norris et al. 2013). Nonpharmacological interventions, including chronotherapy using light or dark therapy or social rhythms to synchronize biological rhythms, have also shown to be helpful in bipolar disorder (Anderson and Bradley 2013).

Sleep-disordered breathing has not been systematically studied in bipolar disorder but can result in sleep fragmentation and sleep debt as a result of reduced sleep quality. One study found a high risk of OSA in 54% of patients with bipolar I disorder based on a self-assessment tool (Soreca et al. 2012).

GENERALIZED ANXIETY DISORDER

Among anxiety disorders, the relation between generalized anxiety disorder (GAD) and sleep has been the most studied. One of the core features of GAD is a complaint of insomnia. Difficulty falling or staying asleep—that is, initiation or maintenance insomnia—manifests in more than half of patients with this disorder (Krystal 2012). Conversely, insomnia is associated with a twofold increased risk of developing anxiety disorders later in life (Breslau et al. 1996). In contrast to isolated insomnia, which is characterized by worrying about sleep quality, in GAD, anxiety focuses on other matters. Anxiety-provoking dreams are another frequent complaint associated with anxiety disorders.

Polysomnographic studies in GAD show increased sleep latency, greater number of arousals, and more waking after sleep onset. Patients with GAD have reduced SWS and a relative increase in stage N1 sleep, which is consistent with self-perception of a lighter sleep (Fuller et al. 1997). Unlike mood disorders, no changes in REM architecture are observed in GAD.

Treatment of insomnia results in better outcomes in GAD; however, the therapeutic benefit in GAD may vary according to the hypnotic agent used. For instance, trials using eszopiclone versus extended-release zolpidem combined with escitalopram resulted in improved outcomes on anxiety only with eszopiclone (Fava et al. 2009; Pollack et al. 2008). Similar results were found when testing combination treatments in insomnia and MDD.

POSTTRAUMATIC STRESS DISORDER

Recurrent distressing dreams related to a traumatic event and difficulty with falling or staying asleep are part of the diagnostic criteria in

PTSD (American Psychiatric Association 2013), and sleep complaints in general are found in nearly all patients with PTSD (Ross et al. 1989). Trauma-related flashbacks and hallucinations around sleep are common in PTSD, as well as sleep talking, excessive movements during sleep, and dream-enactment-like phenomena that can mimic REM sleep behavior disorder (RBD), especially in combat veterans (see Chapter 15). Differentiating between PTSD-related nocturnal behaviors and RBD dream enactment requires polysomnography to determine whether REM atonia is preserved (in PTSD) or lost (in RBD). Differentiating PTSD from RBD can be challenging, because both disorders share common clinical features, and a subset of patients with trauma-associated nocturnal behaviors can present with a loss of normal REM atonia. This rare condition, reported in young adults after combat, was coined "trauma-associated sleep disorder" (Rachakonda et al. 2018). Insomnia can develop due to a fear of sleeping and experiencing nightmares as well as a general hyperarousal and hypervigilant state in PTSD, which is thought to be related to heightened noradrenergic tone (Berridge et al. 2012).

Polysomnographic studies in PTSD show reduced SWS and REM sleep but increased eye movement density during REM, with increased REM-related arousals. They less consistently show reduced TST and increased sleep fragmentation (Krystal 2012), although these are common complaints in patients with PTSD. The same disconnect between subjective experience and objective findings can be seen in patients with insomnia, a phenomenon known as "paradoxical insomnia."

Daytime and nighttime sleep complaints before deployment predict future onset of PTSD and depression, according to a large prospective longitudinal study in soldiers (Koffel et al. 2013). Studies show that the treatment of sleep symptoms with pharmacotherapy (eszopiclone, prazosin) or behavioral therapy is associated with a reduction of daytime PTSD symptoms (Krystal 2012). Whether this result is merely a consequence of improved sleep or due to specific action on PTSD is unclear. The α_1-adrenergic antagonist prazosin has been widely used to reduce daytime symptoms of PTSD and PTSD-related nightmares when taken at bedtime; however, its efficacy on sleep symptoms could not be confirmed in a recent, larger randomized controlled study (Raskind et al. 2018).

SCHIZOPHRENIA

Although sleep disturbances are not among the core symptoms of schizophrenia, they are common in this disorder. Schizophrenia is associated with a reduced need for sleep, daytime sleepiness, and insomnia, which can be severe during the acute phase of the illness. Nightmares and frightening dreams are often reported in schizophrenia. Some studies have reported circadian abnormalities in individuals with schizophrenia, with a tendency to experience a reversed sleep-wake cycle (i.e., being awake during the night and sleeping during the day) (Hofstetter et al. 2003; Martin et al. 2005). Sleep-disordered breathing and RLS/periodic limb movement (PLM) are also overrepresented in schizophrenia, which can be due to the iatrogenic effects of psychotropic treatments as well as to alcohol and illicit drugs (Kalucy et al. 2013). As discussed later, benzodiazepines increase upper airway collapsibility and thus the risk of OSA via muscle relaxation (see Chapter 8), and most antipsychotic drugs increase the risk of RLS/PLM (see Chapter 17).

As in other psychiatric disorders, the relationship between sleep abnormalities and clinical relapse n schizophrenia may be bidirectional. Sleep disturbances are common findings in the weeks to months preceding psychotic exacerbations in patients with schizophrenia; however, it is unclear whether these abnormalities are early manifestations of clinical relapse or contribute to psychotic decompensation (Krystal 2012).

Polysomnographic studies in schizophrenia have shown a number of abnormalities, most of which are shared with other psychiatric disorders: increased sleep fragmentation, decreased amount of SWS with reduced delta power (reduced amplitude of slow oscillations in stage 3 non-REM sleep), and reduced REM sleep, REM sleep latency, and eye movement density in REM sleep when untreated (Krystal 2012). Among these abnormalities, some studies suggest that increased sleep fragmentation correlates with positive symptoms of schizophrenia (hallucinations, delusions, disorganized thoughts) and reduced SWS density with negative symptoms (affective blunting, aboulia, alogia).

Psychotropic Drugs and Sleep

Most psychotropic drugs have consequences on sleep and wake states, ranging from insomnia and disturbed sleep to excessive daytime sedation, nightmares, dream enactment, RLS, and sleep-disordered breathing. These effects vary according to medication class and specific pharmacological profiles and are summarized in Table 1–1.

ANTIDEPRESSANTS

Due to their serotonergic or noradrenergic and anticholinergic effects, most antidepressants inhibit REM sleep, which manifests in prolonged REM sleep latency and overall reduced REM sleep duration. The thera-

TABLE 1–1.   Relation between psychotropic drugs and sleep disturbances

	Antidepressants	Anxiolytics	Antipsychotics
Insomnia	Most (nonsedating) antidepressants can disrupt sleep.	β-Blockers inhibit melatonin release and can cause insomnia.	
Hypersomnia	Sedative antidepressants (mirtazapine, trazodone, amitriptyline, nortriptyline) can cause sleepiness; bupropion, desipramine, and MAOIs can reduce hypersomnia.	Benzodiazepines cause sedation.	Most antipsychotic drugs are sedative.
Sleep-disordered breathing		Benzodiazepines increase risk of OSA via upper airway muscle relaxation.	Antipsychotic drugs that result in weight gain increase risk of OSA.
Parasomnia	Serotonergic and anticholinergic drugs can trigger or worsen RBD (potentially injurious dream enactment); REM sleep rebound and excessive/vivid dreams can occur upon cessation of most antidepressants.	β-Blockers can cause nightmares.	
Sleep-related movement disorders	Serotonergic and antihistaminic agents can trigger or worsen RLS.		Antidopaminergic drugs can trigger or worsen RLS, which must be distinguished from akathisia.

Note.   MAOIs=monoamine oxidase inhibitors; OSA=obstructive sleep apnea; RBD=REM sleep behavior disorder; RLS=restless legs syndrome.

peutic effect of these drugs may, to some extent, be related to this outcome, because selective REM suppression protocols in the laboratory setting can yield clinical benefit of similar magnitude (Vogel et al. 1975). Few antidepressants, including mirtazapine, trazodone, and doxepin, promote both SWS density (slow wave amplitudes) and duration (Krystal 2012).

TST varies across drugs, according to their class and individual properties. For instance, when considering tricyclic antidepressants (TCAs) as a class, amitriptyline, nortriptyline, and clomipramine result in sleep consolidation and increased TST, but most other TCAs, especially desipramine, and monoamine oxidase inhibitors can be activating and used as mild stimulants, thus potentially contributing to insomnia. More commonly prescribed, most selective serotonin reuptake inhibitors (SSRIs) and serotonin-norepinephrine reuptake inhibitors (SNRIs) result in insomnia at a rate of up to three times that of placebo (Lam et al. 1990). Among the SSRIs, however, citalopram has a lower rate of treatment-emergent insomnia, whereas fluvoxamine has a higher rate (about 30%) and can also result in daytime sedation.

Bupropion holds a unique place due to its different pharmacological mechanism—dopamine and norepinephrine reuptake inhibition—with an overall mild but consistent activating effect. Bupropion is often used off-label by sleep specialists to reduce excessive daytime sleepiness and can result in difficulty with sleep onset if it is taken later in the day. This unique mechanism of action is shared with a newer agent, solriamfetol, which has been approved for the indication of excessive daytime sleepiness in narcolepsy and residual sleepiness associated with OSA despite treatment.

Low-dose doxepin (3–6 mg) is the only antidepressant approved by the FDA for the treatment of insomnia and promotes sleep via selective histamine (H_1) blockade. Sedative TCAs (amitriptyline, nortriptyline), trazodone, and mirtazapine also promote sleep via H_1 but also via serotonin-2A ($5\text{-}HT_{2A}$) receptor blockade (see Chapter 4).

Due to their serotonergic properties, all TCAs, SSRIs, and SNRIs can result in a new onset or exacerbation of RLS symptoms or PLMs, as observed on polysomnogram (Hoque and Chesson 2010; see Chapter 17). This is a higher concern with antidepressants that have antihistamine properties (H_1 antagonists), such as mirtazapine, or with low-dose doxepin. Treatment-induced RLS can occur in up to 28% of patients taking mirtazapine (Rottach et al. 2008). Preexisting or new symptoms of RLS should ideally be screened in patients prescribed these drugs, especially if a complaint of insomnia paradoxically worsens despite their use.

Dream recall can be reduced with certain TCAs but not typically with SSRIs and SNRIs. Cessation of antidepressant treatments, especially if abrupt, can result in significant REM sleep rebound and exacerbation of unpleasant vivid dreams or nightmares (Wilson and Argyropoulos 2005). Importantly, as many as 6% of patients treated with antidepressants can experience abnormal dream enactment during REM sleep, also known as RBD (see Chapter 15) (Teman et al. 2009). This condition can lead to serious injuries to self and bed partners and in many adult cases can progress to a neurodegenerative disorder, sometimes after decades (Bodkin 2018; Högl et al. 2018; Postuma et al. 2013). This side effect is likely due to the serotonergic properties of antidepressants and is characterized on polysomnography by increased chin and limb electromyographic activity during REM sleep instead of the normal muscle atonia that usually defines this stage of sleep.

MOOD STABILIZERS

Data are limited for most newer agents used for mood stabilization. Lithium is associated with increased SWS and, like antidepressants, REM sleep inhibition.

ANXIOLYTICS

Benzodiazepine drugs produce a sedative effect via activation of the $GABA_A$ receptor (see Chapter 4). Although often used to improve sleep quality and reduce sleep fragmentation, benzodiazepines reduce SWS and increase in proportion the amount of stage N2 sleep, a lighter stage of sleep. They also increase sleep spindle activity. Benzodiazepines can potentially aggravate any underlying OSA via relaxation of the upper airway dilator muscles (see Chapter 8).

β-Blockers, which are sometimes used to treat event-related (performance) anxiety, are known to inhibit melatonin production via inhibition of adrenergic $β_1$ receptors. β-Blockers reduce SWS and REM sleep and can provoke disturbed sleep, nightmares, and insomnia.

ANTIPSYCHOTICS

Most antipsychotic drugs can have sedative effects, which can be used to consolidate sleep and reduce sleep complaints. The agents found to have lower rates of daytime sedation (less than 30%) are quetiapine, ziprasidone, and aripiprazole, whereas those with higher rates of excessive daytime sleepiness include clozapine, thioridazine, and chlorpromazine, followed by risperidone and olanzapine (Krystal et al. 2008).

Newer antipsychotics such as quetiapine and ziprasidone were shown not only to reduce REM sleep and consolidate sleep but also to promote SWS (Cohrs et al. 2005). Sleep consolidation and SWS enhancement are also observed with olanzapine and clozapine (Krystal 2012), whereas low-dose risperidone reduces REM sleep (Sharpley et al. 2003).

As discussed earlier, all antidopaminergic drugs, and thus most antipsychotics, can result in new-onset or exacerbation of RLS (see Chapter 17). This potentially severe and debilitating symptom can interfere with the ability to sleep and significantly impact quality of life. It is important to distinguish RLS from akathisia, which does not have a circadian pattern and tends to affect the entire body. RLS mostly or only occurs in the second part of the day, evening, or night and in most cases affects the legs more than arms or other body parts.

Several antipsychotic drugs can result in weight gain, thus increasing the risk of obstructive sleep-disordered breathing (see Chapters 8–10). This risk is particularly important with olanzapine.

Conclusion

Sleep and mental health are in a relationship of mutual causality. As summarized in this chapter, current evidence supports the following:

1. Psychiatric disorders affect sleep; hence, sleep symptoms can provide a window into the psychiatric status of an individual.
2. Impaired sleep contributes to mental illness; therefore, addressing sleep disturbances as part of a comprehensive and integrated management plan is not only relevant but also necessary, because most sleep issues can be treated.
3. In practice, many drugs used to treat psychiatric conditions potentially affect sleep and wake.

The effects of psychotropic drugs on sleep are not limited to the promotion of sleep or wake. Psychotropic drugs can result in altered dream experiences, nightmares, potentially injurious parasomnias as seen with RBD, exacerbation of RLS, and obstructive sleep-disordered breathing such as OSA. We recommend mental health practitioners take a mindful and systematic approach grounded in a basic understanding of drug mechanisms and the psychopharmacology of sleep and wake (see Chapters 4, 6, and 7). This should yield success in most clinical situations. Referral to a sleep specialist is indicated in more challenging situations or in treatment-resistant sleep disorders.

KEY CLINICAL POINTS

- Sleep disturbances such as insomnia and hypersomnia are associated with up to 90% cases of major depressive disorder. Treating both mood and sleep symptoms synergically improves clinical outcomes.

- Acute sleep deprivation has beneficial effects on depression but can also precipitate manic episodes in patients with bipolar disorder.

- Although most antidepressants can negatively affect sleep, sedative tricyclic agents (nortriptyline, amitriptyline), low-dose doxepin, mirtazapine, and trazodone can promote sleep.

- Due to their mild stimulant effect, desipramine, bupropion, and monoamine oxidase inhibitors can reduce hypersomnia.

- All serotonergic drugs can potentially exacerbate restless legs syndrome—which should be distinguished from akathisia due to its circadian pattern—as well as REM sleep behavior disorder, which can result in injurious dream enactment.

- Due to their myorelaxant effect on the upper airway dilator muscles, all benzodiazepine drugs can worsen obstructive sleep apnea.

References

American Psychiatric Association: Diagnostic and Statistical Manual of Mental Disorders, 5th Edition. Arlington, VA, American Psychiatric Association, 2013

Anderson KN, Bradley AJ: Sleep disturbance in mental health problems and neurodegenerative disease. Nat Sci Sleep 5:61–75, 2013 23761983

Baglioni C, Battagliese G, Feige B, et al: Insomnia as a predictor of depression: a meta-analytic evaluation of longitudinal epidemiological studies. J Affect Disord 135(1–3):10–19, 2011 21300408

Berridge CW, Schmeichel BE, España RA: Noradrenergic modulation of wakefulness/arousal. Sleep Med Rev 16(2):187–197, 2012 22296742

Bodkin C: Gender implications, in Rapid-Eye-Movement Sleep Behavior Disorder. Edited by Schenck WC, Högl B, Videnovic A. Cham, Switzerland, Springer, 2018, pp 215–222

Breslau N, Roth T, Rosenthal L, et al: Sleep disturbance and psychiatric disorders: a longitudinal epidemiological study of young adults. Biol Psychiatry 39(6):411–418, 1996 8679786

Cohrs S, Meier A, Neumann AC, et al: Improved sleep continuity and increased slow wave sleep and REM latency during ziprasidone treatment: a randomized, controlled, crossover trial of 12 healthy male subjects. J Clin Psychiatry 66(8):989–996, 2005 16086613

Dew MA, Reynolds CF III, Houck PR, et al: Temporal profiles of the course of depression during treatment. Predictors of pathways toward recovery in the elderly. Arch Gen Psychiatry 54(11):1016–1024, 1997 9366658

Earley CJ, Silber MH: Restless legs syndrome: understanding its consequences and the need for better treatment. Sleep Med 11(9):807–815, 2010 20817595

Etain B, Dumaine A, Bellivier F, et al: Genetic and functional abnormalities of the melatonin biosynthesis pathway in patients with bipolar disorder. Hum Mol Genet 21(18):4030–4037, 2012 22694957

Fava M, Asnis GM, Shrivastava R, et al: Zolpidem extended-release improves sleep and next-day symptoms in comorbid insomnia and generalized anxiety disorder. J Clin Psychopharmacol 29(3):222–230, 2009 19440075

Fava M, Asnis GM, Shrivastava RK, et al: Improved insomnia symptoms and sleep-related next-day functioning in patients with comorbid major depressive disorder and insomnia following concomitant zolpidem extended-release 12.5 mg and escitalopram treatment: a randomized controlled trial. J Clin Psychiatry 72(7):914–928, 2011 21208597

Ford DE, Kamerow DB: Epidemiologic study of sleep disturbances and psychiatric disorders. An opportunity for prevention? JAMA 262(11):1479–1484, 1989 2769898

Fuller KH, Waters WF, Binks PG, et al: Generalized anxiety and sleep architecture: a polysomnographic investigation. Sleep 20(5):370–376, 1997 9381061

Giese M, Beck J, Brand S, et al: Fast BDNF serum level increase and diurnal BDNF oscillations are associated with therapeutic response after partial sleep deprivation. J Psychiatr Res 59:1–7, 2014 25258340

Harvey AG, Schmidt DA, Scarnà A, et al: Sleep-related functioning in euthymic patients with bipolar disorder, patients with insomnia, and subjects without sleep problems. Am J Psychiatry 162(1):50–57, 2005 15625201

Hofstetter JR, Mayeda AR, Happel CG, et al: Sleep and daily activity preferences in schizophrenia: associations with neurocognition and symptoms. J Nerv Ment Dis 191(6):408–410, 2003 12826923

Högl B, Stefani A, Videnovic A: Idiopathic REM sleep behaviour disorder and neurodegeneration—an update. Nat Rev Neurol 14(1):40–55, 2018 29170501

Hoque R, Chesson AL Jr: Pharmacologically induced/exacerbated restless legs syndrome, periodic limb movements of sleep, and REM behavior disorder/REM sleep without atonia: literature review, qualitative scoring, and comparative analysis. J Clin Sleep Med 6(1):79–83, 2010 20191944

Kalucy MJ, Grunstein R, Lambert T, et al: Obstructive sleep apnoea and schizophrenia: a research agenda. Sleep Med Rev 17(5):357–365, 2013 23528272

Kaplan KA, Gruber J, Eidelman P, et al: Hypersomnia in inter-episode bipolar disorder: does it have prognostic significance? J Affect Disord 132(3):438–444, 2011 21489637

Koffel E, Polusny MA, Arbisi PA, et al: Pre-deployment daytime and nighttime sleep complaints as predictors of post-deployment PTSD and depression in national guard troops. J Anxiety Disord 27(5):512–519, 2013 23939336

Krystal AD: Psychiatric disorders and sleep. Neurol Clin 30(4):1389–1413, 2012 23099143

Krystal AD, Goforth HW, Roth T: Effects of antipsychotic medications on sleep in schizophrenia. Int Clin Psychopharmacol 23(3):150–160, 2008 18408529

Lam RW, Berkowitz AL, Berga SL, et al: Melatonin suppression in bipolar and unipolar mood disorders. Psychiatry Res 33(2):129–134, 1990 2243889

Lauer CJ, Schreiber W, Holsboer F, et al: In quest of identifying vulnerability markers for psychiatric disorders by all-night polysomnography. Arch Gen Psychiatry 52(2):145–153, 1995 7848050

Martin JL, Jeste DV, Ancoli-Israel S: Older schizophrenia patients have more disrupted sleep and circadian rhythms than age-matched comparison subjects. J Psychiatr Res 39(3):251–259, 2005 15725423

McCall WV, Reboussin BA, Cohen W: Subjective measurement of insomnia and quality of life in depressed inpatients. J Sleep Res 9(1):43–48, 2000 10733688

Minkel JD, Krystal AD, Benca RM: Unipolar major depression, in Principles and Practice of Sleep Medicine, 6th Edition. Edited by Kryger M, Roth T, Dement WC. Philadelphia, PA, Elsevier, 2017, pp 1352–1362

Nofzinger EA, Thase ME, Reynolds CF III, et al: Hypersomnia in bipolar depression: a comparison with narcolepsy using the multiple sleep latency test. Am J Psychiatry 148(9):1177–1181, 1991 1882995

Norris ER, Burke K, Correll JR, et al: A double-blind, randomized, placebo-controlled trial of adjunctive ramelteon for the treatment of insomnia and mood stability in patients with euthymic bipolar disorder. J Affect Disord 144(1–2):141–147, 2013 22963894

Nurnberger JI Jr, Adkins S, Lahiri DK, et al: Melatonin suppression by light in euthymic bipolar and unipolar patients. Arch Gen Psychiatry 57(6):572–579, 2000 10839335

Partonen T, Lönnqvist J: Seasonal affective disorder. Lancet 352(9137):1369–1374, 1998 9802288

Pollack M, Kinrys G, Krystal A, et al: Eszopiclone coadministered with escitalopram in patients with insomnia and comorbid generalized anxiety disorder. Arch Gen Psychiatry 65(5):551–562, 2008 18458207

Postuma RB, Gagnon JF, Tuineaig M, et al: Antidepressants and REM sleep behavior disorder: isolated side effect or neurodegenerative signal? Sleep 36(11):1579–1585, 2013 24179289

Rachakonda TD, Balba NM, Lim MM: Trauma-associated sleep disturbances: a distinct sleep disorder? Curr Sleep Med Rep 4(2):143–148, 2018 30656131

Raskind MA, Peskind ER, Chow B, et al: Trial of prazosin for post-traumatic stress disorder in military veterans. N Engl J Med 378(6):507–517, 2018 29414272

Reynolds CF III, Frank E, Houck PR, et al: Which elderly patients with remitted depression remain well with continued interpersonal psychotherapy after discontinuation of antidepressant medication? Am J Psychiatry 154(7):958–962, 1997 9210746

Ross RJ, Ball WA, Sullivan KA, et al: Sleep disturbance as the hallmark of post-traumatic stress disorder. Am J Psychiatry 146(6):697–707, 1989 2658624

Rottach KG, Schaner BM, Kirch MH, et al: Restless legs syndrome as side effect of second generation antidepressants. J Psychiatr Res 43(1):70–75, 2008 18468624

Sharafkhaneh A, Giray N, Richardson P, et al: Association of psychiatric disorders and sleep apnea in a large cohort. Sleep 28(11):1405–1411, 2005 16335330

Sharpley AL, Bhagwagar Z, Hafizi S, et al: Risperidone augmentation decreases rapid eye movement sleep and decreases wake in treatment-resistant depressed patients. J Clin Psychiatry 64(2):192–196, 2003 12633128

Soreca I, Levenson J, Lotz M, et al: Sleep apnea risk and clinical correlates in patients with bipolar disorder. Bipolar Disord 14(6):672–676, 2012 22938169

St-Amand J, Provencher MD, Bélanger L, et al: Sleep disturbances in bipolar disorder during remission. J Affect Disord 146(1):112–119, 2013 22884237

Szklo-Coxe M, Young T, Peppard PE, et al: Prospective associations of insomnia markers and symptoms with depression. Am J Epidemiol 171(6):709–720, 2010 20167581

Teman PT, Tippmann-Peikert M, Silber MH, et al: Idiopathic rapid-eye-movement sleep disorder: associations with antidepressants, psychiatric diagnoses, and other factors, in relation to age of onset. Sleep Med 10(1):60–65, 2009 18226952

Vogel GW, Thurmond A, Gibbons P, et al: REM sleep reduction effects on depression syndromes. Arch Gen Psychiatry 32(6):765–777, 1975 165796

Wehr TA: Sleep-loss as a possible mediator of diverse causes of mania. Br J Psychiatry 159:576–578, 1991 1751874

Wehr TA, Sack DA, Rosenthal NE: Sleep reduction as a final common pathway in the genesis of mania. Am J Psychiatry 144(2):201–204, 1987 3812788

Wiegand M, Berger M, Zulley J, et al: The influence of daytime naps on the therapeutic effect of sleep deprivation. Biol Psychiatry 22(3):389–392, 1987 3814687

Wilson S, Argyropoulos S: Antidepressants and sleep: a qualitative review of the literature. Drugs 65(7):927–947, 2005 15892588

Wirz-Justice A, Van den Hoofdakker RH: Sleep deprivation in depression: what do we know, where do we go? Biol Psychiatry 46(4):445–453, 1999 10459393

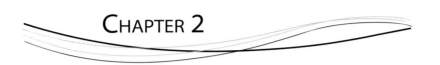
Clinical History and Physical Examination in Sleep Medicine

Logan Schneider, M.D.

Sleep is a unique field because it draws on the expertise of a multitude of subspecialties for insights into pathophysiology, diagnosis, and management, which is a reflection of the complex interplay between sleep and health or disease. Sleep serves as a biomarker of a host of medical conditions (e.g., heart failure, neurodegenerative disease) and influences the physical and mental resiliency of both healthy individuals and those with disease. Moreover, sleep often affects not only patients but also—and sometimes disproportionately—their bed partners and family members. As a result, patients often present to the sleep clinic through referrals from other first-line care providers or specialists as well as at the behest of someone else.

Given that sleep is generally an unobserved state, and that many sleep- and wake-related phenomena vary just as dramatically as the circadian cycle, subjective sleep reports often require collateral information gathering through partner reports, diagnostic testing, or, more recently, consumer sleep tracking devices/services. However, the fundamentals of a thorough history and physical examination can lead to appropriately applied diagnostic testing. This chapter provides a general overview of the approach to patients with concerns related to sleep disorders, whereas subsequent chapters explore specific conditions in greater depth.

Clinical History

BEFORE THE VISIT

The clinical sleep history often begins before the patient encounter; clues to the ultimate diagnosis may be provided by the origin of the consultation. Additionally, screening questionnaires may not only serve to improve clinical efficiency but also provide a measure of baseline symptom severity that can be tracked over time. A host of sleep questionnaires have been validated in the assessment and monitoring of sleep disorders; Table 2–1 provides a limited subset of questionnaires that are often encountered in the practice of sleep medicine. In addition to individual questionnaires, some efforts have focused on providing batteries—some with branching logic, such as the Alliance Sleep Questionnaire (see https://mysleep.stanford.edu) (Kushida et al. 2015)—that allow for broad coverage of disorders while limiting the amount of time patients spend filling in questionnaires.

PATIENT INTERVIEW

Most sleep concerns fit into one of three major categories: insomnia, abnormal sleep-related events, and excessive daytime sleepiness. Each has a broad differential of sleep-related and associated considerations (Figures 2–1, 2–2, and 2–3). Thus, begin the sleep history with the patient's chief concern. Given that most sleep issues are long-standing (and may have already been investigated by others), determining the reason for the current presentation often adds value to the clinical encounter by eliciting the patient's objective, which can guide the rest of the encounter. Whether or not the patient is aware of the sleep problem for which he or she has been referred, a quick screening of sleep practices, sleep-influencing factors, and sleep disorders can help determine if further investigation or treatment is warranted. Because sleep is often unobserved, gather collateral information from bed partners or caregivers to gain much-needed insights into next steps.

Patients can present with a variety of symptoms or concerns; thus, we invite the reader to learn about clinical presentations (signs and symptoms) for each sleep disorder in its dedicated chapter. Once the chief concern is elaborated, elucidate the patient's sleep schedule and habits. Most sleep schedules vary from day to day and from workdays to days off, so approach data collection using representative estimates—averages and ranges are often the most helpful. Also, because sleep habits are often artificially constrained by social circumstances, determine whether external influences (e.g., work or family obligations, technology) play a role in the sleep-related concern by assessing sleep schedule changes during brief (non-workdays/weekends) and prolonged (holidays/vacations) absences from schedule constraints. By comparing these schedules, or explicitly asking, you can determine whether the sleep schedule is aligning with the natural biorhythm (particularly relevant to circadian rhythm

TABLE 2–1. Some questionnaires commonly used in sleep-wake and circadian disorders

Sleep domain and questionnaires	Screen	Monitor
Excessive daytime sleepiness		
Epworth Sleepiness Scale (Johns 1992)	X	X
Pediatric Daytime Sleepiness Scale (Johns 1992)	X	X
Fatigue and functional status		
Fatigue severity scale (Krupp et al. 1989)	X	X
Functional outcomes of sleep questionnaire (Weaver et al. 1997)	X	X
Sleep quality		
Pittsburgh Sleep Quality Index (Levenson et al. 2013)	X	X
PROMIS Sleep Disturbance Questionnaire (Yu et al. 2011)	X	
Narcolepsy		
Swiss Narcolepsy Scale (Sturzenegger et al. 2018)	X	X
Ullanlinna Narcolepsy Scale (Hublin et al. 1994)		X
Insomnia		
Insomnia Severity Index (Bastien et al. 2001)	X	X
Insomnia Symptom Questionnaire (Okun et al. 2009)	X	
Sleep apnea		
Multivariate Apnea Index (Maislin et al. 1995)	X	
STOP-BANG (Nagappa et al. 2015)	X	
Berlin Questionnaire (Netzer et al. 1999)	X	
OSA50 (Chai-Coetzer et al. 2011)	X	
Nasal Obstruction Symptom Evaluation (Ishii et al. 2011)	X	X
Restless legs syndrome		
International Restless Legs Syndrome Scale (Walters et al. 2003)	X	X
Parasomnias and REM sleep behavior disorder		
Frontal Lobe Epilepsy and Parasomnias Scale (Manni et al. 2008)	X	
REM Sleep Behavior Disorder Single-Question Screen (Postuma et al. 2012)	X	
Circadian phase		
Reduced Morningness-Eveningness Questionnaire (Adan and Almirall 1991)	X	

TABLE 2–1.   Some questionnaires commonly used in sleep-wake and circadian disorders *(continued)*

Sleep domain and questionnaires	Screen	Monitor
Sleep schedule		
Consensus Sleep Diary (Carney et al. 2012)	X	X
Psychiatric disorders		
Generalized Anxiety Disorder-7 (Spitzer et al. 2006)	X	X
Patient Health Questionnaire-9 for depressive symptoms (Kroenke et al. 2001)	X	X

disorders; see Chapters 12 and 13). Focus the questioning on major areas of the sleep and wake periods that can indicate potential sleep disorders to explore. Guided by an awareness of sleep and circadian physiology, begin the sleep history with an exploration of the patient's pre-bedtime routine. This should capture at least the 2 hours before habitual bedtime, because that is the approximate time of the dim-light melatonin onset (Pandi-Perumal et al. 2007). Next, explore the timing of sleep intention ("lights off") and the perceived latency to sleep onset, because this is the period in which the homeostatic drive for sleep ought to be maximal (Borbély 1982). In individuals with sleep maintenance issues, gather an estimate of the frequency, perceived cause, timing/distribution, and duration of wake-after-sleep-onset periods, because this information may point to specific disorders. For instance, somnambulism (see Chapter 14) tends to occur earlier in the night compared with REM sleep behavior disorder (RBD; see Chapter 15), and nocturia every 2 hours may indicate REM-related obstructive sleep apnea (OSA) (Ben Mansour et al. 2015).

After getting a general impression of the quantity and, to a lesser degree, the quality of sleep during the major sleep period, explore the most significant modifying factors, daytime function, and a sleep problem–specific review of systems. Some of the most obvious influences on sleep include elements of the social history, such as caffeine, nicotine, and alcohol, because timing of the consumption of these substances in relation to the major sleep period can reveal easily modifiable risk factors for sleep disruptions. Evening alcohol consumption can result in ease of sleep onset but invariably fragments sleep once the alcohol is metabolized (about 1 hour to eliminate one standard drink) (Cederbaum 2012); about one-quarter of caffeine consumed after noon will still be unmetabolized by bedtime (although metabolic phenotypes can have significant genetic differences) (Statland and Demas 1980; Yang et al. 2010); and nicotine is particularly detrimental to sleep quality due to its stimulating ef-

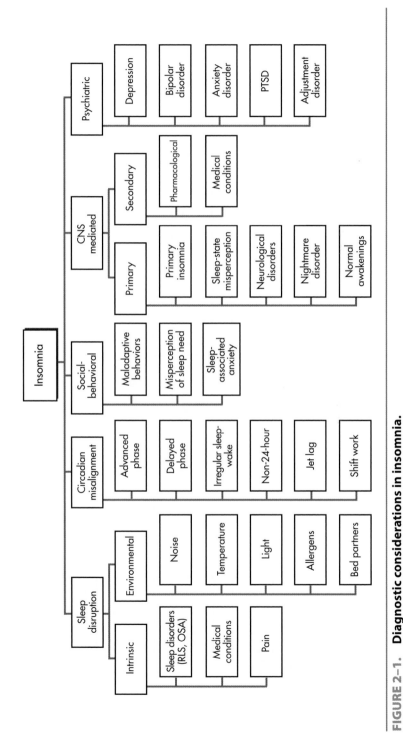

FIGURE 2–1. Diagnostic considerations in insomnia.

Note. OSA=obstructive sleep apnea; RLS=restless legs syndrome.

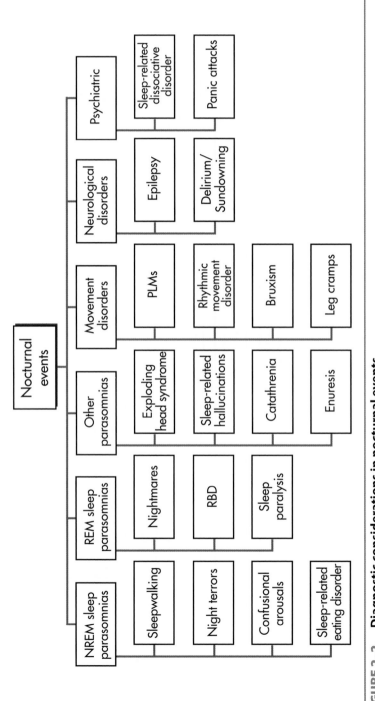

FIGURE 2–2. Diagnostic considerations in nocturnal events.

Note. NREM=non-REM; PLMs=periodic limb movements; RBD=REM sleep behavior disorder.

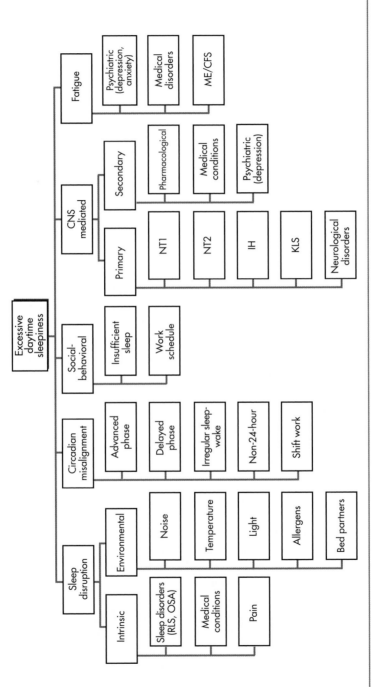

FIGURE 2–3.   Diagnostic considerations in excessive daytime sleepiness.

Note.   IH=idiopathic hypersomnia; KLS=Kleine-Levin syndrome; ME/CFS=myalgic encephalomyelitis/chronic fatigue syndrome; NT1=narcolepsy type 1; NT2=narcolepsy type 2; OSA=obstructive sleep apnea; RLS=restless legs syndrome.

fects (Caviness et al. 2018). Assess for reductions in homeostatic drive as well as insufficient sleep evinced by daytime napping or inadvertent dozing. Nap durations and timing are valuable indicators of sleepiness, and the efficacy/restoration of naps can also point to the nature of a hypersomnolence (e.g., individuals with idiopathic hypersomnia [see Chapter 7] often report that even long naps are nonrestorative, resulting in waking to a state of "sleep drunkenness" [Trotti 2017]). Finally, a host of psychosocial factors act as *zeitgebers*—"time givers"—that warrant interrogation. The most prominent influences from daytime routines are the timing of physical activity (Youngstedt et al. 2016) and the timing and macronutrient mix of meals (St-Onge et al. 2016). The social history provides insights into additional daytime and nocturnal stressors, environmental conditions, and behavioral adaptations likely to impact sleep. Generally, the most relevant areas on which to focus are employment-related activity, bed-partner relationships and habits, and family-member (including pet) interactions with the sleep environment.

Once you have a general impression of the pattern of sleep-wake issues affecting the patient, perform a sleep problem–specific review of systems focused on the most likely contributing to sleep disorders and the associated comorbidities (Table 2–2). When approaching the review of systems, focus on the symptoms and conditions that are most likely to affect the sleep-wake and circadian systems or to be comorbid with sleep disorders. Complementary to the review of systems, the currency and history of medical, surgical, and psychiatric illnesses are sources of important information, because a multitude of disorders can directly result in sleep disorders or be part of the differential diagnosis. In any endorsed medical or psychiatric disorders, determine any temporal relationships of symptoms and severity to the primary sleep concern. Although a number of sleep disorders may be linked to associated conditions, such as restless legs syndrome (RLS) exacerbation or onset during pregnancy or central sleep apnea development during a vacation at altitude, the condition most amenable to correlation to longitudinal variations in biopsychosocial phenomena is insomnia (see Chapters 3–5), given the proposed neurocognitive basis (Buysse et al. 2011) and the fact that most patients fixate on daily cause-effect relationships.

Family history also highlights important predispositions to certain sleep disorders. Having a family history of RLS (see Chapter 17) increases the population prevalence up to fourfold, from 9.4%–15% to 18.5%–63% (Ohayon et al. 2012). Even the complex, multifactorial disorder of OSA (see Chapters 8–9) has an estimated heritability of 35%–40%, with odds ratios >2 consistently reported for individuals who have an affected blood relative (Redline 2016). Beyond these more deeply explored disor-

TABLE 2–2. Review of systems

Sleep-specific	General, sleep-related comorbidities
Morning symptoms	**General and constitutional complaints**
Headache	Chronic pain
Jaw pain	Fevers, chills, sweats, shakes
Nasal congestion	Weight gain or loss (intentional?)
Xerostomia	**Vision**
Daytime functioning	Floppy eyelids
Concentration difficulties	Visual loss—transient, progressive
Fatigue	**Head and neck**
Irritability	Nasal congestion, postnasal drip
Memory problems	Dysarthria, changes in voice or hoarseness
Sleep-disordered breathing	
Awakening with snorts, gasping, choking	Dentition and TMJ function
Cyanosis	**Pulmonary**
Mouth breathing	Cough
Pauses in breathing	Shortness of breath
Snoring	Wheezing
Sleep-related movements	**Cardiovascular**
Bruxism	Orthopnea
Leg cramps	Palpitations
Periodic limb movements	Paroxysmal nocturnal dyspnea
Restless legs symptoms	Pedal edema
Insomnias	**Gastrointestinal**
Chronic pain	Constipation
Environmental disturbance (e.g., light, sound)	Diarrhea
	Heartburn
Fear or anxiety related to bed or sleep	**Genitourinary**
	Erectile dysfunction or dyspareunia
Racing thoughts	Incontinence
Triggers (e.g., stress, argument)	Nocturia (volumes and frequency)
Hypersomnias	**Hematological and immunological**
Cataplexy	Allergies and atopy
Disrupted sleep	Arthritis
Hypnagogic or hypnopompic hallucinations	New or growing lumps/bumps
	Obstetric and gynecological
	Menopausal status
Sleep attacks	Pregnancy status (in relation to sleep issues)

TABLE 2–2. Review of systems (continued)

Sleep-specific	General, sleep-related comorbidities
Hypersomnias (continued)	**Neurological**
Sleep paralysis	Numbness/Paresthesias
Infectious exposures (e.g., H1N1, Streptococcus pyogenes, mononucleosis)	Seizures (bowel/bladder incontinence, tongue biting, amnesia, stereotyped)
	Stroke/Transient ischemic attack
TBI with or without LOC	Tremors/Parkinsonism
Parasomnias	Weakness
Loud noises/flashing lights	**Endocrine**
Nightmares (e.g., themes, emotions, frequency)	Polyuria, polydipsia, polyphagia
	Psychiatric
Sleep walking, talking, or eating (dangerous or embarrassing?)	Depression
	Anxiety (including PTSD)
Dream enactment (injury?)	Substance abuse
Anosmia	**Integumentary**
	Changes in hair, skin, or nails
	Mucosal lesions
	Pruritis

Note.   These are some of the more generally relevant review-of-systems questions pertaining to sleep disorders.
LOC=loss of consciousness; TBI=traumatic brain injury; TMJ=temporomandibular joint.

ders, multiple other sleep disorders have known patterns of heritability due to the genetic architecture of the circadian and sleep neurocircuitry as well as the genetic underpinnings of associated medical and psychiatric conditions (Sehgal and Mignot 2011). With regard to narcolepsy (see Chapter 6), multiplex families with multiple generations affected are rare (Hor et al. 2011), yet a higher prevalence of hypersomnias is found among family members (Billiard et al. 1994; Ohayon et al. 2005).

A medication reconciliation is essential to the collection of the sleep history, because many prescription and nonprescription medications affect sleep and wake (Table 2–3). Many prescription medications have the side effect of drowsiness (Pagel 2009), notably any medications that augment inhibitory GABAergic tone or suppress the wake-promoting monoaminergic (e.g., dopamine, histamine, norepinephrine, serotonin) or cholinergic systems. Similarly, enumerable medications result in the side effect of insomnia (Doufas et al. 2017), often through interactions with the same sleep-wake neurotransmitter systems. Sometimes, simply adjusting the timing of medications can diminish their impact on sleep-

TABLE 2–3.   Medication classes commonly affecting sleep and wake*

Commonly sedating medication classes

    Antiadrenergics (α and β)

    Anticonvulsants

    Anticholinergics (antidiarrheal agents, antiemetics, genitourinary antispasmodics)

    Antihistamines (particularly first generation)

    Antitussives

    Barbiturates

    Benzodiazepines

    Narcotics

    Antiparkinsonian agents (e.g., dopamine agonists)

    Psychiatric medications (antidepressants [certain MAOIs, TCAs, SSRIs] and most antipsychotics)

    Skeletal muscle relaxants and antispasmodics

Commonly insomnogenic medication classes

    Acetylcholinesterase inhibitors

    Catechol O-methyltransferase inhibitors

    Corticosteroids

    Nicotinic receptor agonists

    Antiparkinsonian agents (e.g., dopamine agonists)

    Psychiatric medications (SSRIs, SNRIs, certain TCAs, DNRIs)

    Stimulants (amphetamine salts and amphetaminoids)

*Medication classes commonly associated with drowsiness or insomnia.
DNRI=dopamine norepinephrine reuptake inhibitor; MAOI=monoamine oxidase inhibitor; SSRI=selective serotonin reuptake inhibitor; TCA=tricyclic antidepressant.

wake function, particularly if alternate therapies are not available. Get an accurate list of the current and past attempts at pharmacological management of the patient's sleep concerns in order to gauge the impact on the patient, as evinced by the duration of experimentation, variety and dosages of substances tried, and misconceptions about proper usage (melatonin dosing being notoriously misapplied by patients and clinicians alike).

COLLATERAL DATA

As mentioned earlier, sleep is generally an unobserved phenomenon, which necessitates the collection of collateral information. This is most evident in the case of pediatric patients, because younger children are often unable to accurately report on sleep-related issues. In these circumstances, gather not only family member observations but also historical elements from both school (teacher reports) and social (e.g., other parents, coaches) contexts. Also, as compared with nocturnal events, such as sleepwalking and enuresis (see Chapters 14 and 16, respectively), daytime dysfunction may manifest atypically (i.e., without daytime sleepiness) and may not obviously be linked to an underlying sleep quality impairment unless properly interrogated. In such circumstances, diminishing school performance, hyperactivity, and behavioral or mood disturbances are common symptoms that may warrant further diagnostic investigations.

Additionally, as a complement to the subjective collateral, a profusion of applications and devices are available that can monitor sleep or activity (Choi et al. 2018; Mansukhani and Kolla 2017; Ong and Gillespie 2016). Despite numerous inherent limitations to the technology (Mansukhani and Kolla 2017)—not the least of which is their ever-changing, proprietary algorithms—these devices may still provide meaningful information due to a reasonable degree of internal consistency that can offer a more accurate picture of an individual's sleep-wake activity over time. As these technologies continue to propagate and improve, they will inevitably become more integrated into the diagnosis and monitoring of clinical populations, particularly because sleep clinicians regularly rely upon objective verification of notoriously inaccurate subjective reports (Lauderdale et al. 2008; Lawrence and Muza 2018). As such, the most valuable part of the clinical physical examination often remains the actual monitoring of the patient's sleep; however, several elements of the in-clinic physical examination can assist in the diagnostic process.

Physical Examination

Sleep resides at the crossroads of virtually every medical specialty. Because of the plethora of conditions that influence sleep and wake function or can decompensate in the setting of poor-quality sleep, the sleep clinician must be competent in performing a thorough examination. This section outlines some of the more sleep-relevant physical examination elements that should be evaluated.

VITAL SIGNS

First, focusing on the patient's vital signs can provide insights into potential comorbidities and risk factors. Hypertension can be an indicator of untreated OSA or, when coupled with tachycardia, may indicate sympathetic overactivity from anxiety or toxicity from medications (e.g., stimulants). Autonomic function assessments (including a proper evaluation of orthostatic vital signs) (Agency for Healthcare Research and Quality 2018) are valuable when assessing for possible neurodegenerative conditions that predispose to RBD, as well as in patients with idiopathic hypersomnia (Trotti 2017) or suspected upper-airway resistance syndrome, a distinct nonhypoxic phenotype of OSA (Guilleminault et al. 2005). Deficits in daytime oxygenation in patients with chronic obstructive pulmonary disease, pulmonary artery hypertension, pulmonary fibrosis, or heart failure will also be valuable to note when deciding upon proper diagnostic testing strategies.

Anthropometric measures are easily integrated into the workflow as well. The patient's BMI has clear connections to OSA risk, as do patterns of fat mass distribution such as neck circumference and hip-to-waist ratio (Avidan and Kryger 2016; Chung et al. 2016).

GENERAL

In all patients, observe and document a general impression of their level of alertness as a first step in the examination. Patients present with a range of behaviors, from the patient with Pickwickian syndrome falling asleep mid-conversation (see Chapter 10) to the hypersomniac who is asleep on the examination table when the clinician enters the room (see Chapters 6 and 7) to the fidgety patient with RLS (see Chapter 17) to the hyperactive child who is "bouncing off the walls," as is sometimes seen in pediatric sleep apnea (see Chapter 9). All of these presentations add to the clinical impression, particularly when incongruent with other subjective reports or clinical questionnaires.

PSYCHIATRIC

Although an extensive mental status examination is generally beyond the scope of the sleep clinic encounter, focus on the most relevant comorbid disorders: mood and anxiety disorders. Observations of psychomotor activation or depression and affect congruence with reported mood are complementary to symptomatic reports. Concerning signs, such as pressured speech, tearful affect, or attending to stimuli that are not present, may indicate decompensated psychiatric illness (possibly as a result of or contributing to the primary sleep complaint) and should prompt further questioning and appropriate referral.

INTEGUMENTARY

Although they are not common biomarkers of sleep or sleep-related comorbidities, take note of findings that reflect metabolic (acanthosis nigricans), cardiovascular (hairless or hemosiderin-stained lower extrem-

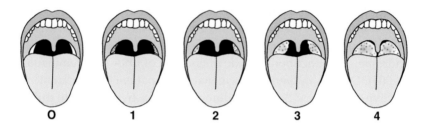

FIGURE 2–4. Grading of tonsillar hypertrophy.

This graphic demonstrates the numeric grading scale used to quantify the relative size of the palatine tonsils based on visual appearance within the oropharynx. Grade 0=no tonsillar tissue (removed); Grade 1=tonsils barely visible behind anterior pillars; Grade 2=tonsils visible beyond anterior pillars; Grade 3=tonsils extend three-quarters (75%) of the distance to midline; Grade 4=tonsils touch and completely obstruct airway.

ities), autonomic (cold, clammy, discolored extremities), rheumatological (nail pitting), hepatic (telangiectasias, palmar erythema), or other systemic diseases that affect sleep-wake function. Also, occult iron deficiency predisposing to RLS (see Chapter 17) may be indicated by pallor within the creases of the palm or of the palpebral conjunctiva.

HEAD AND NECK

The head and neck examination is quite possibly the most valuable in the investigation of sleep disorders, particularly in light of the high prevalence of OSA. Progress logically along the path of natural airflow by examining nasal, pharyngeal, and oral patency. Inferior nasal turbinate hypertrophy, nasal septal deviation or single nostril airflow limitation, and a high arched hard palate all indicate possible increased risk of OSA from high nasal resistance (Avidan and Kryger 2016). Physiologically compounded anatomical risk may be noted in children with signs of atopy, such as nasal crease, allergic shiners, and the nasal salute (Avidan and Kryger 2016). During the oral examination, several features highlight increased risk of OSA: macroglossia (identified by tooth impressions/scalloping), maxillary or mandibular exostoses, ample redundant tissue (noted through sclerotic bite marks on the buccal mucosa), and tonsillar hypertrophy (Figure 2–4) (Avidan and Kryger 2016).

In addition to obstructions, anatomical orientation can even make patients with nonhypertrophic or nonhyperplastic anatomy predisposed to airway collapse. Notably, an aerodynamically disadvantaged posterior aperture of the nasopharynx (evidenced by a particularly low-riding palate) or retropositioned tongue caused by maxillary or mandibular mi-

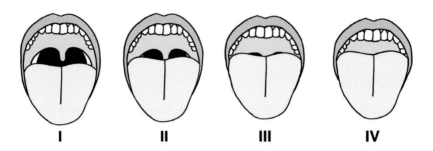

FIGURE 2–5.   Modified Mallampati classification.

Classification based on modified Mallampati. Class I=soft palate, uvula, fauces (opening between the pharynx and the tongue), faucial pillars (anterior and posterior arches that form the tonsillar fossae laterally) visible; Class II=soft palate, major part of uvula, fauces visible; Class III=soft palate, base of uvula visible; Class IV=only hard palate visible.

crogenia (noted via dental malocclusion and degree of incisor overjet) will likely result in a Mallampati (tongue protruded; Figure 2–5) or Friedman (tongue resting in its neutral, mandibular position) airway evaluation highlighting risk of collapse (Avidan and Kryger 2016).

Furthermore, cephalometrics, such as a reduced cricomental space, are external features that suggest additional anatomic predispositions to airflow limitation (Avidan and Kryger 2016). Finally, masseter hypertrophy and a temporomandibular joint click on jaw range of motion are potential signs of bruxism, which may affect management decisions in patients with OSA (see Chapter 8).

CARDIOVASCULAR

Focus the cardiovascular examination on clinical findings that might indicate sleep disorders beyond isolated OSA or might suggest a need for more advanced diagnostic strategies. In the former case, signs of advanced heart failure, such as bibasilar wet crackles, S3 gallop, jugular venous distention with or without a hepatojugular reflex, and pedal edema, might suggest a loop gain–related diathesis for insufficient respiratory drive (i.e., central apneas and hypopneas or frank Cheyne-Stokes respiratory patterns; see Chapter 11). Additionally, murmurs of valvular insufficiency or stenosis or changes in heart sounds (e.g., an additional S4 gallop or a persistently split S2) can help localize cardiopulmonary pathologies that may impact nocturnal gas exchange beyond simple obstructed breathing. Atrial fibrillation and other discernible arrhythmias not only suggest possible complex sleep-related breathing disorders but also highlight an underlying cardiovascular risk that could impact diagnostic and treatment decisions. Along these lines, other signs of cardiovascular disease that may be impacted by untreated sleep disorders (e.g., systemic peripheral vascular disease) can weigh into clinical decision making.

PULMONARY

Beyond the cardiovascular effects on pulmonary function, intrinsic and extrinsic factors resulting in obstructive and restrictive pathologies may indicate complex sleep-disordered breathing issues. Specifically, document aspects of breathing effort, inspiration-expiration ratio, fine crackles, rhonchi, and wheezes, because they pertain to pulmonary diseases that are likely to worsen during sleep. Additionally, among the OSA population, steric forces from obesity may result in sleep-related or daytime hypoventilation (see Chapter 10).

GASTROINTESTINAL

The gastrointestinal examination is not a cornerstone of the sleep examination, but it still can provide indirect evidence of conditions that may impact sleep-wake function. A pulsatile, distended liver may point to diastolic right heart failure. Moreover, diminished bowel sounds might suggest dysautonomia in the context of neurodegenerative disease or a primary autonomic dysfunction. Also, stigmata of cirrhosis with or without ascites certainly may identify risk of encephalopathy-related neurocognitive dysfunction or physiological respiratory abnormalities.

MUSCULOSKELETAL AND EXTREMITIES

Examine the extremities for signs of other systemic diseases that may contribute to or worsen sleep-wake disorders (e.g., digital clubbing, cyanosis in pulmonary diseases). Results consistent with osteoarthritis of large joints (crepitus), degenerative disc disease causing radiculopathy (e.g., positive straight leg raise sign), soft-tissue pathology (e.g., limitations of movement of the rotator cuff, positive Phalen and Tinel maneuvers in carpal tunnel), or inflammatory arthropathies (e.g., rheumatoid arthritis) may explain chronic pain–associated insomnia or RLS (see Chapters 3 and 17). Of particular note, the kyphosis related to ankylosing spondylitis results in a restrictive lung disease that contributes to nocturnal obstructive and hypoventilatory breathing disturbances (see Chapter 10). Additionally, connective tissue disorders such as Ehlers-Danlos and Marfan syndromes appear to represent nontraditional phenotypes of sleep-disordered breathing and dysautonomia (Bohora 2010; De Wandele et al. 2014).

NEUROLOGICAL

Virtually all categories of sleep disorders are affected by or associated with neurological function—so intimately, in fact, that disorders such as RBD can be presymptomatic biomarkers of neurological dysfunction (see Chapter 15). Although an effective screening neurological examination can identify red flags that warrant further investigation, certain clusters of examination findings or neurological syndromes can highlight specific sleep disorders.

Sleep-disordered breathing is traditionally thought of as an anatomical and pulmonary disease; however, respiratory drive is under brain stem, autonomic, and neuromuscular control while sleeping. Although a host of CNS focal lesions from the brain stem to the cortex can contribute to aberrant breathing patterns, neuromuscular disorders are most notable for their association with sleep-disordered breathing. Muscular strength in the extremities is easily assessed both proximally and distally, but the additional ascertainment of neck and bulbar weakness (e.g., facial nerve paresis, dysphonia) and respiratory weakness should prompt further pulmonary function and neuromuscular testing. Additionally, because respiratory function is under autonomic control at night, individuals with autonomic symptoms should have orthostatic vital signs and a cranial nerve assessment (due to the confluence of tracts originating from the diencephalon as well as the pupillary reflex arc providing high-yield autonomic assessments), at the very least. Among the population of individuals suspected to have obesity hypoventilation syndrome (see Chapter 10), reports of morning headaches may suggest idiopathic intracranial hypertension due to carbon dioxide retention, in which case, persistently increased intracranial pressure may be elucidated by papilledema, lateral gaze palsy (cranial nerve VI), and constricted peripheral vision. Finally, given the increased risk of strokes in individuals with untreated OSA, occasional occult neurological deficits are uncovered through a proper screening neurological examination.

In the exploration of parasomnias, specifically RBD (see Chapter 15), a host of neurological conditions on the differential must be investigated. Most obvious is an assessment of neurodegenerative diseases, specifically the α-synucleinopathies, which can present with motor symptoms, namely classic parkinsonism (i.e., bradykinesia, masked facies with reduced blink rate, cogwheel rigidity, usually unilateral low-frequency/high-amplitude resting tremor, postural instability on retropulsion, and walking with a stooped posture and diminished arm swing), or atypical features in Parkinson's disease plus syndromes such as multiple systems atrophy (often manifesting with cerebellar dysfunction, such as ataxia) or the cognitive impairment (initially affecting visuospatial function) in dementia with Lewy bodies. However, in the differentiation of parasomnias from seizures, exploration for an occult mass lesion (specifically cortical) can aid the clinical suspicion derived from the reported history.

Sleep-related movement disorders such as RLS and periodic limb movements (see Chapter 17) may also have objective neurological abnormalities, the most notable of which are the peripheral neuropathies (most commonly stocking-glove dysesthesias associated with diabetes), but they have been associated with neuronal injury anywhere along the nerve (frequently due to compression of nerve roots from degenerative disc disease) and even at sites within the CNS. A screening of neuronal function should include at least a quick assessment of sensory function.

Also, as their name implies, central disorders of hypersomnolence are likely derived from primary CNS pathologies. Although focal neurological deficits are seldom found in association with the hypersomnias (see Chapters 6 and 7), a host of conditions, including traumatic brain injury, autoimmune encephalitides, multiple sclerosis, neuromyelitis optica, and neurodegenerative conditions, may present with neurological or cognitive deficits ranging from the syndromic to the nonspecific.

Conclusion

In summary, much supportive evidence of the presence of sleep-wake disorders and associated comorbidities can be gleaned from a thorough examination. After performing a thorough sleep history and physical examination, formulate a clinical impression of which condition(s) are of sufficient pretest probability to investigate. Ultimately, when deciding to apply a test, ensure that the outcome of a positive or negative result will meaningfully modify your clinical impression, and have a plan in place for how to deal with an unexpected result.

KEY CLINICAL POINTS

- The sleep history often relies upon collateral data: referral documentation, family/bed partner, screening questionnaires, and, more recently, applications and wearable technology.

- Due to overlap of sleep disorders with most other areas of medicine, a thorough screening physical examination provides insight into appropriate diagnostic and management strategies.

- From the first visit, integrate the patient's values system and perspective into the decision-making process as a means of setting the patient–provider team up for successful outcomes.

References

Adan A, Almirall H: Horne and Östberg morningness-eveningness questionnaire: a reduced scale. Pers Individ Dif 12(3):241–253, 1991

Agency for Healthcare Research and Quality: Tool 3F: Orthostatic Vital Sign Measurement. Available at: www.ahrq.gov/professionals/systems/hospital/fallpxtoolkit/fallpxtk-tool3f.html. Accessed November 27, 2018.

Avidan AY, Kryger MH: Physical examination in sleep medicine, in Principles and Practice of Sleep Medicine, 6th Edition. Edited by Kryger MH, Roth T, Dement WC. Philadelphia, PA, Elsevier, 2016, pp 587–606

Bastien CH, Vallières A, Morin CM: Validation of the Insomnia Severity Index as an outcome measure for insomnia research. Sleep Med 2(4):297–307, 2001, 11438246

Ben Mansour A, Zaibi H, Ben Ammar J, et al: Prevalence of nocturia in obstructive sleep apnea syndrome. Eur Respiratory J 46:PA2380, 2015

Billiard M, Pasquié-Magnetto V, Heckman M, et al: Family studies in narcolepsy. Sleep 17(suppl 8): S54–S59, 1994

Bohora S: Joint hypermobility syndrome and dysautonomia: expanding spectrum of disease presentation and manifestation. Indian Pacing Electrophysiol J 10(4):158–161, 2010 20376182

Borbély AA: A two process model of sleep regulation. Hum Neurobiol 1(3):195–204, 1982 7185792

Buysse DJ, Germain A, Hall M, et al: A neurobiological model of insomnia. Drug Discov Today Dis Models 8(4):129–137, 2011 22081772

Carney CE, Buysse DJ, Ancoli-Israel S, et al: The consensus sleep diary: standardizing prospective sleep self-monitoring. Sleep (Basel) 35(2):287–302, 2012 22294820

Caviness CM, Anderson BJ, Stein MD: Impact of nicotine and other stimulants on sleep in young adults. J Addict Med 13(3):209–214, 2018 30461442

Cederbaum AI: Alcohol metabolism. Clin Liver Dis 16(4):667–685, 2012 23101976

Chai-Coetzer CL, Antic NA, Rowland LS, et al: A simplified model of screening questionnaire and home monitoring for obstructive sleep apnoea in primary care. Thorax 66(3):213–219, 2011 21252389

Choi YK, Demiris G, Lin S-Y, et al: Smartphone applications to support sleep self-management: review and evaluation. J Clin Sleep Med 14(10):1783–1790, 2018 30353814

Chung F, Abdullah HR, Liao P: STOP-Bang Questionnaire: a practical approach to screen for obstructive sleep apnea. Chest 149(3):631–638, 2016 26378880

De Wandele I, Rombaut L, Leybaert L, et al: Dysautonomia and its underlying mechanisms in the hypermobility type of Ehlers-Danlos syndrome. Semin Arthritis Rheum 44(1):93–100, 2014 24507822

Doufas AG, Panagiotou OA, Panousis P, et al: Insomnia from drug treatments: evidence from meta-analyses of randomized trials and concordance with prescribing information. Mayo Clin Proc 92(1):72–87, 2017 27842706

Guilleminault C, Poyares D, Rosa A, et al: Heart rate variability, sympathetic and vagal balance and EEG arousals in upper airway resistance and mild obstructive sleep apnea syndromes. Sleep Med 6(5):451–457, 2005 15994124

Hor H, Bartesaghi L, Kutalik Z, et al: A missense mutation in myelin oligodendrocyte glycoprotein as a cause of familial narcolepsy with cataplexy. Am J Hum Genet 89(3):474–479, 2011 21907016

Hublin C, Kaprio J, Partinen M, et al: The Ullanlinna Narcolepsy Scale: validation of a measure of symptoms in the narcoleptic syndrome. J Sleep Res 3(1):52–59, 1994 10607109

Ishii L, Godoy A, Ishman SL, et al: The nasal obstruction symptom evaluation survey as a screening tool for obstructive sleep apnea. Arch Otolaryngol Head Neck Surg 137(2):119–123, 2011 21339396

Johns MW: Reliability and factor analysis of the Epworth Sleepiness Scale. Sleep 15(4):376–381, 1992 1519015

Kroenke K, Spitzer RL, Williams JB: The PHQ-9: validity of a brief depression severity measure. J Gen Intern Med 16(9):606–613, 2001 11556941

Krupp LB, LaRocca NG, Muir-Nash J, et al: The fatigue severity scale. Application to patients with multiple sclerosis and systemic lupus erythematosus. Arch Neurol 46(10):1121–1123, 1989 2803071

Kushida CA, Nichols DA, Holmes TH, et al: SMART DOCS: a new patient-centered outcomes and coordinated-care management approach for the future practice of sleep medicine. Sleep (Basel) 38(2):315–326, 2015 25409112

Lauderdale DS, Knutson KL, Yan LL, et al: Self-reported and measured sleep duration: how similar are they? Epidemiology 19(6):838–845, 2008 18854708

Lawrence G, Muza R: Assessing the sleeping habits of patients in a sleep disorder centre: a review of sleep diary accuracy. J Thorac Dis 10(suppl 1):S177–S183, 2018 29445542

Levenson JC, Troxel WM, Begley A, et al: A quantitative approach to distinguishing older adults with insomnia from good sleeper controls. J Clin Sleep Med 9(2):125–131, 2013 23372464

Maislin G, Pack AI, Kribbs NB, et al: A survey screen for prediction of apnea. Sleep 18(3):158–166, 1995 7610311

Manni R, Terzaghi M, Repetto A: The FLEP scale in diagnosing nocturnal frontal lobe epilepsy, NREM and REM parasomnias: data from a tertiary sleep and epilepsy unit. Epilepsia 49(9):1581–1585, 2008 18410366

Mansukhani MP, Kolla BP: Apps and fitness trackers that measure sleep: are they useful? Cleve Clin J Med 84(6):451–456, 2017 28628429

Nagappa M, Liao P, Wong J, et al: Validation of the STOP-Bang questionnaire as a screening tool for obstructive sleep apnea among different populations: a systematic review and meta-analysis. PLoS One 10(12):e0143697, 2015 26658438

Netzer NC, Stoohs RA, Netzer CM, et al: Using the Berlin Questionnaire to identify patients at risk for the sleep apnea syndrome. Ann Intern Med 131(7):485–491, 1999 10507956

Ohayon MM, Ferini-Strambi L, Plazzi G, et al: Frequency of narcolepsy symptoms and other sleep disorders in narcoleptic patients and their first-degree relatives. J Sleep Res 14(4):437–445, 2005 16364145

Ohayon MM, O'Hara R, Vitiello MV: Epidemiology of restless legs syndrome: a synthesis of the literature. Sleep Med Rev 16(4):283–295, 2012 21795081

Okun ML, Kravitz HM, Sowers MF, et al: Psychometric evaluation of the Insomnia Symptom Questionnaire: a self-report measure to identify chronic insomnia. J Clin Sleep Med 5(1):41–51, 2009 19317380

Ong AA, Gillespie MB: Overview of smartphone applications for sleep analysis. World J Otorhinolaryngol Head Neck Surg 2(1):45–49, 2016 29204548

Pagel JF: Excessive daytime sleepiness. Am Fam Physician 79(5):391–396, 2009 19275068

Pandi-Perumal SR, Smits M, Spence W, et al: Dim light melatonin onset (DLMO): a tool for the analysis of circadian phase in human sleep and chronobiological disorders. Prog Neuropsychopharmacol Biol Psychiatry 31(1):1–11, 2007 16884842

Postuma RB, Arnulf I, Hogl B, et al: A single-question screen for rapid eye movement sleep behavior disorder: a multicenter validation study. Mov Disord 27(7):913–916, 2012 22729987

Redline S: Obstructive sleep apnea: phenotypes and genetics, in Principles and Practice of Sleep Medicine, 6th Edition. Edited by Kryger MH, Roth T, Dement WC. Philadelphia, PA, Elsevier, 2016, pp 1102–1109

Sehgal A, Mignot E: Genetics of sleep and sleep disorders. Cell 146(2):194–207, 2011 21784243

Spitzer RL, Kroenke K, Williams JBW, et al: A brief measure for assessing generalized anxiety disorder: the GAD-7. Arch Intern Med 166(10):1092–1097, 2006 16717171

St-Onge M-P, Roberts A, Shechter A, et al: Fiber and saturated fat are associated with sleep arousals and slow wave sleep. J Clin Sleep Med 12(1):19–24, 2016 26156950

Statland BE, Demas TJ: Serum caffeine half-lives. Healthy subjects vs. patients having alcoholic hepatic disease. Am J Clin Pathol 73(3):390–393, 1980 7361718

Sturzenegger C, Baumann CR, Lammers GJ, et al: Swiss Narcolepsy Scale: a simple screening tool for hypocretin-deficient narcolepsy with cataplexy. Clin Translational Neurosci 2(2):1–5, 2018

Trotti LM: Idiopathic hypersomnia. Sleep Med Clin 12(3):331–344, 2017 28778232

Walters AS, LeBrocq C, Dhar A, et al: Validation of the International Restless Legs Syndrome Study Group rating scale for restless legs syndrome. Sleep Med 4(2):121–132, 2003 14592342

Weaver TE, Laizner AM, Evans LK, et al: An instrument to measure functional status outcomes for disorders of excessive sleepiness. Sleep 20(10):835–843, 1997 9415942

Yang A, Palmer AA, de Wit H: Genetics of caffeine consumption and responses to caffeine. Psychopharmacology (Berl) 211(3):245–257, 2010 20532872

Youngstedt SD, Kline CE, Elliott JA, et al: Circadian phase-shifting effects of bright light, exercise, and bright light + exercise. J Circadian Rhythms 14:2, 2016 27103935

Yu L, Buysse DJ, Germain A, et al: Development of short forms from the PROMIS™ Sleep Disturbance and Sleep-Related Impairment item banks. Behav Sleep Med 10(1):6–24, 2011 22250775

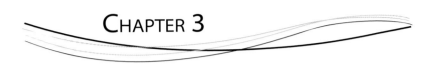

CHAPTER 3

Diagnosis of Insomnia

David N. Neubauer, M.D.

Three major nosologies incorporating insomnia diagnoses are in common use. Each employs different diagnostic criteria, although they do overlap somewhat (Table 3–1). The most detailed categorization of sleep disorders generally and of insomnia specifically is the *International Classification of Sleep Disorders*, 3rd Edition (ICSD-3), published by the American Academy of Sleep Medicine (2014). DSM-5 (American Psychiatric Association 2013) incorporates a sleep disorders section that includes an insomnia disorder diagnosis. Finally, the *International Classification of Diseases*, 10th Revision (ICD-10), published by the World Health Organization and widely used for billing and coding purposes, specifies several sleep disorder diagnoses, including insomnia disorders (World Health Organization 1992).

The key feature shared among these insomnia diagnostic criteria is the subjective complaint element. The foundation of an insomnia disorder diagnosis is dissatisfaction with the quality or quantity of sleep. In addition, adequate opportunity for sleep and the presence of associated daytime consequences may be required. Insomnia disorder criteria do not include objective requirements, such as the number of minutes it takes to fall asleep, the length of time awake during the night, or the estimated total number of hours of sleep.

The recent ICSD-3 and DSM-5 insomnia disorder diagnoses represent major revisions from previous versions. Both are simplified and more globally applicable. They have abandoned the conceptual differentiation between primary and secondary insomnia in favor of the recognition of comorbid insomnia without specific causal attribution. Insomnia should be diagnosed when it warrants independent clinical attention, regardless of whether other medical, mental health, or substance use disorders are present. In addition, past primary insomnia diagnostic subtypes (e.g., psychophysiological insomnia, idiopathic insomnia, inadequate sleep

TABLE 3–1. Key features of the DSM-5 and ICSD-3 insomnia disorder diagnoses

Criteria	DSM-5 insomnia disorder	ICSD-3 short-term insomnia disorder	ICSD-3 chronic insomnia disorder
Sleep complaint	One or more of the following: Difficulty initiating sleep Difficulty maintaining sleep Early morning awakening with inability to return to sleep	One or more of the following: Difficulty initiating sleep Difficulty maintaining sleep Waking up earlier than desired Resistance to going to bed on appropriate schedule Difficulty sleeping without parent/caregiver intervention	One or more of the following: Difficulty initiating sleep Difficulty maintaining sleep Waking up earlier than desired Resistance to going to bed on appropriate schedule Difficulty sleeping without parent/caregiver intervention
Associations with sleep difficulty	Clinically significant distress or impairment in Social Occupational Educational Academic Behavioral Other important areas of functioning	One or more problems/impairments associated with nighttime sleep difficulty: Fatigue/Malaise Attention, concentration, or memory Social, family, occupational, or academic performance Mood disturbance/irritability Daytime sleepiness Behavioral issues (hyperactivity, impulsivity, aggression) Motivation/energy/initiative Concerns or dissatisfaction with sleep	One or more problems/impairments associated with nighttime sleep difficulty: Fatigue/Malaise Attention, concentration, or memory Social, family, occupational, or academic performance Mood disturbance/irritability Daytime sleepiness Behavioral issues (hyperactivity, impulsivity, aggression) Motivation/energy/initiative Concerns or dissatisfaction with sleep

TABLE 3–1. Key features of the DSM-5 and ICSD-3 insomnia disorder diagnoses (*continued*)

Criteria	DSM-5 insomnia disorder	ICSD-3 short-term insomnia disorder	ICSD-3 chronic insomnia disorder
Adequate opportunity	Sleep difficulty occurs despite adequate opportunity for sleep	Sleep difficulty cannot be explained by inadequate opportunity or circumstances for sleep	Sleep difficulty cannot be explained by inadequate opportunity or circumstances for sleep
Frequency	At least 3 nights per week	No requirement	At least three times per week
Duration	At least 3 months	Less than 3 months	At least 3 months
Not attributable to or better explained by	Another sleep-wake disorder Effects of a substance (e.g., drug of abuse, medication) Coexisting mental disorders and medical conditions	Another sleep disorder	Another sleep disorder

Note. ICSD-3 = *International Classification of Sleep Disorders*, 3rd Edition.
Source. American Academy of Sleep Medicine 2014; American Psychiatric Association 2013.

hygiene, and paradoxical insomnia) have been eliminated due to the lack of evidence supporting their existence as distinct clinical entities.

Diagnostic Criteria

INTERNATIONAL CLASSIFICATION OF SLEEP DISORDERS, 3RD EDITION

ICSD-3 is a comprehensive nosology of sleep disorders that lists criteria for insomnia disorders as well as sleep-related breathing disorders, central disorders of hypersomnolence, parasomnias, circadian rhythm sleep-wake disorders, and sleep-related movement disorders. It recognizes three insomnia categories: 1) chronic, 2) short-term, and 3) other. The chronic and short-term insomnia disorders have similar criteria and differ primarily in the duration of the symptoms: <3 months for short-term and ≥3 months for chronic. Also, ICSD-3 does not specify a nights-per-week frequency criterion for short-term insomnia. The "other insomnia" diagnostic category is intended for individuals who warrant clinical attention for their symptoms despite not meeting the full short-term insomnia criteria. Although the insomnia history most typically is reported by the patient, a parent or caregiver may be the primary informant in the case of children or older adults with significant functional impairment.

Six criteria must be met for the ICSD-3 chronic insomnia disorder diagnosis (see Table 3–1). A sleep complaint must be reported, with options that include difficulty with sleep onset or maintenance or waking earlier than desired, resistance going to bed at an appropriate time, or sleep difficulty without the intervention of a parent or caregiver. Although some individuals exclusively have difficulty with falling asleep or remaining asleep, many people experience both problems in patterns that may vary over time. Daytime problems must be reported, presumably associated with the nighttime sleep difficulty. The sleep or wake complaints cannot be due to inadequate opportunity or circumstances for sleep. Accordingly, sufficient time should be allotted for sleep in a comfortable environment that is conducive to sleep. The sleep and wake problems must occur at least three times per week and must have persisted for at least 3 months. Finally, the sleep and waking complaints should not be better explained by another sleep disorder. The "chronic insomnia" designation may be used with patients who have recurrent insomnia symptoms lasting several weeks over a period of several years, despite never having a single 3-month episode. "Chronic insomnia" also may be used with patients who are sleeping adequately with the use of hypnotic medications but would meet the disorder criteria without the medication.

The complaints presumably related to the sleep difficulty that contribute to both the chronic and short-term insomnia diagnoses include multiple options, of which patients must endorse at least one, although typically multiple problems are present. Fatigue or malaise is often reported. Sometimes patients with insomnia describe daytime sleepiness, although more typically they say that they feel "tired and wired" and are unable to sleep during the daytime. Patients may report difficulty with memory, attention, and concentration. Their academic, occupational, family, and social functioning may be impaired. Patients may describe irritability or a mood disturbance. Behavioral problems may include impulsivity, aggressiveness, or hyperactivity. Patients may report low energy, motivation, and initiative as well as an increase in proneness to accidents and errors. Finally, they may have concerns about or dissatisfaction with their sleep.

ICSD-3 notes that insomnia in young children often is associated with inappropriate sleep associations or inadequate limit setting. Children may have significantly delayed sleep onset due to dependency on particular objects or settings or a specific stimulation. Examples include wanting a bottle, to be rocked, or to sleep with a parent. Inadequate limit setting may result in bedtime stalling or refusal, as well as prolonged nighttime awakenings.

Short-term insomnia disorder shares these criteria domains with chronic insomnia disorder, with the exception of requiring <3 months' duration and the absence of the nights-per-week frequency. For many, insomnia symptoms occur in the context of acute stressors; however, the short-term insomnia diagnosis should be reserved for circumstances in which independent clinical attention is warranted. The sleep and related symptoms may improve with treatment or spontaneously with resolution of the stressors, although for some people, persistent sleep difficulty will evolve into a chronic insomnia disorder.

DIAGNOSTIC AND STATISTICAL MANUAL OF MENTAL DISORDERS, 5TH EDITION

DSM-5 includes a single insomnia disorder that is similar to the ICSD-3 chronic insomnia disorder. Dissatisfaction with sleep quality or quantity is a fundamental element that may manifest as difficulty initiating or maintaining sleep or early morning awakening with an inability to return to sleep. With children, the sleep difficulties are present in the absence of caregiver intervention. The second key criterion is clinically significant distress or impairment in important areas of functioning (e.g., social, occupational, educational, academic, behavioral). Adequate opportunity for sleep must be available. The sleep complaint and associated difficulties must be present at least 3 nights per week for a duration of ≥3 months. The insomnia symptoms should not be better explained by another sleep disorder, physiological effects of a substance, or a coexisting medical condition or mental disorder; however, comorbidity with mental, medical, and sleep disorders may be specified. In addition, insomnia disorder may be specified as episodic (symptoms persisting between 1 and 3 months), persistent (symptoms lasting at least 3 months), or recurrent (two or more episodes within a 1-year period). The DSM-5 nosology allows for an "unspecified" insomnia disorder and an "other specified" insomnia disorder that may be coded for brief (<3 months) insomnia symptoms or sleep complaints restricted to nonrestorative sleep.

INTERNATIONAL CLASSIFICATION OF DISORDERS, 10TH REVISION

ICD-10 represents the World Health Organization's comprehensive and hierarchical organization of health conditions, including diseases, disorders, and injuries. Although ICD-10 is important for reimbursement, research, and health policy, it is limited in providing insomnia diagnostic criteria. Insomnia diagnoses are listed with brief descriptions in both the "F" (mental and behavioral disorders) and "G" (diseases of the nervous system) categories. Insomnia not due to a substance or physiological condition is coded as F51.0, with the option of further specification for primary insomnia, adjustment insomnia, paradoxical insomnia, psychophysiological insomnia, insomnia due to other mental disorder, and other insomnia not due to a substance or known physiological condition. The G47 code section includes various sleep disorders, including G47.0 for insomnia, with additional optional coding for unspecified, due to a medical condition, and other insomnias.

Pathophysiology

No single disease pathology has been identified in insomnia disorder; however, several proposed models have supportive evidence and are valuable in guiding treatment and research (Morin and Benca 2012). Insomnia is most usefully viewed as having multiple contributory factors that exert shifting influence over time. The development and continuation of insomnia symptoms may be influenced by genetic vulnerabilities and epigenetic processes, cultural perspectives, personality features, life circumstances, daily behaviors and routines, bedroom environment, use of medications or abused substances, comorbid health conditions, and maladaptive thinking, attitudes, and beliefs about sleep. Overarching themes in insomnia explanatory models emphasize excess physiological and cognitive arousal, and psychological conditioning (American Academy of Sleep Medicine 2014; American Psychiatric Association 2013).

Psychological and cognitive perspectives on insomnia focus on increased vulnerability in people with heightened anxiety, a tendency to worry excessively, a strong somatic focus, and an internalizing personality style. People with persistent insomnia often are preoccupied with their sleep difficulty and the perceived consequences (American Psychiatric Association 2013). They are described as having a selective attention bias in their experience of internal and external sleep-related cues (Harvey 2002). During the daytime, they may require greater effort to maintain normal cognitive functioning. Psychological conditioning of arousal associated with the bed, bedroom, and bedtime routines is posited as a primary factor reinforcing insomnia over time, potentially leading to chronic insomnia (American Psychiatric Association 2013).

The idea of hyperarousal during sleep and waking throughout the day and night is a central element of current insomnia explanatory models, typified by the common complaint of the insomnia patient describing feeling "tired and wired" (Riemann et al. 2015). Despite the lack of a single underlying pathological abnormality causing insomnia disorder, abundant evidence representing diverse physiological measures supports hyperarousal as a common denominator among people with insomnia disorder. Domains of evidence showing excessive arousal among insomnia subjects include heart rate and heart rate variability, core body temperature, basal skin resistance, phasic vasoconstriction, metabolic rate, hypothalamic-pituitary-adrenal axis activity (e.g., cortisol, adrenocorticotropic hormone, and corticotropin releasing factor), and immune function and cytokine levels. Electroencephalographic studies during sleep show increased beta and gamma activity and decreased slow-wave activity among insomnia subjects. Brain imaging studies comparing insomnia subjects with control subjects show heightened metabolic activity during sleep and wake and diminished reductions in metabolic activity during sleep in specific brain regions associated with wake promotion.

Several studies support the argument for a genetic vulnerability to insomnia. Familial aggregation has been observed (Riemann et al. 2015); twin studies have found a heritability coefficient between 42% and 57%. Specific candidate genes investigated relate to a circadian clock gene

(*PER3*), the β3 GABA$_A$ receptor subunit, and the serotonin transporter. Stressful life events could trigger epigenetic mechanisms affecting stress regulatory processes and possibly long-term brain structure changes that perpetuate sleep difficulty.

The "Three-P" (predisposing, precipitating, and perpetuating) insomnia model emphasizes the multitude of influences that can undermine sleep quality and quantity over time, including the transition from acute to chronic insomnia (Ebben and Spielman 2009). This model incorporates a hypothetical insomnia threshold beyond which sleep is disturbed. Everyone has some degree of predisposition to insomnia, with factors such as personality characteristics and biological processes elevating a person's baseline vulnerability. Precipitants that might move an individual beyond the insomnia threshold include acute stressors, schedule changes, and medical or mental health illness episodes. As the precipitant or its effect diminishes, sleep may shift back to the baseline condition of adequate sleep. However, new perpetuating factors may emerge that promote ongoing sleep difficulty. Maladaptive behaviors, such as daytime napping or the use of alcohol as a hypnotic, or the development of conditioned arousal associated with attempts to sleep at night, can result in chronic insomnia even in the absence of the acute precipitants.

Epidemiology

The reported prevalence of insomnia depends on the population examined and the insomnia definition employed in the survey. In the general population, about 30%–35% of individuals endorse at least transient insomnia symptoms (e.g., difficulty falling asleep, difficulty staying asleep, or early morning awakening). Complaints exclusively of difficulty with sleep maintenance are more common than those of difficulty with sleep onset, although many patients report both. Approximately 15%–20% of people meet the diagnostic criteria for short-term insomnia disorder. Finally, about 6%–10% of the general population meets criteria for chronic insomnia disorder (American Academy of Sleep Medicine 2014; American Psychiatric Association 2013; Ohayon 2002).

The risk for significant insomnia complaints is higher among women, at a rate 1.44 times greater than that for men. The prevalence of insomnia is higher among older individuals, perhaps due to age-related sleep changes, increasing comorbidities and disabilities, and greater medication use. In general, people with chronic medical and mental health disorders have higher rates of insomnia symptoms. Approximately 50% of people treated for chronic conditions are estimated to have persistent insomnia. Epidemiological studies also show that lower socioeconomic status is associated with an increased insomnia risk (American Psychiatric Association 2013).

Clinical Presentation, Course, and Complications

CLINICAL PRESENTATION

The DSM-5 and ICSD-3 insomnia disorder diagnostic criteria encompass the features of typical patient presentations: dissatisfaction with sleep quantity or quality in association with one or more complaints about how the patient feels or functions during the daytime. Concerns regarding daytime consequences or impairment usually are key components of the chief complaint and lead to the patient seeking help from a health care provider. Patients may report difficulty falling or remaining asleep, perhaps with a sense of very light sleep or multiple arousals from sleep, and they also describe problems, such as fatigue, poor concentration, decreased productivity, and irritability. Although no precipitant for an insomnia episode may be apparent, patients frequently describe stressful life events (e.g., separation or divorce, loss of job, or death of a loved one) in relation to their initial or recurrent sleep difficulties. Co-occurring schedule or environmental changes also may be offered as causes. In addition, people may explain their sleep problems in relation to comorbid conditions, such as pain, anxiety, or depression.

Although insomnia may begin at any age, initial episodes most commonly occur in young adulthood. An increased insomnia incidence also is observed among older adults and among women at the time of menopause. Complaints of sleep onset difficulty are typical for young adults, whereas sleep maintenance problems are more frequently described by older adults, perhaps in part due to circadian influences and different precipitating and perpetuating factors.

Comorbidity of insomnia symptoms with medical conditions and mental health disorders is reported at a high rate. Insomnia occurs at an increased frequency in patients diagnosed with diabetes, cardiovascular disease, numerous neurological conditions (e.g., Parkinson's disease), chronic obstructive pulmonary disease, arthritis, fibromyalgia, and other pain conditions. Sleep complaints are highly prevalent among patients with mood, anxiety, substance use, and trauma- and stressor-related disorders.

COURSE

Duration of reported sleep difficulty may range from days to decades, with symptom patterns including acute and situational, chronic, and recurrent sleep-related problems. Acute insomnia often resolves as precipitating factors decline or as individuals adapt to their situation, although they may remain vulnerable to recurrences when stressors return. Although insomnia follows no predictable course, past and current episodes do increase the likelihood of future insomnia (Ohayon 2009). One study found that 1 year after a baseline assessment documenting insomnia, 70% of the subjects continued to experience insomnia, and after 3 years, 50% still reported insomnia (American Academy of Sleep Medicine 2014). For many patients with chronic insomnia, the predominance of sleep onset or sleep maintenance difficulty varies over time. Moreover, sleep may vary considerably from night to night.

COMPLICATIONS

Complications of insomnia may be evident early in the course of an episode or emerge later with chronic insomnia symptoms. Although aspects of daytime impairment are fundamental to the insomnia disorder diagnosis, these may worsen as the sleep disturbance persists. For example, complaints of fatigue, irritability, functional impairment, low motivation and energy, and worry about poor sleep and its consequences may become more prominent over time. In addition, although insomnia frequently evolves in people with a variety of comorbid conditions, abundant evidence demonstrates an increased future risk of the new onset or recurrence of various mental health and medical disorders. Numerous longitudinal studies show that a history of insomnia is associated with a greater risk of future depressive, anxiety, and substance use disorders. Persistent insomnia has been shown to be an independent risk factor for suicidal behavior. Future hypertension and myocardial infarction are increased in people with insomnia. The strongest evidence for cardiovascular and metabolic complications has been found in the insomnia disorder phenotype of individuals with objective short sleep duration (<6 hours) (Vgontzas et al. 2012).

Additional complications associated with chronic insomnia include absenteeism and work disability, medication and substance misuse, interpersonal and social problems, and reduced quality of life (American Psychiatric Association 2013; Olfson et al. 2018). On a societal level, chronic insomnia accounts for a large economic burden (Daley et al. 2009).

Diagnostic Procedures, Tests, and Questionnaires

CLINICAL HISTORY

The diagnosis of insomnia disorder and the development of a treatment plan should evolve from a comprehensive history (Schutte-Rodin et al. 2008). A complete evaluation includes physical and mental status examinations and may be supplemented with sleep logs or diaries and, possibly, objective testing with actigraphy or sleep recordings. Because multiple factors generally contribute to the initiation and perpetuation of insomnia, the assessment of patients complaining of sleep difficulties should explore the constellation of influences potentially undermining sleep. Input from a bed partner or other household informant can be invaluable. Inquiries also should be made about any family history of sleep-related symptoms or disorders.

A detailed sleep history includes a review of nighttime and daytime symptoms as well as habits and routines throughout the day and night (Table 3–2). Key elements include evening activities, bedtime routines, the bedroom environment, typical bedtime hours, sleep onset latency, nighttime sleep experience (e.g., awakenings, quality, duration), morning awakening time and whether an alarm clock is used, daytime and evening alertness or drowsiness, and daytime sleeping (planned naps or inadvertent sleep episodes). Does the patient snore, breathe irregularly, or move excessively while asleep? More specific questioning may depend on the patient's chief complaint. Special attention should be given to possible daytime consequences, because these represent diagnostic criteria for insomnia disorder. Patients should be asked about any associations with the onset or recurrence of their sleep difficulties. Questions also should explore the variability of routines and any differences associated with work, school, or vacation schedules. Many people follow nonconventional schedules due to work requirements or lifestyle choices, so sleep-wake symptoms may need to be considered in multiple contexts.

The sleep history for insomnia should include any details of past treatment approaches and associated benefits or adverse experiences. What does the patient currently do when attempting to optimize sleep? Has the patient participated in cognitive or behavioral therapies for insomnia? Has the patient used alcohol, dietary supplements, over-the-counter sleep aids, or prescription medications specifically for the sleep complaints? Does the patient use any medications or other substances

TABLE 3–2.   Insomnia history assessment inventory

Primary insomnia complaint

Nighttime symptoms

  Sleep onset difficulty

  Awakenings

    Frequency and duration

    Associated symptoms and experiences

    Difficulty returning to sleep

    Behaviors during the night

  Early morning awakening

  Estimated sleep amount

  Sleep quality

Daytime/evening symptoms

  Fatigue

  Sleepiness and napping or inadvertent sleep episodes

  Reduced motivation, energy, or initiative

  Mood disturbance or irritability

  Cognitive dysfunction (attention, concentration, memory)

  Proneness to errors and accidents

  Diminished quality of life

  Functional and performance impairment

    Social

    Occupational

    Educational

    Academic

    Behavioral

Course of sleep disturbance

Premorbid sleep pattern

Onset (abrupt or gradual)

Associated circumstances

  Precipitating factors

    Physical or mental conditions

    Life circumstances (stressful events)

  Perpetuating factors

Frequency when affected by insomnia symptoms (days per week)

Duration (weeks, months, years)

Pattern of insomnia symptoms

  Acute

  Episodic

  Persistent

TABLE 3–2.   Insomnia history assessment inventory *(continued)*

Course of sleep disturbance (*continued*)

Severity

Intensity

Impact on functioning

Sleep-wake schedule

Opportunity and circumstances for adequate sleep

Bedtime and typical sleep latency

Time of final awakening and rise time

Schedule regularity and variations

School

Work (including shift work) and days off

Lifestyle choices affecting sleep-wake time

Vacation

Transmeridian travel

Pre-sleep conditions

Usual evening routines

Mental state (e.g., worry about sleep)

Bedroom environment

Light

Noise

Temperature

Sleep surface (bed, sofa, other)

Activities in bed (e.g., reading, television, electronic screens)

Bed partners (including pets)

Daytime or evening napping

Typical daytime activities

Exercise

Light exposure (natural sunlight, bright workplace lighting)

Fatigue/sleepiness countermeasures

Additional sleep-related symptoms

Breathing

Snoring, gasping, or coughing

Witnessed cessation of breathing

Body movements

Kicking or twitching

Restlessness (evening or nighttime)

Urinary frequency

Gastroesophageal reflux

Pain

TABLE 3–2.   Insomnia history assessment inventory *(continued)*

Medication and substance use (amount and timing)

Prescription and over-the-counter medications

Dietary supplement use (including melatonin)

Alcohol

Caffeine

Nicotine

Other substances (e.g., cannabis)

Previous and current treatments and responses (effectiveness and side effects)

Coexisting sleep-wake disorders

Mental health and medical histories (including comprehensive review of systems)

Family history of sleep-related symptoms and disorders

Source.   American Psychiatric Association 2013; Morin and Benca 2012; Schutte-Rodin et al. 2008.

(e.g., caffeine) to promote daytime alertness? Has the patient made any lifestyle modifications to improve sleep?

Comorbid conditions that might influence insomnia symptoms should be explored. The patient's review of systems and problem list should be examined. Sleep disorders commonly associated with sleep disruption and daytime impairment include sleep-disordered breathing, circadian rhythm abnormalities, parasomnias, and restless legs syndrome (RLS). It will be important to determine whether the individual has a prominent advanced or delayed sleep phase tendency. Mood, anxiety, stress-related, psychotic, and substance use disorders are among the many psychiatric conditions with increased risk for sleep disruption. Any medical problems causing pain or discomfort may undermine sleep quality. A list of all prescribed medications, over-the-counter products, and dietary supplements should be reviewed with regard to possible effects on sleep.

Both physical and mental status examinations may provide findings that are helpful diagnostically and in guiding aspects of treatment. Optimizing the management of comorbid conditions may be important for improving sleep. A routine physical examination may reveal findings of cardiovascular or neurological disorders. A focused examination of the neck and the oral and nasal airways may provide evidence suggestive of obstructive sleep apnea (OSA). The mental status examination may reveal symptoms of the various psychiatric disorders associated with sleep complaints. Routine laboratory studies (e.g., blood and urine) may aid with medical diagnoses relevant to insomnia symptoms; however, no findings are specific for the diagnosis of insomnia disorder.

Sleep logs and diaries are available in a variety of formats. Some are designed to highlight sleep time on a grid, with multiple daily rows representing each hour of the day and night (typically centered around midnight), for individuals to fill in when they have slept. Others ask daily questions such as bedtime, latency to sleep, number of awakenings, total sleep, wakeup time, daytime activities, and medication use. Each format has strengths and weaknesses, but both can offer useful information, especially if the data have been collected over a period of several weeks. These sleep logs and diaries can aid in the initial diagnostic process, as well as in monitoring therapeutic progress over time.

DIAGNOSTIC TESTS FOR INSOMNIA

The core insomnia disorder diagnostic criteria are subjective; accordingly, the diagnosis does not depend on objective measures of sleep. However, sleep testing may be indicated to investigate comorbid sleep disorders that may contribute to sleep-wake complaints or to identify alternate conditions within the differential diagnosis (Schutte-Rodin et al. 2008). An overnight laboratory clinical polysomnographic study monitors electroencephalographic activity, eye movements, snoring, airflow, respiratory effort, oxygen saturation, heart rhythm, chin and leg muscle activity, and body movements via video recording. Patients at high risk for OSA may be evaluated with a more limited home sleep study. Usually, these studies are performed during a single night.

Activity monitoring can be done over a period of days to weeks with a small device typically worn on the nondominant wrist. Actigraphy, which is especially useful in assessing possible circadian rhythm sleep-wake disorders, can estimate the timing of sleep and reflect nighttime awakenings (Smith et al. 2018). Numerous consumer-oriented devices and apps offer estimates of sleep, sleep stages, and sleep quality; however, these currently are of limited value for diagnostic purposes.

QUESTIONNAIRES

Several questionnaires and scales target aspects of sleep and sleep disturbances, as well as possible daytime consequences and risk factors for common sleep disorders. Questionnaires may be employed to screen for insomnia symptoms and other sleep disorders and may be used to assess symptoms and sleep quality over time. The most commonly used questionnaire that focuses specifically on insomnia symptoms is the Insomnia Severity Index, which is a self-reported seven-item list of questions related to nighttime sleep characteristics, daytime functioning and impairment, and level of distress regarding sleep difficulty (Morin et al. 2011). The Dysfunctional Beliefs and Attitudes About Sleep Scale (Morin et al. 2002) can help direct therapeutic strategies for insomnia patients. A useful general screening instrument for sleep disturbances and sleep disorders is the Pittsburgh Sleep Quality Index (Buysse et al. 1989), which includes 19 items to create a single global score and 7 component scores representing sleep quality, latency, quality, efficiency, and disturbance as well as medication use and daytime dysfunction. The STOP-BANG is an eight-item scale including signs and symptoms representing risk factors for OSA and may be helpful in the differential diagnosis of persistent sleep disturbance (Nagappa et al. 2015). The Epworth Sleepiness Scale, which assesses sleep propensity in eight different circumstances, can aid in evaluating daytime sleepiness and help direct further evaluation of sleep-related complaints (Johns 1991).

Differential Diagnosis

Difficulty falling asleep and remaining asleep occurs commonly and in various circumstances. Diagnosis and effective management necessitate the differentiation of a criteria-based insomnia disorder from the presence of various sleep complaints. The insomnia evaluation process should identify whether an insomnia disorder diagnosis is warranted and reveal the presence of any comorbid conditions that may be causing or contributing to the sleep disturbance and related symptoms. The evaluation may reveal an alternate diagnosis or additional conditions that should be addressed to improve a patient's sleep (American Academy of Sleep Medicine 2014; American Psychiatric Association 2013).

ACUTE (OR SITUATIONAL) VERSUS CHRONIC INSOMNIA

When people report the triad of nighttime sleep difficulty with daytime consequences in the context of an adequate opportunity for sleep, the frequency and duration of the symptoms then must be reviewed. When the sleep disturbance has occurred for <3 months, the insomnia symptoms may be considered acute or situational. Appropriate diagnoses may include *short-term insomnia disorder* (ICSD-3) and *other specified insomnia disorder* (DSM-5), although *chronic insomnia disorder* (ICSD-3) or *insomnia disorder* (DSM-5) may become warranted if symptoms persist.

SHORT SLEEPERS

Some individuals routinely experience relatively short sleep duration but do not report any daytime impairment or consequences. This short sleep may be considered a normal variant that does not require treatment, although education and reassurance may be helpful.

BEHAVIORALLY INDUCED SLEEP RESTRICTION

In contrast, people may complain of inadequate nighttime sleep with daytime impairment when they do not allot sufficient time in bed due to their school or work schedule or other lifestyle choices. This condition may be described as *chronic volitional sleep restriction* or *insufficient sleep syndrome*.

SLEEP-DISRUPTIVE ENVIRONMENTAL CIRCUMSTANCES

The evaluation also may reveal circumstances in which a person's sleep is disturbed exclusively due to identifiable external environmental conditions, such that sleep and daytime functioning are normal when sleep occurs away from the typical bedroom. A label of *sleep-disruptive environmental circumstances* may be appropriate in these cases.

COMORBID PSYCHIATRIC OR MEDICAL CONDITIONS

A large proportion of patients with insomnia symptoms are diagnosed with one or more comorbid psychiatric or medical conditions, some of which very frequently are associated with sleep difficulty. For example, sleep disturbances are among the diagnostic criteria options for major depressive disorder, generalized anxiety disorder, and PTSD and often are associated with painful physical conditions. Assuming the individuals satisfy the required insomnia disorder criteria, should they additionally be given an insomnia disorder diagnosis, or should their sleep complaints be considered elements of comorbid disorders? The answer is that an insomnia disorder should be diagnosed when the sleep disturbance warrants independent attention and management.

OTHER SLEEP DISORDERS

Difficulty with sleep onset and maintenance and any associated daytime symptoms may result from several different sleep disorders. The insomnia differential diagnosis should determine whether a patient has one or more sleep disorders and whether the insomnia complaints represent an independent insomnia disorder or are better explained by another sleep disorder.

Circadian Rhythm Sleep-Wake Disorders

Circadian rhythm sleep-wake disorders (see Chapters 12 and 13) inherently involve persistent or recurrent sleep disturbance with insomnia symptoms or excessive sleepiness, or both. *Delayed sleep-wake phase disorder* should be considered in patients with chronic sleep onset difficulty. Similarly, *advanced sleep-wake phase disorder* should be considered in those with chronic early morning awakening. Rarely, people may have an *irregular sleep-wake rhythm disorder* with no discernible circadian cycle of sleep and wake periods. *Non-24-hour sleep-wake rhythm disorder*, most common among totally blind individuals, involves alternating periods of nighttime sleep and daytime alertness gradually shifting into nighttime sleep difficulty and daytime sleepiness due to the relative alignment and misalignment of the patient's nonentrained circadian system to the day-night cycle. *Shift work disorder* and *jet lag disorder*, which may be associated with impaired sleep and alertness at desired times, should be evident by the history and temporal relationship.

Sleep-Related Breathing Disorders

Sleep-related breathing disorders (or sleep-disordered breathing; see Chapters 8–11) should be considered when people describe difficulty with sleep onset or sleep maintenance. *Obstructive sleep apnea disorders* are common and underdiagnosed (Krakow et al. 2014). OSA results from upper airway collapsibility during sleep and leads to snoring, breathing pauses, and gasping arousals. Daytime sleepiness and nighttime awakenings often are associated with OSA. Although the risk for OSA increases with obesity, abnormalities of the upper airway independently contribute to the airway collapse. *Central sleep apnea syndromes* may occur in the presence of impaired respiratory effort, possibly related to a medical condition, such as congestive heart failure. They also should be considered in the context of opioid use, whether as an abused substance, maintenance agonist therapy, or prescribed analgesic.

Restless Legs Syndrome

RLS often involves sleep onset difficulty (Chapter 17). Key features of RLS are uncomfortable akathisia-like sensations, urges to move the legs while inactive or at rest, transient relief with movement, and usual temporal occurrence in the evening or nighttime. Nighttime sleep quality may be impaired by periodic limb movements that commonly accompany RLS.

Parasomnias

Difficulty with sleep onset or sleep maintenance often occurs in conjunction with parasomnias, abnormal behaviors, or experiences that may arise as a person falls asleep or later in the sleep period during REM or non-REM (NREM) sleep (see Chapters 14–16). *Nightmare disorder* and *REM sleep behavior disorder* emerge from REM sleep, whereas *sleepwalking*, *sleep terrors*, and *confusional arousals* occur during NREM sleep. *Sleep paralysis* may be associated with sleep onset and awakenings.

Narcolepsy

Narcolepsy (see Chapter 6) is characterized by persistent excessive daytime sleepiness and possibly cataplexy, sleep paralysis, and hypnagogic hallucinations; however, complaints of difficulty falling and remaining asleep also are common. Nighttime (polysomnography) and daytime nap (multiple sleep latency test) laboratory sleep studies confirm the diagnosis of narcolepsy in a patient with the necessary clinical history.

Substance/Medication-Induced Sleep Disorder, Insomnia Type

Substance/medication-induced sleep disorder, insomnia type, may be diagnosed when a patient has sleep complaints in temporal association with the intoxication or withdrawal of a substance or medication with known potential effects on sleep.

Conclusion

Identification and proper diagnosis of sleep-related symptoms are essential for effective patient care as well as for epidemiology, health care economics, and research targeting insomnia pathophysiology. Currently, subjective sleep complaints are the basis of insomnia disorder diagnoses. Although selected evidence supports insomnia explanatory models of hyperarousal and psychological processes, no objective test for insomnia disorder is available. Future insomnia nosologies likely will benefit from advances in the understanding of the regulation of sleep and waking and perhaps will allow definitions of evidence-based insomnia phenotypes, with corresponding guidance for effective treatment.

KEY CLINICAL POINTS

- Insomnia disorder diagnoses require the triad of a sleep complaint, daytime consequences, and adequate opportunity for sleep.

- Insomnia disorder diagnoses are based on subjective dissatisfaction with sleep quality or quantity, with complaints involving difficulty with sleep onset or maintenance or early morning awakening with difficulty returning to sleep.

- Common daytime consequences of insomnia are fatigue, poor concentration, impaired performance, irritability, and proneness to errors and accidents.

- Parents and caregivers may serve as primary informants in the case of children and older adults with cognitive impairment.

- The insomnia diagnosis should be based on a comprehensive history that considers comorbid mental health and medical conditions that may influence a patient's sleep-wake cycle.

- A key element of the insomnia disorder differential diagnosis is the identification of any other sleep disorders that might be causing or contributing to the sleep-wake difficulties.

- DSM-5 and ICSD-3 provide comprehensive insomnia disorder diagnostic criteria and valuable discussions of the essential features, typical course, prevalence, risk factors, and differential diagnosis.

- DSM-5 insomnia disorder and ICSD-3 chronic insomnia disorder criteria require a minimum 3-month duration of sleep complaints and a frequency of at least 3 nights per week.

- Although insomnia symptoms occur commonly in association with comorbid conditions (i.e., anxiety, mood, and pain-related disorders), insomnia disorder should be diagnosed when the symptoms require independent attention and management.

References

American Academy of Sleep Medicine: International Classification of Sleep Disorders, 3rd Edition. Darien, IL, American Academy of Sleep Medicine, 2014

American Psychiatric Association: Diagnostic and Statistical Manual of Mental Disorders, 5th Edition. Arlington, VA, American Psychiatric Association, 2013

Buysse DJ, Reynolds CF III, Monk TH, et al: The Pittsburgh Sleep Quality Index: a new instrument for psychiatric practice and research. Psychiatry Res 28(2):193–213, 1989 2748771

Daley M, Morin CM, LeBlanc M, et al: The economic burden of insomnia: direct and indirect costs for individuals with insomnia syndrome, insomnia symptoms, and good sleepers. Sleep 32(1):55–64, 2009 19189779

Ebben MR, Spielman AJ: Non-pharmacological treatments for insomnia. J Behav Med 32(3):244–254, 2009 19169804

Harvey AG: A cognitive model of insomnia. Behav Res Ther 40(8):869–893, 2002 12186352

Johns MW: A new method for measuring daytime sleepiness: the Epworth Sleepiness Scale. Sleep 14(6):540–545, 1991 1798888

Krakow B, Ulibarri VA, McIver ND: Pharmacotherapeutic failure in a large cohort of patients with insomnia presenting to a sleep medicine center and laboratory: subjective pretest predictions and objective diagnoses. Mayo Clin Proc 89(12):1608–1620, 2014 25236429

Morin CM, Benca R: Chronic insomnia. Lancet 379(9821):1129–1141, 2012 22265700

Morin CM, Blais F, Savard J: Are changes in beliefs and attitudes about sleep related to sleep improvements in the treatment of insomnia? Behav Res Ther 40(7):741–752, 2002 12074370

Morin CM, Belleville G, Bélanger L, Ivers H: The Insomnia Severity Index: psychometric indicators to detect insomnia cases and evaluate treatment response. Sleep (Basel) 34(5):601–608, 2011 21532953

Nagappa M, Liao P, Wong J, et al: Validation of the STOP-Bang questionnaire as a screening tool for obstructive sleep apnea among different populations: a systematic review and meta-analysis. PLoS One 10(12):e0143697, 2015 26658438

Ohayon MM: Epidemiology of insomnia: what we know and what we still need to learn. Sleep Med Rev 6(2):97–111, 2002 12531146

Ohayon MM: Observation of the natural evolution of insomnia in the American general population cohort. Sleep Med Clin 4(1):87–92, 2009 20161295

Olfson M, Wall M, Liu SM, et al: Insomnia and impaired quality of life in the United States. J Clin Psychiatry 79(5), 2018 30256547

Riemann D, Nissen C, Palagini L, et al: The neurobiology, investigation, and treatment of chronic insomnia. Lancet Neurol 14(5):547–558, 2015 25895933

Schutte-Rodin S, Broch L, Buysse D, et al: Clinical guideline for the evaluation and management of chronic insomnia in adults. J Clin Sleep Med 4(5):487–504, 2008 18853708

Smith MT, McCrae CS, Cheung J, et al: Use of actigraphy for the evaluation of sleep disorders and circadian rhythm sleep-wake disorders: an American Academy of Sleep Medicine clinical practice guideline. J Clin Sleep Med 14(7):1231–1237, 2018 29991437

Vgontzas AN, Fernandez-Mendoza J, Bixler EO, et al: Persistent insomnia: the role of objective short sleep duration and mental health. Sleep (Basel) 35(1):61–68, 2012 22215919

World Health Organization: International Statistical Classification of Diseases and Related Health Problems, 10th Revision (ICD-10). Geneva, Switzerland, World Health Organization, 1992

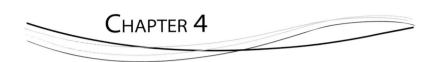

CHAPTER 4

Pharmacological Treatment of Insomnia

Emmanuel H. During, M.D.

Chronic insomnia is estimated to affect 22.1% of the U.S. population, approximately 70.7 million individuals (Roth et al. 2011). Insomnia has a crippling impact on productivity, causing an estimated annual loss of $63.2 billion (Kessler et al. 2011). Effective treatment of insomnia should always address the treatable causes and perpetuating factors. These may include underlying medical or psychiatric disorders, any environmental stressors, and other modifiable factors. When therapy for insomnia is required, cognitive-behavioral therapy for insomnia (CBT-I) should be recommended as first-line treatment when available (see Chapter 5). In this setting, a limited course of pharmacotherapy can be an adjunctive treatment. Some patients, however, may not have access or be amenable to CBT-I and may require pharmacotherapy. This chapter reviews the mechanism of action, evidence on efficacy, and side effects of the wide range of pharmacological agents used to treat insomnia, including FDA-approved drugs for insomnia, prescription drugs used off-label, over-the-counter sleep aids, and some common dietary supplements.

The Sleep-Wake Regulation Circuitry

Pharmacological agents used to treat insomnia promote sleep either via activation of sleep-promoting pathways or through inhibition of wake-promoting pathways. Sleep-inducing circuits are mostly represented by the GABAergic (referring to the neurotransmitter GABA) and melatonergic pathways (Figure 4–1). Benzodiazepines and benzodiazepine receptor agonist hypnotics activate the GABAergic system, while melatonin and the prescription drug ramelteon activate the melatonergic pathway. Circuits that promote arousal are represented by the monoaminergic sys-

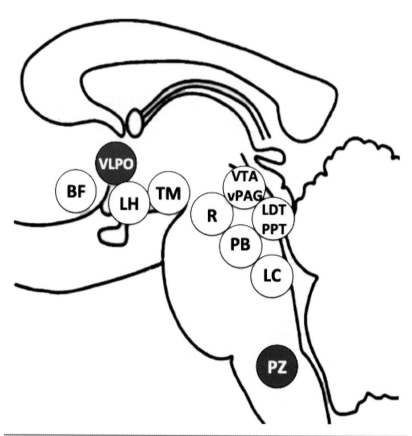

FIGURE 4–1.   The sleep-promoting and arousal systems.

Schematic representation of the main nuclei and centers promoting arousal (*white*) and sleep (*dark gray*) in the brain stem, diencephalon, and basal forebrain of the CNS and their respective neurotransmitters (sagittal view; left is anterior, right is posterior).
BF=basal forebrain (acetylcholine); LC=locus coeruleus (norepinephrine); LDT= laterodorsal tegmentum (acetylcholine); LH=lateral hypothalamus (orexin/hypocretin); PB= parabrachial nucleus (glutamate); PPT=pedunculopontine tegmentum (acetylcholine); PZ= parafacial zone (GABA); R=raphe nucleus (serotonin); TM=tuberomammillary nucleus (histamine); VLPO=ventrolateral preoptic area of the hypothalamus (GABA and galanin); vPAG=ventral periaqueductal gray (dopamine); VTA=ventral tegmental area (dopamine).

tem (the monoamine neurotransmitters include histamine, dopamine, norepinephrine, and serotonin), acetylcholine, hypocretin/orexin, and glutamate. Within the wake-promoting system, hypocretin/orexin acts as a modulator enhancing the action of monoamines. A number of the prescription sedative agents discussed in this chapter act by inhibiting the arousal system at one or multiple levels.

FDA-Approved Prescription Hypnotics

The drugs approved by the FDA for the treatment of insomnia belong to five pharmacological classes: benzodiazepines, nonbenzodiazepine benzodiazepine receptor agonists, melatonin receptor agonists (ramelteon), antihistamines (doxepin), and hypocretin/orexin receptor antagonists (suvorexant) (Table 4–1).

BENZODIAZEPINES

The efficacy of benzodiazepine drugs relies on the strong inhibitory effect of GABAergic projections from the median ventrolateral preoptic nucleus of the hypothalamus to the wake-promoting centers in the brain stem and diencephalon, capable of "switching off" the arousal system. Benzodiazepines bind to the $GABA_A$ receptor at a different site (the interface of the α and γ subunits) than do GABA, nonbenzodiazepine drugs, barbiturates, and alcohol. Benzodiazepines act as a positive allosteric modulator of the chloride channel, facilitating influx of chloride and subsequent inhibition of neuronal activity via hyperpolarization of the membrane potential. Introduced on the U.S. market in 1963, benzodiazepines have been widely used for treating anxiety, seizures, alcohol withdrawal, and other states of psychomotor agitation, in addition to insomnia. They have anxiolytic properties at low doses, and they induce sleep at higher doses.

When prescribing a benzodiazepine, attention should be given to onset of action (time to peak concentration, or T_{max}) and half-life of the drug (see Table 4–1). A benzodiazepine with a shorter onset of action should be favored in cases of initiation insomnia, whereas one with a longer half-life may be more appropriate in maintenance or early morning insomnia. Treatment should be started at a low dose and adjusted based on clinical response and tolerance.

The most common side effects of benzodiazepine drugs include confusion, ataxia, increased risk of falls, and residual morning grogginess. These side effects pose a higher safety risk in the elderly. In addition, benzodiazepines have the potential for CNS and respiratory depression, adverse effects potentiated by other commonly prescribed drugs, such as opioids, in addition to alcohol. Benzodiazepines are U.S. Drug Enforcement Administration Schedule IV controlled substances due to their associated risk of abuse and dependence (Vinkers and Olivier 2012). In addition to transient rebound insomnia and return of prior insomnia (Schutte-Rodin et al. 2008), abrupt discontinuation of benzodiazepines can result in anxiety and seizures, particularly with drugs that have a short half-life. This risk is also more often observed with use at higher

TABLE 4–1.   FDA-approved hypnotic drugs for the treatment of chronic insomnia

Drug	Dosage, mg	Onset of action	Elimination half-life, hours	Common side effects	U.S. DEA schedule
Benzodiazepines (GABA$_A$ receptor positive allosteric modulator)					
Triazolam	0.125–0.25	Very rapid	2–4	Headache, nausea	IV
Temazepam	7.5–30	Rapid	4–20	Hangover effect	IV
Estazolam	1–2	Intermediate	10–24	Hangover effect	IV
Quazepam	7.5–15	Rapid	40–70	Daytime sedation, headache	IV
Flurazepam	15–30	Rapid	48–120	Daytime sedation	IV
Nonbenzodiazepine benzodiazepine receptor agonists (GABA$_A$ receptor positive allosteric modulator)					
Zaleplon	5–10	Very rapid	1	Headache, paresthesia, nausea	IV
Zolpidem (SL)	1.75–3.5	Very rapid	2–3	Amnesia, headache, nausea	IV
Zolpidem	5–10	Rapid	2–3	NREM parasomnias, amnesia, headache, nausea	IV
Zolpidem (XR)	6.25–12.5	Rapid	3	NREM parasomnias, amnesia, headache, nausea	IV
Eszopiclone	1–3	Rapid	6	Unpleasant metallic taste, headache	IV
Melatonin receptor agonist (MT$_1$ and MT$_2$ receptor agonist)					
Ramelteon	8	Very rapid	1–2.6	Well tolerated	None
Antihistamine (H$_1$ receptor antagonist)					
Doxepin	3–6	Intermediate	15	Nausea, upper respiratory infections	None
Orexin receptor antagonist (OX$_1$ and OX$_2$ receptor antagonist)					
Suvorexant	5–20	Rapid	12	Hypnagogic/Hypnopompic hallucinations, headache	IV

Note.   Generic side effects of excessive sedation, daytime grogginess, and dizziness were not listed. Only specific or other common side effects were listed for each drug. DEA=Drug Enforcement Administration; NREM=non-REM; SL=sublingual; XR=extended release.

doses. Several observational studies have shown an association between long-term use of benzodiazepines and cognitive decline or dementia (Billioti de Gage et al. 2014; Gallacher et al. 2012; Wu et al. 2009). Studies are needed to elucidate whether chronic use of these medications independently increases neurodegenerative risk, because insomnia can also be an early symptom of neurodegeneration.

NONBENZODIAZEPINE BENZODIAZEPINE RECEPTOR AGONISTS ("Z DRUGS")

First introduced to the U.S. market in 1992, the so-called Z drugs are among the most widely prescribed drugs for insomnia (Gottesmann 2002; Sanger 2004). Nonbenzodiazepines bind at the same site as benzodiazepines on the $GABA_A$ receptor between the α and γ subunits, but do so more selectively to certain α subunits. This selectivity accounts for their hypnotic and amnestic effects and lack of anxiolytic, myorelaxant, or antiepileptic effects. Other differences exist within the nonbenzodiazepine group as well; for instance, eszopiclone has greater selectivity for the α_3 receptor subtype, which may result in different clinical properties. The three nonbenzodiazepine drugs available in the United States—zaleplon, zolpidem, and eszopiclone—have unique pharmacokinetic profiles that make them more suited for certain types of insomnia and have short, intermediate, and long durations of action, respectively (see Table 4–1). Additionally, the sublingual formulation of zolpidem has a rapid onset of action that may be appropriate for occasional middle-of-the-night use, whereas its controlled-release formulation provides a longer sedative effect that may be appropriate for late insomnia.

Like benzodiazepines, the nonbenzodiazepines should be initiated at a lower dose and titrated based on response. In females, zolpidem should be prescribed at a maximum dose of 5 mg, whereas the maximum FDA-approved dose for males is 10 mg. Other nonbenzodiazepines have no sex difference when prescribing.

Nonbenzodiazepines present similar side effects and risks as benzodiazepines, including residual morning grogginess, confusion, risk of imbalance, and falls (Drake et al. 2017). They may, however, present a lower risk of tolerance. For this reason, they are often preferred (Zammit et al. 2004). Nonbenzodiazepines are nonetheless Schedule IV controlled substances due to a risk of tolerance and abuse. The American Geriatric Society (AGS) approves a limited course of a nonbenzodiazepine or melatonin receptor agonist over most other sedative-hypnotics (Bloom et al. 2009; Gooneratne and Vitiello 2014). In some individuals, nonbenzodiazepines and benzodiazepines can result in complex parasomnias (see Chapter 14) that sometimes have medicolegal implications (Gunja 2013; Pressman 2011). The FDA recently added a black box warning to the prescribing information and patient medication guides for eszopiclone, zaleplon, and zolpidem because rare but serious injuries and death have occurred as a result of sleep behaviors, including sleepwalking, sleep driving, and other activities during sleep. The FDA also requires a contraindication to avoid use of eszopiclone, zaleplon, and zolpidem in patients who have previously experienced an episode of complex sleep behavior with these medications. In addition, caution should be used when prescribing these drugs in patients with restless legs syndrome (RLS) because they may induce sleepwalking and sleep-related eating disorder (Howell and Schenck 2012; Provini et al. 2009). Lastly, there is limited evidence of an association between zolpidem and dementia (Cheng et al. 2017; Shih et al. 2015).

MELATONIN RECEPTOR AGONIST RAMELTEON

The melatonin receptor agonist class has emerged in the past decade and is used for treating insomnia and certain circadian disorders. Ramelteon is a melatonin-1 and -2 (MT_1 and MT_2) receptor agonist with higher affinity than melatonin itself. Sleep initiation is mediated by binding at MT_1, counteracting the wake-promoting effect of the suprachiasmatic nucleus (SCN). The SCN, known as the central or master clock, promotes arousal to counteract the natural effect of fatigue and accumulated sleep drive in the late hours of the day. Although ramelteon does not appear to significantly increase total sleep time, it has shown to reduce sleep latency by several minutes (Kuriyama et al. 2014). Due to its short elimination half-life, this drug is suitable for initiation insomnia (see Table 4–1). Ramelteon is metabolized by the hepatic CYP1A2, which is inhibited by the antidepressant fluvoxamine; therefore, these drugs should not be prescribed together. Unlike benzodiazepines and nonbenzodiazepines, the melatonin receptor agonist ramelteon does not present a risk of abuse potential or dependence. Per the AGS, ramelteon is an acceptable option for treatment of insomnia in the elderly.

ANTIHISTAMINE DOXEPIN

Doxepin belongs to the class of tricyclic antidepressants (TCAs). At doses of 75 mg and higher, doxepin has some antidepressant properties. Below 10 mg, however, this drug selectively blocks the histamine-1 (H_1) receptor, with 4 times the potency of amitriptyline and 800 times the potency of diphenhydramine. Unlike several other sedative TCA agents and over-the-counter antihistamine sedatives, at such a low dose, doxepin has no antimuscarinic (anticholinergic) side effects. Due to a slow onset of action, doxepin is not suited for initiation insomnia; however, its long elimination half-life of 15 hours is appropriate for the treatment of maintenance and late insomnia (Atkin et al. 2018; Yeung et al. 2015). It can, however, cause weight gain and nausea, in addition to morning sedation. Lower (3 mg) doses should therefore be tried first and titrated up if needed. Doxepin presents no risk of abuse or dependence. It has a relatively favorable safety profile in the elderly per the 2015 Beers criteria issued by the AGS (Samuel 2015), and the American College of Physicians (ACP) favors doxepin over nonbenzodiazepine drugs in this population. A study comparing ambulation and coordination at peak plasma concentration for doxepin, zolpidem, or placebo showed an increased risk of falls with zolpidem but no difference between doxepin and placebo (Drake et al. 2017).

DUAL OREXIN/HYPOCRETIN RECEPTOR ANTAGONIST SUVOREXANT

The dual orexin-1 and -2 (OX_1 and OX_2) receptor antagonist suvorexant induces sedation via inhibition of the wake-promoting neurotransmitter orexin. Among other functions, orexin, also called hypocretin, secreted by the posterior lateral hypothalamus inhibits REM sleep and is a potent enhancer of the arousal system (de Lecea et al. 1998). Orexin is deficient in individuals with narcolepsy, resulting in excessive daytime sleepiness, and is therefore an obvious target for the development of hypnotic drugs for treating insomnia. Inhibition of the OX_2 receptor likely has a more important role than OX_1 in promoting sleep. Suvorexant has an intermediate half-life of 12 hours, with a relatively rapid onset of action, which makes it a suitable agent for both initiation and maintenance insomnia. Suvorexant has higher efficacy at higher doses; however, due to safety concerns over morning sedation, the maximum FDA-approved dose is 20 mg (Patel et al. 2015; Vermeeren et al. 2015). Other side effects can include sleep-related hallucinations. Due to its mechanism of action, suvorexant should not be used in individuals with narcolepsy. Although the risk of abuse and dependence is lower for suvorexant than for a benzodiazepine or nonbenzodiazepine, it is a Schedule IV controlled substance. The ACP considers suvorexant safe for use in elderly patients with insomnia. A pooled analysis from five trials comparing suvorexant with placebo in the elderly showed no additional risk of falls, no effect on morning psychomotor performance, and only a mildly higher rate (5.4% vs. 3.2% for 15 mg suvorexant dose and placebo, respectively) of reported residual somnolence (Herring et al. 2017). Other dual orexin receptor antagonists such as lemborexant and almorexant are becoming available and may represent as a "class" a more suitable option in the elderly or cognitively impaired, compared to benzodiazepines and non-benzodiazepine receptor agonists (Neylan et al. 2020).

Off-Label Prescription Drugs for Insomnia

Several drugs have been used off-label for the treatment of insomnia. These include other benzodiazepine drugs, sedative antidepressants, the $\alpha_2\delta$ ligand gabapentin, and some antipsychotic drugs (Table 4–2).

OTHER BENZODIAZEPINES

Due to their positive allosteric action at the $GABA_A$ receptor, all benzodiazepines can potentially induce sleep and be used as hypnotic agents. Consideration should be given to the half-life of a drug, however, because those with longer half-lives (e.g., clonazepam, diazepam) may result in more daytime side effects. Conversely, benzodiazepines with a shorter half-life result in a higher risk of rebound symptoms of insomnia, anxiety, or even seizures upon discontinuation.

TRAZODONE

Trazodone was marketed in the United States in the early 1980s. Although it belongs to the group of antidepressants, it is more often used for insomnia. Trazodone is a serotonin antagonist ($5\text{-}HT_{2A}$ blockade) and reuptake inhibitor. Serotonin reuptake, and thus antidepressant effect, is only achieved at higher doses (Stahl 2013). At lower doses of 25–150 mg, trazodone induces sleep via selective H_1, noradrenergic α_1, and serotonergic $5\text{-}HT_{2A}$ blockade. Serotonin $5\text{-}HT_{2A}$ receptors are present in GABAergic cells of the thalamus that promote sleep (Rodriguez et al. 2011). Trazodone promotes slow-wave sleep and reduces the number of arousals. It is usually well tolerated; however, be aware of a rare risk of priapism with this drug (Rhodes 2001). Despite a possible association between trazodone and increased falls in elderly patients (Ruxton et al. 2015), trazodone is generally considered safe in this population, including patients with Alzheimer's dementia (Camargos et al. 2014; Miller et al. 2019).

MIRTAZAPINE

Mirtazapine has an overlapping mechanism of action with trazodone because it blocks the H_1 and $5\text{-}HT_{2A}$ receptors at low doses (up to 30 mg)

TABLE 4–2. Sedative drugs used off-label for the treatment of chronic insomnia

Drug	Dosage, mg	Onset of action	Elimination half-life, hours	Common side effects	U.S. DEA schedule
Benzodiazepines (GABA$_A$ receptor positive allosteric modulator)					
Alprazolam	0.25–0.5	Rapid	10–12	Hangover effect, skin rash, reduced plasma concentrations with smoking	IV
Lorazepam	0.5–2	Rapid-intermediate	12	Hangover effect	IV
Diazepam	2–10	Rapid-intermediate	44–48*	Hangover effect	IV
Sedative antidepressant drugs					
Mirtazapine (H$_1$ and 5-HT$_{2A}$)	15–45	Intermediate	20–40	Weight gain, increased appetite, gastrointestinal symptoms, hangover effect	None
Trazodone (H$_1$, α_1, and 5-HT$_{2A}$ antagonists)	25–100	Rapid-intermediate	5–9	Nausea, priapism	None
Amitriptyline, nortriptyline (H$_1$, M$_1$, and 5-HT$_{2A}$ antagonists)	10–30	Intermediate-slow	13–36	Dry mouth, blurry vision, constipation, weight gain, QT interval prolongation, hangover effect	None

TABLE 4–2. Sedative drugs used off-label for the treatment of chronic insomnia *(continued)*

Drug	Dosage, *mg*	Onset of action	Elimination half-life, *hours*	Common side effects	U.S. DEA schedule
$\alpha_2\delta$ **Ligand of the voltage-gated calcium channel**					
Gabapentin (reduces release of excitatory neurotransmitters)	300–1,200	Intermediate-slow	5–7	Weight gain, lower extremity edema	None
Sedative antipsychotics (H$_1$, M$_1$, and α_1 antagonist)					
Quetiapine	25–75	Rapid-intermediate	6	Dry mouth, weight gain, QT interval prolongation	None
Olanzapine	1–5	Slow	20–50	Insulin resistance, hypertriglyceridemia	None

Note. Generic side effects of excessive sedation, daytime grogginess, and dizziness were not listed. Only specific or other common side effects were listed for each drug.

DEA=Drug Enforcement Administration; H=histamine; M=muscarinic.

*Metabolized into desmethyldiazepam, temazepam, and oxazepam.

in addition to being a potent noradrenergic α_2 antagonist, resulting in an activating effect at higher doses. Although effective for some patients, tolerance is often limited by increased appetite and weight gain.

LOW-DOSE TRICYCLIC ANTIDEPRESSANTS

The two most commonly used TCA agents in insomnia are amitriptyline and nortriptyline, due to their triple inhibitory action at the H_1, M_1 (anticholinergic), and $5-HT_{2A}$ receptors at low doses (10–30 mg). Of these two agents, amitriptyline has the most sedating effect. A relatively slow onset of action and prolonged half-life make these agents more suitable for maintenance insomnia. Residual morning sedation is a common side effect of TCAs. This adverse effect should be screened for and often resolves after advancing nighttime dosing. Although TCAs are effective for many patients, their utility is limited by their antimuscarinic side effects: confusion, memory loss, blurry vision, urinary retention, and constipation. Due to these side effects, TCAs can pose a risk in the elderly and should be avoided in this population (Samuel 2015). Low-dose TCAs nevertheless remain an interesting option in young or middle-aged adults who may also have chronic pain (Liu et al. 2017).

GABAPENTIN

Introduced on the market in 1993 as an antiepileptic agent, gabapentin has been widely used for several indications, including for its hypnotic properties (Lo et al. 2010). Although the mechanism of action of gabapentin is not entirely clear, it binds at the $\alpha_2\delta$ subunit of the presynaptic voltage-gated calcium channel, reducing the release of excitatory neurotransmitters. Gabapentin also modulates the synthesis of GABA and glutamate, an important excitatory neurotransmitter. Gabapentin has shown to reduce sleep latency and promote slow-wave sleep. An important characteristic of gabapentin resides in its erratic, nonlinear gastric absorption and availability. As a result, doses required to achieve sedation vary greatly among individuals (between 300 mg and 1,200 mg). However, a newer gabapentin prodrug (gabapentin enacarbil) increases the bioavailability of gabapentin by its absorption through high-capacity rapid intestinal transporters. Most common side effects include residual morning sedation, which can be resolved by advancing nighttime dosing, and weight gain, although gabapentin can on occasion cause lower extremity edema. Early concerns regarding psychiatric side effects (e.g., depression, suicidal thoughts) have been contradicted by a large retrospective study in more than 130,000 patients that showed no increased risk of suicide in nonpsychiatric populations and reduced rate of suicide attempts in those with a mood or other psychiatric disorder (Gibbons et al. 2010). Gabapentin is a particularly interesting treatment option in patients with chronic pain or RLS who also have insomnia.

SEDATIVE ANTIPSYCHOTIC AGENTS

Several antipsychotic drugs have been used off-label for the treatment of insomnia, including quetiapine and olanzapine. These two drugs promote sleep via H_1, M_1, and α_1 blockade (Tassniyom et al. 2010). Quetiapine has sedative properties at low doses ≤50 mg, whereas its effect on mood and psychosis is achieved at moderate and high doses, respectively. Olanzapine and quetiapine can result in nausea and weight gain due to their antihistaminic action, as well as residual sedation (hangover feeling) due to their long half-life. Although the exact underlying mechanism is not understood, olanzapine is associated with a significant cardiovascular risk via insulin resistance and hypertriglyceridemia. A systematic review and meta-analysis including more than 124,000 elderly individuals showed an increased risk of falls in those taking olanzapine (Ruxton et al. 2015). In addition, due to their anticholinergic properties, these drugs should be used with extreme caution in elderly patients (Samuel 2015). Quetiapine also presents a risk of QT-interval prolongation.

Over-the-Counter Sleep Aids

Over-the-counter sleep aids available in the United States are limited to diphenhydramine and doxylamine, which are both antihistamines. These two drugs are marketed as single compounds or combined with an analgesic (acetaminophen, ibuprofen, naproxen). They belong to the first generation of antihistamines, which induce sleep through H_1 receptor blockade, in addition to having potent muscarinic anticholinergic action. The sleep-inducing effect of diphenhydramine remains modest, reducing sleep latency by <10 minutes compared with placebo (Morin et al. 2005). The intermediate to long elimination half-life of antihistamines makes them more suitable for maintenance insomnia, but their effect remains modest (about 12 minutes' increase in total sleep time for diphenhydramine). In addition, they present the inconvenience of rapid tolerance and need for dose escalation (Richardson et al. 2002). Their anticholinergic properties can cause a number of side effects such as dry mouth, constipation, urinary retention, and confusion, all of which pose a safety risk in elderly patients. They should generally be avoided in this vulnerable population (Samuel 2015).

Dietary Supplements Used for Insomnia

Several dietary supplements are marketed as sleep-promoting agents. This category of compounds is not regulated and encompasses various natural and synthetic agents, such as melatonin; GABA; tryptophan or 5-hydroxytryptophan, both precursors of serotonin and melatonin; chamomile; valerian extract; kava kava; and tart cherry juice. Among them, melatonin has the best evidence, because its role in sleep physiology is well established and its efficacy has been demonstrated in the treatment of circadian rhythm disorders. Melatonin is physiologically synthesized by the pineal gland and released every 24 hours, just a few hours before usual bedtime, acting as a synchronizing hormone in the brain. Melatonin synthesis reduces with aging and likely decreases further in some neurodegenerative diseases. A 2-mg dose of melatonin is estimated to induce sleep 9 minutes faster than placebo (Sateia et al. 2017). Although extended-release formulations are now available and may have an additional benefit in consolidating sleep, due to its short half-life of <1 hour, melatonin may otherwise only be suitable for initiation insomnia. Although idiosyncratic reactions are occasionally seen, studies have not consistently shown a difference in terms of adverse effects between melatonin and placebo. Although its efficacy may be limited, melatonin remains a safe treatment option in elderly patients.

Kava kava has been associated with risk of liver failure (Stickel et al. 2003). Other supplements generally have low-quality evidence in terms of efficacy and safety. Based on one study, tryptophan 250 mg may mildly reduce sleep fragmentation (<10-minute reduction in wake after sleep onset) and subjectively improve sleep quality compared with placebo; however, potential harmful effects have not been studied (Hudson et al. 2005). Valerian extract also has limited efficacy data, with only one study reporting an objective increase in sleep duration after a nighttime dose of valerian 375 mg (Morin et al. 2005) and no evidence suggesting improvement in subjective sleep quality (Sateia et al. 2017). Other herbal supplements have even weaker evidence.

Emerging Therapies for Insomnia

Novel pharmacological agents, such as adenosine receptor inhibitors and casein kinase inhibitors, have gained increasing interest in recent years (for a review, see Atkin et al. 2018). In addition, drugs specifically binding to the MT_1 receptor could promote sleep without altering sleep architecture, as is seen with dual MT_1/MT_2 agonists. In addition, several selective (OX_2) or dual (OX_1/OX_2) orexin receptor agonists, such as almorexant, could soon become available and interesting options in elderly patients. Piromelatine, an agent that has melatonergic and serotonergic action, is being investigated in patients with mild Alzheimer's disease. Finally, lumateperone is a new antipsychotic drug and selective antagonist of the $5-HT_{2A}$ receptor at low doses that could become an interesting alternative to the sedative antidepressant drugs currently used off-label for insomnia (Atkin et al. 2018).

KEY CLINICAL POINTS

- Sedative drugs promote sleep via activation of the sleep-inducing pathways or inhibition of the wake-promoting circuits. Knowledge of basic mechanisms of action and pharmacokinetics is essential for prescribers to understand a drug's expected benefit on insomnia as well as common side effects and potential risks.

- A number of sedative drugs such as gabapentin, low-dose tricyclic agents, and other antidepressants have been used off-label to treat insomnia. Although most of their evidence in treating insomnia stems from uncontrolled studies and anecdotal evidence, they can represent interesting treatment options.

- Although nonbenzodiazepine receptor agonists (Z drugs) may more selectively induce sleep than benzodiazepines do, they may also be associated with long-term risk of dementia and cognitive decline with chronic use.

- Melatonergic agents, pure antihistamine doxepin, orexin/hypocretin receptor antagonists, and trazodone have a more favorable profile in elderly or cognitively impaired individuals.

- In contrast, due to their combined anticholinergic effects, over-the-counter antihistamine drugs (diphenhydramine and doxylamine) are associated with a number of side effects and cognitive impairment, which makes them not suitable in elderly or cognitively impaired individuals.

References

Atkin T, Comai S, Gobbi G: Drugs for insomnia beyond benzodiazepines: pharmacology, clinical applications, and discovery. Pharmacol Rev 70(2):197–245, 2018 29487083

Billioti de Gage S, Moride Y, Ducruet T, et al: Benzodiazepine use and risk of Alzheimer's disease: case-control study. BMJ 349(2):g5205, 2014

Bloom HG, Ahmed I, Alessi CA, et al: Evidence-based recommendations for the assessment and management of sleep disorders in older persons. J Am Geriatr Soc 57(5):761–789, 2009 19484833

Camargos EF, Louzada LL, Quintas JL, et al: Trazodone improves sleep parameters in Alzheimer disease patients: a randomized, double-blind, and placebo-controlled study. Am J Geriatr Psychiatry 22(12):1565–1574, 2014 24495406

Cheng HT, Lin FJ, Erickson SR, et al: The association between the use of zolpidem and the risk of Alzheimer's disease among older people. J Am Geriatr Soc 65(11):2488–2495, 2017 28884784

de Lecea L, Kilduff TS, Peyron C, et al: The hypocretins: hypothalamus-specific peptides with neuroexcitatory activity. Proc Natl Acad Sci USA 95(1):322–327, 1998

Drake CL, Durrence H, Cheng P, et al: Arousability and fall risk during forced awakenings from nocturnal sleep among healthy males following administration of zolpidem 10 mg and doxepin 6 mg: a randomized, placebo-controlled, four-way crossover trial. Sleep 40(7), 2017 28575467

Gallacher J, Elwood P, Pickering J, et al: Benzodiazepine use and risk of dementia: evidence from the Caerphilly Prospective Study (CaPS). J Epidemiol Community Health 66(10):869–873, 2012 22034632

Gibbons RD, Hur K, Brown CH, Mann JJ: Gabapentin and suicide attempts. Pharmacoepidemiol Drug Saf 19(12):1241–1247, 2010 20922708

Gooneratne NS, Vitiello MV: Sleep in older adults: normative changes, sleep disorders, and treatment options. Clin Geriatr Med 30(3):591–627, 2014 25037297

Gottesmann C: GABA mechanisms and sleep. Neuroscience 111(2):231–239, 2002 11983310

Gunja N: In the Zzz zone: the effects of Z-drugs on human performance and driving. J Med Toxicol 9(2):163–171, 2013 23456542

Herring WJ, Connor KM, Snyder E, et al: Suvorexant in elderly patients with insomnia: pooled analyses of data from phase III randomized controlled clinical trials. Am J Geriatr Psychiatry 25(7):791–802, 2017 28427826

Howell MJ, Schenck CH: Restless nocturnal eating: a common feature of Willis-Ekbom syndrome (RLS). J Clin Sleep Med 8(4):413–419, 2012 22893772

Hudson C, Hudson SP, Hecht T, et al: Protein source tryptophan versus pharmaceutical grade tryptophan as an efficacious treatment for chronic insomnia. Nutr Neurosci 8(2):121–127, 2005 16053244

Kessler RC, Berglund PA, Coulouvrat C, et al: Insomnia and the performance of US workers: results from the America insomnia survey. Sleep (Basel) 34(9):1161–1171, 2011 21886353

Kuriyama A, Honda M, Hayashino Y: Ramelteon for the treatment of insomnia in adults: a systematic review and meta-analysis. Sleep Med 15(4):385–392, 2014 24656909

Liu Y, Xu X, Dong M, et al: Treatment of insomnia with tricyclic antidepressants: a meta-analysis of polysomnographic randomized controlled trials. Sleep Med 34:126–133, 2017 28522080

Lo H-S, Yang C-M, Lo HG, et al: Treatment effects of gabapentin for primary insomnia. Clin Neuropharmacol 33(2):84–90, 2010 20124884

Miller BL, La AL, Krystal AD, et al: Long-term trazodone use and cognition: a potential therapeutic role for slow-wave sleep enhancers. J Alzheimers Dis 67(3):911–921, 2019 30689583

Morin CM, Koetter U, Bastien C, et al: Valerian-hops combination and diphenhydramine for treating insomnia: a randomized placebo-controlled clinical trial. Sleep 28(11):1465–1471, 2005 16335333

Neylan TC, Richards A, Metzler TJ, et al: Acute cognitive effects of the hypocretin receptor antagonist almorexant relative to zolpidem and placebo: a randomized clinical trial. Sleep 2020 32303763 Epub ahead of print

Patel KV, Aspesi AV, Evoy KE: Suvorexant: a dual orexin receptor antagonist for the treatment of sleep onset and sleep maintenance insomnia. Ann Pharmacother 49(4):477–483, 2015 25667197

Pressman MR: Sleep driving: sleepwalking variant or misuse of z-drugs? Sleep Med Rev 15(5):285–292, 2011 21367628

Provini F, Antelmi E, Vignatelli L, et al: Association of restless legs syndrome with nocturnal eating: a case-control study. Mov Disord 24(6):871–877, 2009 19199358

Rhodes CT: Trazodone and priapism—implications for responses to adverse events. Clin Res Regul Aff 18(1–2):47–52, 2001

Richardson GS, Roehrs TA, Rosenthal L, et al: Tolerance to daytime sedative effects of H1 antihistamines. J Clin Psychopharmacol 22(5):511–515, 2002 12352276

Rodriguez JJ, Noristani HN, Hoover WB, et al: Serotonergic projections and serotonin receptor expression in the reticular nucleus of the thalamus in the rat. Synapse 65(9):919–928, 2011 21308802

Roth T, Coulouvrat C, Hajak G, et al: Prevalence and perceived health associated with insomnia based on DSM-IV-TR; International Statistical Classification of Diseases and Related Health Problems, tenth revision; and Research Diagnostic Criteria/International Classification of Sleep Disorders. Biol Psychiatry 69(6):592–600, 2011 21195389

Ruxton K, Woodman RJ, Mangoni AA: Drugs with anticholinergic effects and cognitive impairment, falls and all-cause mortality in older adults: a systematic review and meta-analysis. Br J Clin Pharmacol 80(2):209–220, 2015 25735839

Samuel MJ: American Geriatrics Society 2015 updated Beers criteria for potentially inappropriate medication use in older adults. J Am Geriatr Soc 63(11):2227–2246, 2015 26446832

Sanger DJ: The pharmacology and mechanisms of action of new generation, non-benzodiazepine hypnotic agents. CNS Drugs 18(1):9–15, 2004

Sateia MJ, Buysse DJ, Krystal AD, et al: Clinical practice guideline for the pharmacologic treatment of chronic insomnia in adults: an American Academy of Sleep Medicine clinical practice guideline. J Clin Sleep Med 13(2):307–349, 2017 27998379

Schutte-Rodin S, Broch L, Buysse D, et al: Clinical guideline for the evaluation and management of chronic insomnia in adults. J Clin Sleep Med 4(5):487–504, 2008 2576317

Shih HI, Lin CC, Tu YF, et al: An increased risk of reversible dementia may occur after zolpidem derivative use in the elderly population: a population-based case-control study. Medicine (Baltimore) 94(17):e809, 2015 4603066

Stahl SM: Stahl's Essential Psychopharmacology Neuroscientific Basis and Practical Applications, 4th Edition. Cambridge, UK, Cambridge University Press, 2013

Stickel F, Baumüller HM, Seitz K, et al: Hepatitis induced by kava (Piper methysticum rhizoma). J Hepatol 39(1):62–67, 2003 12821045

Tassniyom K, Paholpak S, Tassniyom S, et al: Quetiapine for primary insomnia: a double blind, randomized controlled trial. J Med Assoc Thailand 93(6):729–734, 2010

Vermeeren A, Sun H, Vuurman EFPM, et al: On-the-road driving performance the morning after bedtime use of suvorexant 20 and 40 mg: a study in non-elderly healthy volunteers. Sleep (Basel) 38(11):1803–1813, 2015 26039969

Vinkers CH, Olivier B: Mechanisms underlying tolerance after long-term benzodiazepine use: a future for subtype-selective GABA$_A$ receptor modulators? Adv Pharmacol Sci 2012:416864, 2012 22536226

Wu C-S, Wang S-C, Chang I-S, et al: The association between dementia and long-term use of benzodiazepine in the elderly: nested case-control study using claims data. Am J Geriatr Psychiatry 17(7):614–620, 2009 19546656

Yeung W-F, Chung K-F, Yung K-P, et al: Doxepin for insomnia: a systematic review of randomized placebo-controlled trials. Sleep Med Rev 19:75–83, 2015 25047681

Zammit GK, McNabb LJ, Caron J, et al: Efficacy and safety of eszopiclone across 6 weeks of treatment for primary insomnia. Curr Med Res Opin 20(12):1979–1991, 2004 15701215

CHAPTER 5

Nonpharmacological Treatment of Insomnia

Fiona Barwick, Ph.D., D.B.S.M.

Insomnia is a 24-hour disorder with a clinical presentation that is often described as "tired but wired" because individuals are unable to nap even when they want to and rarely fall asleep unintentionally, unless insomnia co-occurs with another sleep, medical, or psychiatric disorder (Bonnet and Arand 2010). Problems initiating or maintaining sleep at night are accompanied by daytime symptoms, most commonly fatigue, irritability, anxiety, dysphoria, and concentration or memory difficulties (American Academy of Sleep Medicine 2014). Acute insomnia (lasting <1 month), which often occurs in the context of major life events, usually remits after the precipitating event resolves or as an individual adapts. In chronic insomnia (lasting >3 months), however, sleep problems persist even after the initial precipitant resolves or its impact diminishes. Chronic insomnia typically does not remit without treatment, and symptoms can last for years, with up to 74% of individuals reporting insomnia after 1 year and almost 50% reporting it up to 3 years later (Morin et al. 2009a).

Insomnia Model

A model commonly used to describe the course of insomnia identifies predisposing, precipitating, and perpetuating factors (Morin et al. 2015; Spielman et al. 1987). *Predisposing factors* increase vulnerability to insomnia (e.g., age, sex, anxious temperament, experience of trauma, personal or family history of insomnia). *Precipitating factors* trigger insomnia (e.g., stressful life events related to family, work, school, finances, or health as well as shift work or frequent travel). *Perpetuating* factors prolong insomnia (e.g., irregular sleep-wake schedule, excessive time in bed, inappropriate daytime napping, and worry about or preoccupation with sleep). Cognitive-behavioral therapy for insomnia (CBT-I) targets and

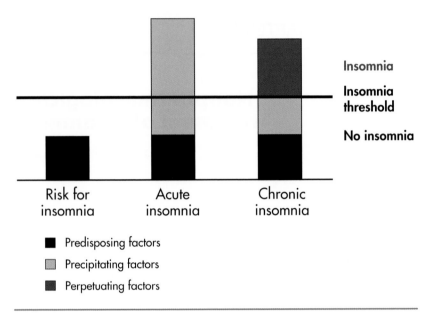

FIGURE 5–1.   Three factors contributing to the course of insomnia.
Source.   Adapted by permission from Springer Nature: *Psychiatric Clinics of North America*, "A Behavioral Perspective on Insomnia Treatment" by Spielman AJ, Caruso LS, Glovinsky PB. Copyright © 1987.

modifies the perpetuating factors, which include the unhelpful beliefs, negative emotions, and maladaptive behaviors that prolong and exacerbate insomnia (Figure 5–1).

Recommended Treatment

CBT-I is the recommended treatment for insomnia. It is a multicomponent therapy with a strong empirical base demonstrating equivalent success to pharmacotherapy over the short term and greater success at sustaining improvements over the long term (Morin et al. 2006a). Equivalent or superior outcomes for CBT-I are important, given patient preference for nonpharmacological treatment (Vincent and Lionberg 2001). Furthermore, FDA-approved prescription drugs for insomnia are minimally supported by weak recommendations due to limited benefit over placebo or inconsistent-quality evidence; off-label prescription drugs and over-the-counter agents used as sleep aids have limited data on efficacy for insomnia; some of these agents have significant side effects (Sateia et al. 2017). Guidelines suggest that behavioral and cognitive treatments should be recommended whenever possible. Medications should be limited to the lowest dose and shortest duration necessary, accompanied by careful monitoring of adverse effects.

Sleep Hygiene

CBT-I is not equivalent to sleep hygiene but rather includes sleep hygiene as one component of treatment. Sleep hygiene comprises environmental factors and lifestyle practices that can influence sleep (Hauri 1991). Environmental factors include establishing a protected sleep environment. Lifestyle practices include appropriate timing and consumption of meals, exercise, alcohol, and caffeine. For example, individuals are encouraged to keep their bedroom comfortable, dark, quiet, and cool (62°F–68°F), although preferences can vary. Recommendations for keeping screens and electronic devices out of the bedroom are becoming increasingly common. Meals, exercise, alcohol, and caffeine should all be timed appropriately so they do not interfere with sleep (i.e., meals, alcohol, and vigorous exercise should be finished 3–4 hours before bedtime; caffeine should be finished 10–14 hours before bedtime). Caffeine and alcohol should be limited or eliminated in individuals who are sensitive to their effects. Nicotine should be discontinued because of adverse effects on sleep and health. Proper sleep hygiene can support good sleep but does not, by itself, correct poor sleep.

Cognitive-Behavioral Therapy for Insomnia

DESCRIPTION AND INDICATION

CBT-I is a brief, collaborative, skills-based, multicomponent treatment that uses a variety of therapies, some of which are effective as stand-alone interventions, to target thoughts and behaviors that interfere with sleep and perpetuate insomnia. Specific therapies include stimulus control, sleep restriction, relaxation, cognitive reframing, sleep hygiene, and sleep education. Changing unhelpful beliefs and behaviors can circumvent the vicious circle that ensues when unhelpful cognitions, negative emotions, and maladaptive behaviors exacerbate and perpetuate insomnia, an understanding that informs CBT treatment for other chronic conditions (Hofmann et al. 2012). CBT-I can be safely implemented with young, middle-aged, and older adults with chronic insomnia. See Table 5–1 for a summary of component therapies and specific techniques.

TABLE 5–1. Components of cognitive-behavioral therapy for insomnia (CBT-I)

Treatment (level of evidence)	Target	Technique
Stimulus control therapy (1a)	Reinforce association between bed, bedroom, bedtime, and sleep	Go to bed only when sleepy
	Extinguish conditioned association between bed or bedroom and wakefulness	Use the bed and bedroom for sleep only (e.g., no reading, no television)
	Reestablish consistent sleep-wake schedule	Get out of bed if awake for what feels like >20 minutes and do something relaxing elsewhere until sleepy again, repeating as often as necessary
		Get up at the same time every day, no matter the sleep quality/quantity
Sleep restriction therapy (1a)	Strengthen homeostatic sleep drive	Use 2 weeks of sleep log data prior to start of treatment to determine average total sleep time
	Reduce time awake at night	Set sleep schedule to match average self-estimated total sleep time
	Improve sleep efficiency (SE)	Avoid napping or dozing before bedtime
		As sleep consolidates (SE >85%), gradually expand time in bed by 15 minutes/week based on perceived sleep need (feeling tired or sleepy during the day) and SE (>85%, add 15 minutes; <80%, subtract 15 minutes)

TABLE 5–1. Components of cognitive-behavioral therapy for insomnia (CBT-I) (continued)

Treatment (level of evidence)	Target	Technique
Relaxation training (1b)	Reduce somatic, cognitive, and emotional hyperarousal that interferes with sleep	Diaphragmatic breathing
		Progressive muscle relaxation
	Shift sympathovagal balance toward sleep at bedtime	Body scan
		Biofeedback
		Autogenic training
		Visualization/imagery training
		Meditation/mindfulness
Cognitive therapy (2b)	Change unhelpful thoughts and beliefs about sleep, insomnia, and daytime consequences	Identify, challenge, and reframe thoughts, feelings, and beliefs that interfere with sleep and sleep regimen
	Reduce excessive worry about sleep and efforts to control sleep	Cognitive reframing
		Mindfulness/acceptance
		Behavioral experiments
Sleep hygiene (insufficient evidence as single therapy)	Environmental factors and lifestyle practices that can help or hinder sleep	Teach healthy lifestyle practices (e.g., regular exercise, diet/meal timing, caffeine intake, alcohol or nicotine use) that support good sleep
		Educate about importance of protecting sleep environment (e.g., light, noise, temperature, screens, clock watching) to maintain good sleep

TABLE 5–1.   Components of cognitive-behavioral therapy for insomnia (CBT-I) *(continued)*

Treatment (level of evidence)	Target	Technique
Psychoeducation (insufficient evidence as single therapy)	Learn to understand normal healthy adult sleep	Understand healthy adult sleep Normal sleep architecture Changes in sleep patterns with aging Systems that affect sleep-wake and circadian rhythms
Cognitive-behavioral therapy (1b)	Improve sleep by identifying and changing un-helpful thoughts, feelings, and behaviors that interfere with establishing and maintaining healthy sleep patterns and habits	Stimulus control Sleep restriction Relaxation Cognitive therapy Sleep hygiene Sleep education

Note. Level of evidence based on University of Oxford Centre for Evidence-Based Medicine (www.cebm.net), as cited in Morin et al. (2015), with 1a–2b referencing higher to lower quality of evidence (e.g., systematic review of randomized controlled trials vs. individual cohort study).
SE calculation=(Total sleep time/total time in bed)×100.

Source.   Morgenthaler et al. 2006; Schutte-Rodin et al. 2008.

BEHAVIORAL TECHNIQUES

Behavioral techniques help individuals with insomnia change unhelpful behaviors that prevent them from establishing and maintaining consistent and healthy sleep-wake patterns.

Stimulus Control

Stimulus control helps extinguish the conditioned arousal that develops over time, consciously or unconsciously, as individuals come to associate bed, bedtime, and sleep with anxiety, frustration, and wakefulness. It often manifests when individuals struggle to sleep at bedtime in their own bed but fall asleep easily at other times or in other settings (e.g., on the sofa, in a hotel room). Stimulus control ensures that individuals fall asleep quickly when they are in bed and that they stay out of bed when they are awake at night. As wakeful associations are extinguished, bed and bedtime once again become cues for sleep (Bootzin et al. 1991).

For example, if an individual reports wakefulness at night for what "feels like" more than 20 minutes, she is instructed to get out of bed and go somewhere other than the bedroom, where she should do something enjoyable and relaxing for 30 minutes or until she feels sleepy, at which time she can return to bed. Time awake in and out of bed should be estimated, because checking the clock time at night can increase distress and tension. The choice of relaxing activities varies according to individual preference but could include listening to calming music, reading a magazine or book in dim light, watching reruns of favorite shows, or doing a guided meditation. These actions should be repeated as often as necessary every night until the individual falls asleep easily when back in bed.

Sleep Restriction

Sleep restriction runs counter to the widely held belief that spending more time in bed will lead to more and better sleep. For individuals with insomnia, spending more time in bed worsens sleep by decreasing the homeostatic drive for sleep (Process S), increasing time awake at night, and exacerbating worries about and compensatory efforts around nighttime sleep and daytime functioning. The paradoxical reality, supported by substantial research, is that decreasing time in bed is the most effective way to improve sleep.

Sleep restriction limits time spent in bed each night (the "sleep window") to an estimated average nightly total sleep time ("sleep ability"), which is best estimated from a 2-week sleep diary completed before treatment begins. Napping or dozing before bedtime should be eliminated or limited to <30 minutes at least 8 hours before bedtime. Restricting time in bed consolidates sleep by removing wakefulness at night, increasing homeostatic sleep pressure during the day, and inducing a state of mild sleep deprivation, because individuals with insomnia tend to underestimate sleep duration and overestimate wakefulness at night compared with results on polysomnography (Perlis et al. 1997). As wakefulness diminishes and sleep quality improves, time in bed is gradually increased until optimal sleep duration is reached without the return of excessive wakefulness at night (Spielman et al. 1987).

For example, if a patient says he is getting 6 hours of sleep a night but spends 9 hours in bed, he is prescribed a 6-hour sleep window with a consistent bedtime and rise time. Some clinicians will add an additional 30 minutes to allow time to fall or return to sleep. In clinical practice, sleep restriction is never <5 hours. With strict adherence to this window, sleep quality typically improves within 2–3 weeks in the absence of comorbid disorders such as sleep apnea or depression. Once sleep has consolidated and sleep efficiency ([total sleep time/total time in bed]×100) has improved to 85% or more, the sleep window is expanded by 15 minutes weekly based on the perceived sleep need (e.g., feeling tired or sleepy during the day). Reports of minimal initiation or maintenance insomnia (<30 minutes), good sleep efficiency (≥85%), perceived adequate nighttime sleep, and good daytime functioning indicate that the optimal sleep window has been achieved.

Relaxation Training

Relaxation training helps counter the physiological hyperarousal that occurs with insomnia. Individuals with insomnia often become increasingly tense and anxious as bedtime approaches because of their concerns about sleep. They can show increased activation of the hypothalamic-pituitary-adrenal axis and the autonomic nervous system, including elevated heart rate, blood pressure, body temperature, and cortisol levels. They also show increases in cerebral glucose metabolism at night and high-frequency electroencephalographic activity prior to and during sleep (e.g., beta 16–32 Hz and gamma 32–48 Hz) (Riemann et al. 2010). They may have more pronounced and maladaptive reactions to stress (Drake et al. 2004). Relaxation reduces sympathetic activation, a fight-or-flight response that is incompatible with sleep, and instead engages a parasympathetic or "rest and digest" response, which calms the mind and body, helping individuals relax into sleep. Relaxation techniques can be included in a 1-hour "wind-down" period before bedtime, when work-related or goal-oriented activities are eschewed in favor of more relaxing and enjoyable pursuits. This allows individuals to "de-stress" from their day, thus shifting their sympathovagal balance toward sleep.

Specific and easily learned techniques include diaphragmatic breathing, which encourages breathing from the abdomen rather than the chest, and progressive muscle relaxation, in which various muscle groups are progressively tensed and then released. Web- and application-based resources describe and demonstrate these along with a wide variety of other relaxation techniques, including body scanning, visual imagery, autogenic training, and meditation. These techniques take time to learn, so practice, persistence, and patience are key. Learning is facilitated by choosing one technique and practicing it daily for several weeks.

When implementing all of the behavioral techniques discussed in this section, particularly sleep restriction, individuals should be advised to anticipate a likely increase in daytime sleepiness, which they should manage as necessary by refraining from driving or operating machinery or from engaging in tasks requiring sustained vigilance. Special caution should be used for those in occupations that require sustained alertness under potentially hazardous conditions (e.g., commercial drivers or air traffic controllers).

COGNITIVE THERAPY

Cognitive techniques help individuals with insomnia correct misconceptions, alter unhelpful beliefs, reduce emotional distress, and reduce cognitive and emotional hyperarousal (e.g., worry, rumination, and negative affect) around bed, bedtime, and sleep (Morin et al. 2002). These techniques are best implemented with individuals who are cognitively intact.

Psychoeducation

Psychoeducation reduces worry about sleep by helping individuals understand healthy adult sleep patterns, normal variability in sleep duration and circadian phase, and changes in sleep with aging. Common misconceptions are that sleep onset should happen quickly, an earlier bedtime is better, waking up at night is abnormal, adults require 8 hours of sleep, and any experience of daytime fatigue or impairment is due solely to poor sleep.

Cognitive Reframing

Cognitive reframing helps individuals challenge inaccurate, overly negative, and unhelpful beliefs about sleep, insomnia, and daytime consequences so they can arrive at more balanced and accurate perspectives. For example, common maladaptive thoughts reflecting worry about the ability to return to sleep at night or to function the following day can be challenged and reframed so individuals recognize they will return to sleep eventually and, even after a night of "poor" sleep, are able to function adequately, as they have done many, many times before.

EVIDENCE FOR RECOMMENDATION

CBT-I is highly effective, with 70%–80% of individuals who report insomnia experiencing a clinically significant reduction in symptoms, 40% of whom achieve total remission. It produces benefits equal to medication in the short term, which are better sustained than medication in the long term (Morin et al. 2017). Treatment yields moderate to large effect sizes for sleep onset latency, wakefulness after sleep onset, and sleep quality and small to moderate effect sizes for total sleep time. Subjective sleep onset latency and wakefulness after sleep onset decrease on average from 60–70 minutes pretreatment to 35 minutes posttreatment. Increase in total sleep time is more modest (30 minutes, from 6 hours to 6.5 hours) but often continues and exceeds 6.5 hours several months after treatment ends. CBT-I can also improve daytime functioning, ameliorating fatigue and enhancing quality of life (Morin et al. 2006a, 2016).

CBT-I can improve sleep, even in the context of medical and psychiatric comorbidities (Wu et al. 2015), and may reduce insomnia symptoms in individuals with chronic pain, cancer, depression, anxiety, and psychosis. It may also improve comorbid symptoms for depression, anxiety, PTSD, and psychosis (Belleville et al. 2011; Cunningham and Shapiro 2018; Freeman et al. 2017; Ho et al. 2016; Johnson et al. 2016). It is recommended as a standard first-line treatment for chronic insomnia in adults of all ages by national and international health-focused organizations (Buscemi et al. 2005; Qaseem et al. 2016; Riemann et al. 2017; Schutte-Rodin et al. 2008; Wilson et al. 2010).

IMPLEMENTATION AND DELIVERY

CBT-I is significantly preferred by patients over pharmacological treatment (Vincent and Lionberg 2001). It is typically delivered in four to eight weekly or biweekly sessions by a qualified psychologist or clinician trained in mental health, with four sessions appearing to yield optimal outcomes (Edinger et al. 2007). It can be delivered effectively in self-help, individual, group, or online formats, an especially important consideration given limited access to and numbers of qualified providers. Individuals with insomnia show improvements across all modalities, but outcomes may be better with face-to-face interventions or additional phone or text message support in self-help and online interventions (van Straten et al. 2018; Zachariae et al. 2016). Alternative delivery modalities are a useful addition to traditional CBT-I formats, especially when used in primary care settings or when integrated into a stepped-care approach (Espie 2009). However, the success of CBT-I ultimately depends on individual motivation and adherence to treatment recommendations.

CBT-I AND PHARMACOTHERAPY

CBT-I and pharmacotherapy may have complementary roles in the management of insomnia, especially as no single treatment modality is effective, acceptable, or tolerated by all patients. Although CBT-I and drugs are equally effective within 4–8 weeks, drugs alone produce more rapid results within the first 2 weeks, whereas CBT-I generates more sustained benefits over subsequent months. Relapse to chronic insomnia is also more common when drugs are used alone, especially after discontinuation. Combining both approaches may optimize outcomes during initial treatment by producing benefits more quickly. However, advantages diminish over time and may even be counterproductive, because some studies suggest gains are maintained more successfully when medications are discontinued within a few weeks and CBT-I techniques alone are used to manage any return of insomnia symptoms (Morin et al. 2009b). Furthermore, individuals may experience insomnia symptoms only in the absence of sleep aids and thus may continue to use drugs far longer than is recommended. In these cases, CBT-I can help individuals discontinue sedative-hypnotic medications (Morgan et al. 2003).

Modifications of CBT-I

MEDICAL AND PSYCHIATRIC COMORBIDITIES

Stimulus control and sleep restriction are most effective when applied strictly, but caution should be used when prescribing these techniques to individuals with bipolar disorder, seizure disorder, persistent migraines, chronic pain, fall risk, or daytime sleepiness, because sleep restriction can further exacerbate these conditions. Stimulus control can be modified by using counter-control, in which individuals are told to stay in bed but create a different set of cues for wakefulness versus sleep (e.g., sitting up on top of the covers with lights on when awake vs. lying down under the covers with lights off when asleep). Sleep restriction can be modified to sleep compression, which allows a more gradual restriction (e.g., reducing time in bed by 30–60 minutes every 1–2 weeks). For individuals with cognitive impairment—those with dementia, brain injury, or intellectual disability—behavioral strategies can be emphasized while cognitive strategies can be minimized.

BRIEF BEHAVIORAL THERAPY FOR INSOMNIA

Brief behavioral therapy for insomnia (BBT-I) typically comprises two sessions that focus on behavioral components for treating insomnia (i.e., stimulus control and sleep restriction), sometimes supplemented with telephone support or take-home materials. BBT-I appears to result in significantly improved sleep based on self-report questionnaires, sleep logs, and actigraphy, with similar outcomes to CBT-I (van Straten et al. 2018). However, research to date is limited and has been conducted mainly in middle-aged and older adults. Of note, a recent dismantling study comparing behavioral therapy, cognitive therapy, and CBT-I concluded that behavioral therapy leads to faster results than cognitive therapy but is less successful at sustaining improvements over time and recommended CBT-I for maximizing short- and long-term treatment effects (Harvey et al. 2014).

CHILDREN

Prepubescent children, generally ages 3–12 years, can experience insomnia as well (Mindell and Owens 2015). Given children's development, behavioral techniques are often emphasized over cognitive techniques when treating sleep problems. Insomnia in children often manifests behaviorally as bedtime resistance (e.g., requesting to watch another show or hear another story), bedtime refusal (e.g., refusing to get ready for bed or coming out of the bedroom frequently after lights out), or difficulty falling asleep or returning to sleep without parental presence. The cause of these behaviors is usually minimal or unpredictable limit setting, so the most effective treatment is for caregivers to set and enforce appropriate and consistent routines, schedules, and limits around bedtime and sleep.

An appropriate schedule includes a regular bedtime that is consistent with a child's circadian rhythm. For very late bedtimes, this schedule can be gradually advanced in 15-minute intervals over several weeks until the desired bedtime is reached (i.e., bedtime fading). For children who come out of the bedroom repeatedly, returning them calmly to bed and closing the bedroom door for progressively longer periods after each "curtain call" can be useful. For children who experience prolonged night waking after normal nighttime arousals, graduated extinction, in which a child is put to bed drowsy but awake and parental check-ins are progressively delayed by 5 minutes, is highly effective. If the child is learning to self-soothe and fall asleep independently, the amount of time between check-ins can be modified based on parental tolerance of, and child response to, treatment. Check-ins should be kept reassuring but brief (1–2 minutes) and neutral (pat on shoulder rather than pick up and cuddle). Pure extinction—that is, leaving children alone to work out their distress until they realize it does not lead to parental presence—achieves faster results but is rarely used because parents have difficulty tolerating it. Positive reinforcement, such as sticker charts and reward systems, can be used to enhance motivation and adherence to desired behaviors, but punishment should be avoided because it is not an effective means of changing behaviors. Extinction bursts, in which behavior worsens before it improves, should be expected. As with most childrearing, clear and consistent routines along with supportive and positive reinforcement are key, and proactive problem solving can increase the likelihood of success.

ADOLESCENTS

Adolescents ages 12–18 years experience sleep problems that also occur in adulthood, including insomnia (Mindell and Owens 2015). Because adolescents have reached almost full cognitive maturity, CBT-I can be used effectively to treat insomnia, including sleep onset problems associated with delayed sleep-wake phase and sleep-related anxiety. When applying sleep restriction for adolescents, however, 6 hours should be the lower limit because of the potential for daytime impairment. Because they are phase delayed, teenagers may have a harder time implementing recommendations such as limiting screen use in the evening or getting up at the same time in the morning. These difficulties can be compounded by excessive socializing and use of electronic media at night as well as high anxiety or depressed mood and consequent school avoidance in the morning. Cognitive-behavioral work is always collaborative, but especially so with teenagers, who may benefit from techniques such as "decisional balance" to explore the reasons they may or may not want to change current behaviors or to enlist their agreement in self-imposing an "electronic curfew" prior to bedtime. Additional cognitive techniques, such as motivation enhancement, dialectical behavior therapy, or acceptance and commitment therapy, can be incorporated to identify ambivalence while eliciting and reinforcing motivation for behavior change.

OLDER ADULTS

Prevalence of insomnia increases with age—not because of age, per se, but rather due to greater incidence of medical and psychiatric comorbidities, more frequent use of medications, and age-related changes such as reduced physical activity and social engagement. More than 40% of adults age 60 years or older report difficulty initiating or maintaining sleep, and sleep problems appear to persist (Ancoli-Israel 2009). Despite increased rates of insomnia, older adults also benefit from CBT-I and its specific components, as evidenced by studies conducted in this population (Lovato et al. 2014). Although improvements might be more modest in the presence of significant medical or psychiatric comorbidities, outcomes for older adults are similar to younger adults. CBT-I is effective even for those with sedative-hypnotic dependency, and long-term gains are sustained more successfully with CBT-I than with medication (Qaseem et al. 2016; Schutte-Rodin et al. 2008). Given age-related changes in pharmacokinetics and pharmacodynamics, as well as the pervasiveness of polypharmacy in older adults, CBT-I is an especially important treatment alternative that enables older adults to improve sleep without adding another medication to their regimen. For older adults with mild or moderate cognitive impairment, treatment focused on behavioral techniques (e.g., stimulus control, sleep restriction) rather than cognitive techniques will be more successful in theory, although little research has been conducted in this population. Similarly, bright light exposure in the evening might help treat advanced circadian sleep phase syndrome and early morning awakenings, both of which are common in older adults, but research support is minimal.

Complementary and Alternative Treatments

Complementary and alternative treatments are not recommended currently for the treatment of insomnia because evidence for their efficacy, risks, and benefits is inadequate.

ACUPUNCTURE

Acupuncture, in which needles or other stimulation is applied to specific areas of the body called "meridian points," is one of the major treatment modalities of traditional Chinese medicine and a popular complementary therapy in Western countries. Although numerous studies have examined the effects of acupuncture on insomnia, study quality is too poor and studies too heterogeneous and biased to draw conclusions about efficacy and safety, except as an adjunct to recommended treatment or in response to patient preference (Cheuk et al. 2012).

HYPNOSIS

Hypnosis, wherein an altered state of consciousness enhances response to suggestion, showed possible modest improvement in sleep in a systematic review, but findings were mixed and the studies were small, of low quality, and focused on sleep as a secondary outcome (Chamine et al. 2018).

NEUROSTIMULATION AND OTHER INTERVENTIONS

Neurostimulation includes noninvasive techniques such as transcranial magnetic stimulation, which uses external magnetic fields to generate weak electrical currents that stimulate the brain cortex, and cranial electrical stimulation, which uses low-intensity alternating electric currents applied to the head. Although evidence indicates possible benefits for depression and chronic pain, almost no studies have looked at effects on insomnia, and those that have showed mixed results (Kirsch and Nichols 2013; Rosenquist et al. 2013). A novel device that uses a water-cooling headband to cool the forehead and theoretically reduce activity in the frontal cortex may reduce sleep latency and promote sleep stability in the early part of the night (Roth et al. 2018).

Conclusion

CBT-I is the recommended approach for treating insomnia because it is so effective at reducing and resolving insomnia symptoms. However, work remains to be done. Despite its effectiveness, CBT-I is not widely available because of the limited number of clinicians qualified to provide this treatment, particularly in rural areas. Internet delivery formats have been developed over the past few years and are likely to become increasingly common in the future, making CBT-I more accessible to all. Availability of CBT-I is especially important given preliminary research showing that CBT-I alone might be effective in improving not only insomnia but also comorbid psychiatric disorders—including depression, anxiety, bipolar disorder, and psychosis—although more evidence is needed. Conversely, recent research indicates that more severe insomnia phenotypes, such as insomnia with short sleep duration (<6 hours on polysomnogram), have a blunted response to CBT-I and, because of significant cardiovascular risk, might benefit from the addition of hypnotics. CBT-I will remain an indispensable treatment in the armamentarium for insomnia, so future clinical and research efforts must continue to develop and disseminate this highly effective therapy to all who might benefit.

KEY CLINICAL POINTS

- Cognitive-behavioral therapy for insomnia (CBT-I) is recommended as a standard first-line treatment for chronic insomnia in adults of all ages by national and international health-focused organizations.

- CBT-I is a brief, collaborative, skills-based, multicomponent treatment that uses various therapies—including sleep restriction, stimulus control, and relaxation—to modify unhelpful beliefs, negative emotions, and maladaptive behaviors that exacerbate and perpetuate insomnia.

- Sleep hygiene, which comprises environmental factors and lifestyle practices that can influence sleep, is a component of, but not equivalent to, CBT-I and is not effective as a stand-alone therapy.

- Among individuals who report insomnia, 70%–80% treated with CBT-I experience a clinically significant reduction in symptoms and 40% of those achieve total remission.

- Preferred by patients, CBT-I demonstrates equivalent success to pharmacotherapy for insomnia over the short term and greater success at sustaining improvements over the long term.

- CBT-I can improve sleep even in the context of medical and psychiatric comorbidities, including chronic pain, cancer, depression, anxiety, and psychosis.

- Insufficient sleep and delayed sleep phase in adolescents can be safely and effectively addressed with CBT-I.

- CBT-I can help adults of all ages, but especially older adults, to decrease and discontinue medications used for sleep.

References

American Academy of Sleep Medicine: International Classification of Sleep Disorders, 3rd Edition. Darien, IL, American Academy of Sleep Medicine, 2014

Ancoli-Israel S: Sleep and its disorders in aging populations. Sleep Med 10(suppl 1):S7–S11, 2009 19647483

Belleville G, Cousineau H, Levrier K, et al: Meta-analytic review of the impact of cognitive-behavior therapy for insomnia on concomitant anxiety. Clin Psychol Rev 31(4):638–652, 2011 21482322

Bonnet MH, Arand DL: Hyperarousal and insomnia: state of the science. Sleep Med Rev 14(1):9–15, 2010 19640748

Bootzin RR, Epstein DR, Wood JM: Stimulus control instructions, in Case Studies in Insomnia. Critical Issues in Psychiatry (An Educational Series for Residents and Clinicians). Edited by Hauri PJ. Boston, MA, Springer, 1991, 19–28

Buscemi N, Vandermeer B, Friesen C, et al: National Institutes of Health State of the Science Conference statement on Manifestations and Management of Chronic Insomnia in Adults, June 13–15, 2005. Sleep 28(9):1049–1057, 2005 16268373

Chamine I, Atchley R, Oken BS: Hypnosis intervention effects on sleep outcomes: a systematic review. J Clin Sleep Med 14(2):271–283, 2018 29198290

Cheuk DK, Yeung WF, Chung KF, et al: Acupuncture for insomnia. Cochrane Database Syst Rev 12(9):CD005472, 2012 22972087

Cunningham JE, Shapiro CM: Cognitive behavioural therapy for insomnia (CBT-I) to treat depression: a systematic review. J Psychosom Res 106:1–12, 2018 29455893

Drake C, Richardson G, Roehrs T, et al: Vulnerability to stress-related sleep disturbance and hyperarousal. Sleep 27(2):285–291, 2004 15124724

Edinger JD, Wohlgemuth WK, Radtke RA, et al: Dose-response effects of cognitive-behavioral insomnia therapy: a randomized clinical trial. Sleep 30(2):203–212, 2007

Espie CA: "Stepped care": a health technology solution for delivering cognitive behavioral therapy as a first line insomnia treatment. Sleep 32(12):1549–1558, 2009 20041590

Freeman D, Sheaves B, Goodwin GM, et al: The effects of improving sleep on mental health (OASIS): a randomised controlled trial with mediation analysis. Lancet Psychiatry 4(10):749–758, 2017 28888927

Harvey AG, Bélanger L, Talbot L, et al: Comparative efficacy of behavior therapy, cognitive therapy, and cognitive behavior therapy for chronic insomnia: a randomized controlled trial. J Consult Clin Psychol 82(4):670–683, 2014 24865869

Hauri PJ: Sleep hygiene, relaxation therapy, and cognitive interventions, in Case Studies in Insomnia. New York, Springer, 1991, pp 65–84

Ho FY-Y, Chan CS, Tang KN-S: Cognitive-behavioral therapy for sleep disturbances in treating posttraumatic stress disorder symptoms: a meta-analysis of randomized controlled trials. Clin Psychol Rev 43(suppl C):90–102, 2016 26439674

Hofmann SG, Asnaani A, Vonk IJ, et al: The efficacy of cognitive behavioral therapy: a review of meta-analyses. Cognit Ther Res 36(5):427–440, 2012 23459093

Johnson JA, Rash JA, Campbell TS, et al: A systematic review and meta-analysis of randomized controlled trials of cognitive behavior therapy for insomnia (CBT-I) in cancer survivors. Sleep Med Rev 27(suppl C):20–28, 2016 26434673

Kirsch DL, Nichols F: Cranial electrotherapy stimulation for treatment of anxiety, depression, and insomnia. Psychiatr Clin North Am 36(1):169–176, 2013 23538086

Lovato N, Lack L, Wright H, et al: Evaluation of a brief treatment program of cognitive behavior therapy for insomnia in older adults. Sleep (Basel) 37(1):117–126, 2014 24470701

Mindell J, Owens J: A Clinical Guide to Pediatric Sleep: Diagnosis and Management of Sleep Problems. Philadelphia, PA, Wolters Kluwer, 2015

Morgan K, Dixon S, Mathers N, et al: Psychological treatment for insomnia in the management of long-term hypnotic drug use: a pragmatic randomised controlled trial. Br J Gen Pract 53(497):923–928, 2003 14960215

Morgenthaler T, Kramer M, Alessi C, et al: Practice parameters for the psychological and behavioral treatment of insomnia: an update. An American Academy of Sleep Medicine report. Sleep 29(11):1415–1419, 2006 17162987

Morin CM, Blais F, Savard J: Are changes in beliefs and attitudes about sleep related to sleep improvements in the treatment of insomnia? Behav Res Ther 40(7):741–752, 2002 12074370

Morin CM, Bootzin RR, Buysse DJ, et al: Psychological and behavioral treatment of insomnia: update of the recent evidence (1998–2004). Sleep 29(11):1398–1414, 2006a 17162986

Morin CM, LeBlanc M, Daley M, et al: Epidemiology of insomnia: prevalence, self-help treatments, consultations, and determinants of help-seeking behaviors. Sleep Med 7(2):123–130, 2006b 16459140

Morin CM, Bélanger L, LeBlanc M, et al: The natural history of insomnia: a population-based 3-year longitudinal study. Arch Intern Med 169(5):447–453, 2009a 19273774

Morin CM, Vallières A, Guay B, et al: Cognitive behavioral therapy, singly and combined with medication, for persistent insomnia: a randomized controlled trial. JAMA 301(19):2005–2015, 2009b 19454639

Morin CM, Drake CL, Harvey AG, et al: Insomnia disorder. Nat Rev Dis Primers 1:15026, 2015 27189779

Morin CM, Beaulieu-Bonneau S, Bélanger L, et al: Cognitive-behavior therapy singly and combined with medication for persistent insomnia: impact on psychological and daytime functioning. Behav Res Ther 87:109–116, 2016 27658218

Morin CM, Davidson JR, Beaulieu-Bonneau S: Cognitive behavior therapies for insomnia I: approaches and efficacy, in Principles and Practice of Sleep Medicine, 6th Edition. Edited by Kryger M, Roth T, Dement W. Philadelphia, PA, Elsevier, 2017, pp 804–813

Perlis ML, Giles DE, Mendelson WB, et al: Psychophysiological insomnia: the behavioural model and a neurocognitive perspective. J Sleep Res 6(3):179–188, 1997 9358396

Qaseem A, Kansagara D, Forciea MA, et al: Management of chronic insomnia disorder in adults: a clinical practice guideline from the American College of Physicians. Ann Intern Med 165(2):125–133, 2016 27136449

Riemann D, Spiegelhalder K, Feige B, et al: The hyperarousal model of insomnia: a review of the concept and its evidence. Sleep Med Rev 14(1):19–31, 2010 19481481

Riemann D, Baglioni C, Bassetti C, et al: European guideline for the diagnosis and treatment of insomnia. J Sleep Res 26(6):675–700, 2017 28875581

Rosenquist PB, Krystal A, Heart KL, et al: Left dorsolateral prefrontal transcranial magnetic stimulation (TMS): sleep factor changes during treatment in patients with pharmacoresistant major depressive disorder. Psychiatry Res 205(1–2):67–73, 2013 23021320

Roth T, Mayleben D, Feldman N, et al: A novel forehead temperature-regulating device for insomnia: a randomized clinical trial. Sleep 41(5):zsy045, 2018 29648642

Sateia MJ, Buysse DJ, Krystal AD, et al: Clinical practice guideline for the pharmacologic treatment of chronic insomnia in adults: an American Academy of Sleep Medicine Clinical Practice Guideline. J Clin Sleep Med 13(2):307–349, 2017 27998379

Schutte-Rodin S, Broch L, Buysse D, et al: Clinical guideline for the evaluation and management of chronic insomnia in adults. J Clin Sleep Med 4(5):487–504, 2008 18853708

Spielman AJ, Caruso LS, Glovinsky PB: A behavioral perspective on insomnia treatment. Psychiatr Clin North Am 10(4):541–553, 1987 3332317

van Straten A, van der Zweerde T, Kleiboer A, et al: Cognitive and behavioral therapies in the treatment of insomnia: a meta-analysis. Sleep Med Rev 38:3–16, 2018 28392168

Vincent N, Lionberg C: Treatment preference and patient satisfaction in chronic insomnia. Sleep 24(4):411–417, 2001 11403525

Wilson SJ, Nutt DJ, Alford C, et al: British Association for Psychopharmacology consensus statement on evidence-based treatment of insomnia, parasomnias and circadian rhythm disorders. J Psychopharmacol 24(11):1577–1601, 2010 20813762

Wu JQ, Appleman ER, Salazar RD, et al: Cognitive behavioral therapy for insomnia comorbid with psychiatric and medical conditions: a meta-analysis. JAMA Intern Med 175(9):1461–1472, 2015 26147487

Zachariae R, Lyby MS, Ritterband LM, et al: Efficacy of internet-delivered cognitive-behavioral therapy for insomnia—a systematic review and meta-analysis of randomized controlled trials. Sleep Med Rev 30(suppl C):1–10, 2016 26615572

CHAPTER 6

Narcolepsy

Taisuke Ono, M.D., Ph.D.
Mari Matsumura, M.P.H.
Seiji Nishino, M.D., Ph.D.

Narcolepsy is a chronic sleep disorder characterized by excessive daytime sleepiness (EDS) and dissociated manifestations of REM sleep including cataplexy, hypnagogic hallucinations, and sleep paralysis (Nishino and Mignot 2011a). Narcolepsy is therefore regarded as a central disorder of hypersomnolence with REM sleep abnormalities. The major pathophysiology of human narcolepsy has been elucidated based on the discovery of narcolepsy genes (hypocretin/orexin ligand and its receptor genes) in animals (Chemelli et al. 1999; Lin et al. 1999). Hypocretins/Orexins are hypothalamic neuropeptides involved in sleep and wake regulation (de Lecea et al. 1998; Sakurai et al. 1998). Mutations in hypocretin-related genes are rare in humans, but hypocretin ligand deficiency is found in many cases (Nishino et al. 2001; Peyron et al. 2000). This discovery refines the etiology of narcolepsy and leads to the development of new diagnostic tests and targeted treatments.

Diagnostic Criteria

The first diagnostic criterion for narcolepsy, according to the 2014 *International Classification of Sleep Disorders*, 3rd Edition (ICSD-3), is that "the patient has daily periods of irrepressible need to sleep or daytime lapses into sleep occurring for at least 3 months" (American Academy of Sleep Medicine 2014). In the ICSD-3, narcolepsy is classified into type 1 (NT1) or type 2 (NT2) based on the pathophysiology of the disease (Table 6–1). *Hypersomnia*, defined as a mean sleep latency of 8 minutes during a mul-

TABLE 6–1.   ICSD-3 diagnostic criteria for narcolepsy

Narcolepsy type 1 (NT1)	Narcolepsy type 2 (NT2)
Criteria A and B must be met:	Criteria A–E must be met:
A. Daily periods of irrepressible need to sleep or daytime lapses into sleep occurring for at least 3 months.	A. Daily periods of irrepressible need to sleep or daytime lapses into sleep occurring for at least 3 months.
B. Presence of one or both of the following:	B. An MSL of ≤8 minutes and two or more SOREMPs are found on an MSLT performed according to standard techniques. A SOREMP on the preceding nocturnal PSG may replace one of the SOREMPs on the MSLT.
1. Cataplexy and an MSL of ≤8 minutes and two or more SOREMPs on an MSLT performed according to standard techniques. A SOREMP (within 15 minutes of sleep onset) on preceding nocturnal PSG may replace one of the SOREMPs on the MSLT.	C. Cataplexy is absent.
2. CSF hypocretin-1 concentration, measured by immunoreactivity, is either ≤110 pg/mL or <1/3 of mean values obtained in normal subjects with the same standardized assay.	D. Either CSF hypocretin-1 concentration has not been measured or CSF hypocretin-1 concentration measured by immunoreactivity is either >110 pg/mL or >1/3 of mean values obtained in normal subjects with the same standardized assay.
	E. The hypersomnolence or MSLT findings are not better explained by other causes, such as insufficient sleep, OSA, delayed sleep phase disorder, or the effect of medication or substances or their withdrawal.

Note.   CSF=cerebrospinal fluid; ICSD-3=*International Classification of Sleep Disorders*, 3rd Edition; MSL=multiple sleep latency; MSLT=multiple sleep latency test; OSA= obstructive sleep apnea; PSG=polysomnography; SOREMP=sleep-onset REM period.

Source.   American Academy of Sleep Medicine 2014. Used with permission.

tiple sleep latency test (MSLT), is another criterion common to NT1 and NT2. Criteria for NT1 also include the presence of cataplexy (a sudden and transient muscle weakness triggered by emotions such as laughing) or hypocretin deficiency (i.e., low cerebrospinal fluid [CSF] hypocretin-1 levels), whereas for NT2, cataplexy is absent and hypocretin levels are normal, but other REM sleep abnormalities (two or more sleep-onset REM periods [SOREMPs] during MSLT) must be present (American Academy of Sleep Medicine 2014).

Pathophysiology

NT1 is caused by deficiencies in hypocretin signaling, likely due to selective and acquired loss of hypothalamic hypocretin/orexin-producing neurons (American Academy of Sleep Medicine 2014). Occurrences of cataplexy are tightly associated with hypocretin deficiency and human leukocyte antigen (HLA) positivity. Animal models lacking hypocretin neurotransmission, acutely or congenitally, exhibit key symptoms of narcolepsy, indicating a causal relationship between hypocretin deficiency and NT1 (Nishino and Mignot 1997).

Most patients (90%–95%) with narcolepsy who have cataplexy have undetectable or low (<110 pg/mL) CSF hypocretin-1 levels (Figure 6–1). In the few subjects with cataplexy who have normal hypocretin-1 levels, the partial loss of hypocretin neurons or impairment of undetermined hypocretin pathways may be involved (American Academy of Sleep Medicine 2014). A very few patients without cataplexy are hypocretin deficient and thus are classified as having NT1. The strong association of HLA (i.e., *HLA-DQB1*06:02*) with narcolepsy has led to the hypothesis that autoimmunity is the likely etiological mechanism that explains the selectivity of neuronal destruction in the hypothalamus (Mahlios et al. 2013), but definitive evidence proving this has not yet been obtained.

Sleep to wakefulness (and vice versa) comes with sharp transitions. The mechanism of this transition is referred to as the "flip-flop switch," named after switches similar in behavior in an electrical circuit (Saper et al. 2005). Hypocretin neurons play an important role in the regulation and stabilization of the sleep/awake and REM/non-REM (NREM) flip-flop switches. Hypocretin neurons enhance activity in the wake-promoting projections arising from neurons in the upper brain stem. On the other hand, sleep is promoted by inhibiting hypocretin neurons and the neurons in the ascending reticular activating system (Saper et al.

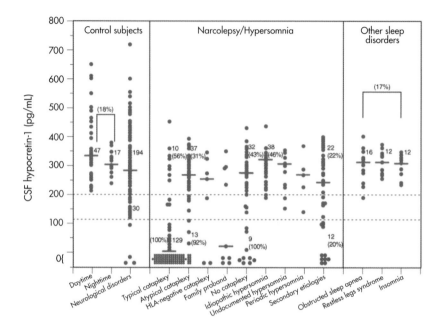

FIGURE 6–1.   CSF hypocretin-1 concentrations are plotted for individuals across various control and sleep disorders.

Each point represents the crude concentration of hypocretin-1 in a single person. Cutoffs for normal (>200 pg/mL) and low (≤110 pg/mL) concentrations are shown. Also noted is total number of subjects in each range. The percentage of *HLA-DQB1*06:02* positivity for a given group in a given range is parenthetically noted for certain disorders. Control carrier frequencies for *DQB1*06:02* are 17%–22% in healthy control subjects and secondary narcolepsy. In other patient groups, values are higher, with almost all hypocretin-deficient narcolepsy being *HLA-DQB1*06:02* positive. The median value in each group is shown by the *horizontal bar*. CSF=cerebrospinal fluid; HLA=human leukocyte antigen.
Source.   Updated from previously published data in Mignot E, Lammers GJ, Ripley B, et al: "The Role of Cerebrospinal Fluid Hypocretin Measurement in the Diagnosis of Narcolepsy and Other Hypersomnias." *Archives of Neurology* 59(10):1553–1562, 2002.

2010). Hypocretin neurons also suppress REM sleep by enhancing activity of the monoaminergic neurons in the locus coeruleus (noradrenergic) and dorsal raphe nucleus (serotonergic), which in turn activate REM sleep–suppressing neurons (Sorensen et al. 2013). Thus, lack of hypocretin results in sleepiness and REM sleep propensity. In comparison, the pathophysiology of NT2 is largely unknown, and NT2 is clinically heterogeneous.

Epidemiology

PREVALENCE AND SEX, CULTURAL, OR RACIAL CONSIDERATIONS

The prevalence of narcolepsy with cataplexy is estimated to be 0.025%–0.05% (Longstreth et al. 2007). On the other hand, the exact prevalence of NT2 is unknown. Although both sexes are affected, the prevalence of NT1 and NT2 may be slightly higher in males (American Academy of Sleep Medicine 2014).

RISK FACTORS

Occurrences of narcolepsy are genetically influenced. *HLA-DQB1*06:02* was the first narcolepsy-susceptible gene to be identified, which led to an autoimmune hypothesis. However, familial occurrences of narcolepsy are rare (see "Familial Patterns, Genetics" section). Polygenic and environmental influences for the etiology have been suggested. History of streptococcal pharyngitis (Koepsell et al. 2010), antibody titer of anti-streptolysin-O within several years after the onset of narcolepsy (Aran et al. 2009), or β-hemolytic group A streptococcal infection (Ambati et al. 2015) has been observed at higher rates. The association between the increase in narcolepsy incidence and the 2009 H1N1 influenza pandemic may be the strongest evidence in support of the autoimmune hypothesis of narcolepsy. In China, the incidence of narcolepsy increased after the outbreak of natural pH1N1 infections (Han et al. 2011). Significant increases in narcolepsy incidences in children were reported after vaccination with Pandemrix, a pH1N1 AS03-adjuvanted vaccine, in northern Europe (Partinen et al. 2012), France (Dauvilliers et al. 2013), England (Winstone et al. 2014), and Ireland (O'Flanagan et al. 2014). In contrast, no increase in narcolepsy incidents was seen in the United States (Duffy et al. 2014), Canada (Montplaisir et al. 2014), and several European countries (Ahmed et al. 2014). Affected subjects were clinically indistinguishable from those with NT1 (i.e., cataplexy, hypocretin deficiency, and HLA positivity). Narcolepsy onset incidences increased in the countries where Pandemrix was used (Sarkanen et al. 2018). Thus, understanding the types of vaccinations and their adjuvants may help bridge the autoimmunity hypothesis of narcolepsy and the loss of hypocretin cells seen in NT1 (Luo et al. 2018).

The risk factors associated with NT2 are unknown. Head trauma and unspecified viral illnesses have been reported as possible triggers for NT2, but associations have been unproven.

FAMILIAL PATTERNS, GENETICS

The morbidity of familial cases is low, at approximately 5% (Nishino et al. 2010). The risk of NT1 in the first-degree relatives of affected individuals is about 1%–2%. However, this is a 10- to 40-fold increase compared with the population prevalence. This increased risk cannot be explained only by the effect of one gene, suggesting a polygenic influence. At the genetic level, NT1 is closely associated with *HLA-DQB1*06:02*, which is found in 95% of patients with narcolepsy with cataplexy and in 41% of patients with narcolepsy without cataplexy, but in only 18%–35% of the general population (Mignot et al. 1997). Similarly, a high association of NT1 with *HLA-DQA1*01:02*, which encodes for a subunit of the antigen presenting heterodimer, suggests that these HLA haplotypes are functionally involved in the disease onset. In addition, genome-wide association studies have demonstrated that NT1 is associated with the T-cell receptor α gene. Taken together, these results suggest that the immune system is activated and the autoimmune process initiated via antigen presentation by the HLA molecules to the T-cells (Toyoda et al. 2015).

Clinical Presentation, Course, and Complications

EXCESSIVE DAYTIME SLEEPINESS

EDS is a core symptom of narcolepsy and is defined as an "irresistible sleepiness in a situation when an individual would be expected to be awake, and alert" (Arand et al. 2005, p. 123; see also Nishino and Mignot 2011a). Even if the patient secures adequate sleep time at night, strong drowsiness repeatedly occurs during the day. In some cases, EDS presents as "sleep attacks," or sudden irresistible sleep, and patients may fall asleep even in situations requiring attention or concentration, such as during meals or while walking. The patients usually wake up naturally after a short time (10–20 minutes). Most patients feel greatly refreshed immediately after awakening, but sleepiness may appear again within several hours. EDS often lasts for a lifetime and has a serious impact on the social ability of the patients.

SLEEP FRAGMENTATION

One-third of patients with narcolepsy experience nighttime fragmentation of sleep (Dauvilliers et al. 2007). These patients generally cannot stay asleep for a long time. Thus, their sleep typically tends to be fragmented, and they often wake up several times during the night. This usually worsens with age. Deficiency of sleep-wake-stabilizing hypocretin is considered a fundamental cause of sleep fragmentation (Schneider and Mignot 2017).

CATAPLEXY

Cataplexy is a sudden loss of skeletal muscle tone that generally occurs in bilateral symmetry and is triggered by strong, typically positive emotions during arousal, such as laughter or excitement (Nishino and Mignot 2011a; Overeem et al. 2011). The episodes can last from a few seconds to at most 2 minutes. If the cause of the attack continues, the attack may continue and appear as a long episode. Patients are conscious throughout the entire episode and can recognize the surrounding situation. Symptoms of cataplexy and sleepiness usually co-occur during the first year of the disease; however, cases have been reported in which cataplexy has appeared approximately 20 years after the patient developed sleepiness (Taddei et al. 2016). Individual differences in the frequency of cataplexy are large and vary from less than once a month to more than 20 times a day. In most cases, loss of muscle tone affects the lower limbs. Weakness in the arms, slurring of speech, and dropping of the jaw or head may also be present. When cataplexy episodes are severe, patients could collapse to the ground. Cataplexy in children can be quite atypical, especially in the acute stage of disease onset. The episodes may occur without clear emotional triggers and often cause facial hypotonia with droopy eyelids, mouth openings, and a protruding tongue (Serra et al. 2008). Recent studies have noted the possibility that atypical features of cataplexy in young children may cause delayed diagnoses and higher estimates of the age at onset (Rocca et al. 2015). Deep tendon reflexes disappear transiently and reversibly in cataplexy, so checking reflexes during an episode can be a valuable diagnostic finding. Frequency of cataplexy is often seen to gradually decrease with age, possibly because patients can empirically recognize the situation in which cataplexy occurs and can avoid the situation on their own.

SLEEP PARALYSIS

Sleep paralysis is an inability to move during transition periods of sleep and arousal, especially during sleep onset, and lasts from a few seconds to a few minutes. In most cases, episodes are described as an inability to move limbs or speak despite being awake (Nishino and Mignot 2011a). The patient recovers spontaneously within a few minutes. Accessory respiratory muscles be inactive during these episodes, and the diaphragm remains the only muscle to support respiration. Therefore, although gas exchange remains adequate, patients may feel pressure on their chests. Sleep paralysis may be caused even in healthy people by sleep deprivation, an irregular sleep schedule, and stress.

SLEEP-RELATED HALLUCINATIONS

Sleep-related hallucinations are vivid, dreamlike experiences that occur in the transition from arousal to sleep (hypnopompic) or sleep to arousal (hypnagogic) and are usually brief but at times continue for a few minutes (Nishino and Mignot 2011a). These are typically visual hallucinations combined with somatosensory hallucinations, although other types of hallucinations are possible. Sleep-related hallucinations are at times difficult to differentiate from nightmares, and these symptoms are not specific to narcolepsy. Thus, sleep-related hallucinations are not useful diagnostic signs.

COMPLICATIONS

Around the time of disease onset, unexplained weight gain is often observed. Obesity (BMI ≥30) occurs more than twice as frequently in patients with narcolepsy as in control subjects (American Academy of Sleep Medicine 2014).

An increased prevalence of depressive symptoms and anxiety disorders has been reported. In addition, narcolepsy often accompanies other sleep disorders. In a cohort study of patients with narcolepsy, comorbidities such as insomnia (28%); sleep-related breathing disorders (24%); parasomnias, including REM sleep behavior disorder (24%) and NREM parasomnias (10%); sleep-related movement disorders, such as bruxism (31%); periodic limb movements of sleep (75%); and restless legs syndrome (24%) were observed (Frauscher et al. 2013).

CLINICAL COURSE

The onset of NT1 typically occurs between the ages of 10 and 25 years. However, age at onset has been bimodal in some populations, in which the first peak was at 14.7 years and the second peak was at 35 years (Dauvilliers et al. 2001). Sleepiness is usually the first symptom to manifest. Cataplexy most often occurs within 1 year of onset, but in rare cases, it may precede the onset of sleepiness or commence up to 40 years later (American Academy of Sleep Medicine 2014). Hypnagogic hallucinations, sleep paralysis, and disturbed nocturnal sleep often manifest later in the course of the disease. In most cases, symptoms gradually develop over several years, and by the time the clinical picture is fully developed, the severity of the symptoms usually has stabilized. Cataplexy may lessen with age or occasionally increase in frequency and severity.

When left untreated, NT1 is a lifelong condition that is socially disabling and isolating. Patients have a tendency to fail in school and are often dismissed from their jobs (American Academy of Sleep Medicine 2014), and they may avoid driving for fear of a motor vehicle accident. Depression and weight gain are also common.

Diagnostic Procedures, Tests, and Questionnaires

Diagnosis of narcolepsy is usually made on clinical grounds, confirmed by polysomnography followed by MSLT. Subjective sleepiness and daily sleeping habits are evaluated by questionnaires and confirmation of a sleep diary. The Epworth Sleepiness Scale is one of the most frequently used questionnaires for assessing subjective sleepiness. Scores from 11 to 24 represent increasing levels of EDS (Johns 1991). Because cataplexy rarely appears during examination, diagnosis is usually made based on medical history. It is helpful to ask patients if anything unusual happens when they hear something funny or when they laugh. In patients with narcolepsy, nighttime sleep tends to be fragmented; therefore, clinicians should inquire about this symptom. CSF hypocretin-1 measurements are not routinely available. A diagnostic algorithm for narcolepsy is shown in Figure 6–2 (Schneider and Mignot 2017).

POLYSOMNOGRAPHY

In patients with narcolepsy, sleep latency is often short on polysomnography (<10 minutes). In healthy subjects, REM sleep does not appear until 60–90 minutes after sleep onset, but in those with narcolepsy, REM sleep often appears within 15 minutes of nocturnal sleep onset. This is referred to as SOREMP. Distinctively in narcolepsy, sleep is divided by frequent arousal reactions during the night, and the time spent in deep slow-wave sleep is short (Roth et al. 2013).

MULTIPLE SLEEP LATENCY TEST

The MSLT measures how quickly a patient falls asleep in a quiet environment during the day and is an objective measure of EDS. This test consists of five scheduled napping opportunities every 2 hours, starting no later than 2 hours after awakening, and is conducted during the day, fol-

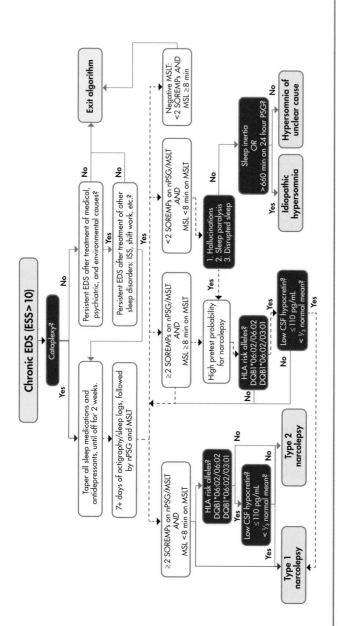

FIGURE 6–2.   Diagnostic algorithm for narcolepsy.

The investigation of a sleepy patient (Epworth Sleepiness Scale [ESS] score >10) varies depending upon the presence of cataplexy. The potential workup is illustrated by the *dark gray path* if cataplexy is endorsed, the *light gray path* if cataplexy is not endorsed, and the *dashed path* where the investigations overlap. CSF=cerebrospinal fluid; EDS=excessive daytime sleepiness; HLA=human leukocyte antigen; ISS=insufficient sleep syndrome; MSL=mean sleep latency; MSLT=multiple sleep latency test; nPSG=nocturnal polysomnogram; PSG=polysomnogram; SOREMP=sleep-onset REM period.

Source.   Reprinted from Schneider L, Mignot E: "Diagnosis and Management of Narcolepsy." *Seminars in Neurology* 37(4):454–455, 2017. Copyright © 2017 Theime (www.thieme.com). Used with permission.

lowing a polysomnogram. Patients are instructed to lie down and sleep. Sleep latency—that is, latency to the first episode of 30 seconds of sleep after lights off—is recorded. If the patient does not fall sleep, the exam is continued for 20 minutes and finished. The ICSD-3 criteria for narcolepsy require two or more SOREMPs with an average sleep latency of <8 minutes but allow replacement of one SOREMP in the MSLT with a SOREMP from the preceding polysomnogram (American Academy of Sleep Medicine 2014).

MEASUREMENT OF CSF HYPOCRETIN-1 CONCENTRATION

A CSF hypocretin-1 level of ≤110 pg/mL, or less than one-third of the mean value obtained in healthy control subjects, is an alternative criterion (to cataplexy and MSLT findings) for diagnosing NT1 (i.e., hypocretin deficiency) according to ICSD-3. CSF hypocretin-1 measurement is also useful to diagnose cataplexy cases with negative MSLT, cases in children, and cases in which it is difficult to judge the existence of cataplexy. Academic centers currently able to test for CSF hypocretin are, unfortunately, rare.

Differential Diagnosis

Narcolepsy is often misdiagnosed as a psychiatric condition, typically depression, or as epilepsy, especially in children (Nishino and Mignot 2011). Other forms of primary or secondary hypersomnia, such as sleep-related breathing disorders (see Chapters 8–11), idiopathic/recurrent hypersomnia (see Chapter 7), or hypersomnia associated with depression, may also confound narcolepsy (Nishino and Mignot 2011a). The presence of cataplexy is useful in diagnosing narcolepsy apart from other forms of hypersomnia. However, when cataplexy is predominant, narcolepsy can also be confused with syncope, drop attacks, atonic attacks, or conversion disorder. Furthermore, some well-informed individuals may mimic the symptoms of narcolepsy in order to benefit from a disability leave from work or to obtain a prescription of psychostimulants.

Narcolepsy without cataplexy (i.e., NT2) may overlap with idiopathic hypersomnia (see Chapter 7), a less common and heterogeneous disorder with chronic sleepiness (Bassetti and Aldrich 1997; Black et al. 2004). By definition, patients with idiopathic hypersomnia lack cataplexy and have fewer than two SOREMPs on the MSLT. Some of these individuals have deep, excessively long periods of sleep; difficulty waking from sleep; and long, unrefreshing naps (Aldrich 1996; Bassetti and Aldrich 1997).

Kleine-Levin syndrome is characterized by relapsing-remitting episodes of severe hypersomnolence. The first episode is triggered by an infection or alcohol intake in many cases, and further episodes recur every 1–12 months for years. Individual episodes generally last a few days to a few weeks, with rare episodes lasting several weeks to months. During these episodes, patients may sleep for as long as 16–20 hours per day and present anterograde amnesia, excessive food intake, hypersexuality, irritability, childishness, or psychotic symptoms (American Academy of Sleep Medicine 2014).

Narcolepsy can also be related to a medical or neurological disorder or discrete brain lesion. Several cases of narcolepsy in association with brain tumors, most often localized in the posterior hypothalamus and the superior part of the brain stem, have been reported (Nishino and Kanbayashi 2005). Narcolepsy has also been reported in patients with multiple sclerosis, encephalitis, cerebral ischemia, cranial trauma, brain tumor, and neurodegeneration. Some symptomatic cases of narcolepsy are reported to be associated with moderate declines in CSF hypocretin levels (Nishino and Kanbayashi 2005). Secondary narcolepsies are also present in children affected by Niemann-Pick type C disease (Nishino and Kanbayashi 2005). The diagnosis of secondary narcolepsy requires that narcolepsy develop in close temporal relationship with the neurological disorder, because the association may be incidental rather than causal. Hypersomnia cases associated with hypocretin deficiency have also been reported in some paraneoplastic anti-Ma antibodies and neuromyelitis optica cases (Nishino and Kanbayashi 2005; Kanbayashi et al. 2009). In ICSD-3, narcolepsy with or without cataplexy associated with these conditions is classified under "narcolepsy due to a medical condition," and a significant underlying medical or neurological disorder must account for the EDS or cataplexy (American Academy of Sleep Medicine 2014). Other diagnostic criteria, namely the symptoms, polysomnography results, and laboratory findings, are the same as for NT1 and NT2.

Treatments

Pharmacological management of NT1 and other hypersomnias is shown in Table 6–2 (Schneider and Mignot 2017). For EDS, nonamphetamine wake-promoting compounds (modafinil/armodafinil) or amphetamine-like CNS stimulants are often used (Nishino 2010; Nishino and Kotorii

TABLE 6–2. Pharmacological management of type 1 narcolepsy and other hypersomnias

Drug	Dosing	Mechanism of action	Side effects
Wake-promoting agents (primarily for excessive daytime sleepiness)			
Caffeine	Titrate to effect	Blocks adenosine receptor	Jitteriness, diuresis
Modafinil	100–400 mg	Exact mechanism unknown; likely related to dopamine transporter blockade	Headache, nausea, dry mouth, Stevens-Johnson syndrome (rare), birth control metabolism
Armodafinil	150–250 mg		
Amphetamines			
Amphetamine/ Dextroamphetamine	10–60 mg	Release and reuptake inhibition; blockade at dopamine and vesicular monoamine transporters (at higher doses) results in increased DA > NE(NA) > 5-HT	Sympathetic activation, psychosis, addiction
Dextroamphetamine	5–60 mg		
Methamphetamine	5–60 mg		
Amphetamine-like			
Methylphenidate	10–60 mg	Dopamine/vesicular monoamine transporter reuptake inhibition	Sympathetic activation, psychosis, addiction
Mazindol	3–8 mg	Not FDA approved	Sympathetic activation, psychosis, addiction
Pemoline	18.75–112.5 mg		

TABLE 6–2.   Pharmacological management of type 1 narcolepsy and other hypersomnias *(continued)*

Drug	Dosing	Mechanism of action	Side effects
Antidepressants (primarily for cataplexy management, with some stimulant effects depending upon class)			
Serotonin-norepinephrine reuptake inhibitors			
Venlafaxine	37.5–300 mg	Serotonin-norepinephrine reuptake inhibition	GI upset (main reason for discontinuation), potential withdrawal with abrupt cessation
Duloxetine	20–60 mg	Serotonin-norepinephrine reuptake inhibition	GI upset (main reason for discontinuation), potential withdrawal with abrupt cessation; rarely associated with hepatotoxicity (avoid if alcohol abuse is an issue)
Selective serotonin reuptake inhibitors			
Fluoxetine	20–80 mg	Selective serotonin reuptake inhibition; beneficial with concomitant depression/anxiety; ideal due to long half-life	Sexual dysfunction (particularly in males), insomnia, weight gain, gastrointestinal upset
Citalopram	20–60 mg		
Sertraline	50–200 mg		
Tricyclic antidepressants (TCAs)			
Clomipramine	25–150 mg	TCA with NE > 5-HT reuptake inhibition, but also antagonizes H_1, α_1, muscarinic, and $5\text{-}HT_{2A}$ receptors	Overdose risk, anticholinergic side effects, cardiac conduction abnormalities, open-angle glaucoma exacerbation
Imipramine	50–200 mg		
Protriptyline	10–60 mg		

TABLE 6–2.   Pharmacological management of type 1 narcolepsy and other hypersomnias *(continued)*

Drug	Dosing	Mechanism of action	Side effects
Sleep modulators (sodium oxybate addresses all symptoms of NT1)			
Sodium oxybate (γ-hydroxybutyrate [GHB])	4.5–9 g divided into two doses nightly	Exact mechanisms unknown; likely agonist at GHB and GABA$_B$ receptors and others; increases slow-wave and REM sleep; approved for treatment of hypersomnia and cataplexy	Nausea, weight loss, parasomnias, sodium overload, abuse, respiratory suppression
Others (off-label, possibly useful for sleepiness in non-NT1)			
Clarithromycin	500–1,000 mg bid	Exact mechanisms unknown; antibiotic that likely reduces GABA signaling via GABA$_A$ receptor block	Chronic antibiotic use leads to reversible hearing loss, GI upset, altered taste, QTc prolongation, CNS excitation/psychotic disorder; P450 3A inhibitor
Flumazenil	6 mg every 6 hours to every 3 hours*	GABA$_A$ receptor block	Possible tolerance, uncertain receptor upregulation

Note.   5-HT=5-hydroxytryptophan (serotonin); DA=dopamine; GI=gastrointestinal; NA=noradrenaline; NE=norepinephrine; NT1=narcolepsy type 1.
*See Rye DB, Bliwise DL, Parker K, et al.: "Modulation of Vigilance in the Primary Hypersomnias by Endogenous Enhancement of GABA$_A$ Receptors."
Science Translational Medicine 4(161):161ra151, 2012.
Source.   Reprinted from Schneider L, Mignot E: "Diagnosis and Management of Narcolepsy." *Seminars in Neurology* 37(4):454–455, 2017. Copyright © 2017
Theime (www.thieme.com). Used with permission.

2010). These compounds possess wake-promoting effects in subjects with narcolepsy as well as in control populations, but high doses are required to normalize abnormal sleep tendencies during the daytime for narcolepsy (Mitler 1994). For consolidating nighttime sleep, sodium oxybate (sodium salt of γ-hydroxybutyric acid [GHB]) is used, and nighttime administration of sodium oxybate reduces EDS and cataplexy during the daytime (Scrima et al. 1989; Lammers et al. 1993). Because of its short half-life, sodium oxybate must be administered twice a night. Sodium oxybate is considered a standard therapy for narcolepsy (Wise et al. 2007).

STIMULANTS

Pharmacology

The most commonly prescribed stimulants are amphetamine and amphetamine-like drugs such as dextroamphetamine, methamphetamine, and methylphenidate, and wake-promoting compounds such as modafinil/armodafinil (R-enantiomer of racemic modafinil, with a longer half-life) (Nishino and Kotorii 2010; Nishino and Mignot 2011b; Nishino and Okuro 2008; Schneider and Mignot 2017; see Table 6–2). The hypocretin system sends strong excitatory projections onto monoaminergic cells, and a lack of excitatory inputs to these systems is likely involved in the pathophysiology of narcolepsy. The main effect of stimulants is to increase the transmission of monoamines such as dopamine and norepinephrine by stimulating monoamine release and blocking their reuptake. The primary mechanism of action for amphetamines is increased dopamine release, although weaker effects on norepinephrine and serotonin release are also observed. Increased release occurs because amphetamines inhibit vesicular storage of monoamines, resulting in exchange diffusion of dopamine via the dopamine transporter. Other compounds such as methylphenidate increase dopamine transmission primarily by inhibiting reuptake of monoamines, and at higher doses norepinephrine, thereby increasing the availability of already-released dopamine.

Abuse and dose escalation can occur with amphetamines, especially in cases without cataplexy. Less abuse is reported with methylphenidate, and modafinil/armodafinil is not believed to be addictive. Studies have shown that the wake-promoting effect of these compounds is secondary to the dopamine release stimulation and dopamine reuptake inhibition (Nishino et al. 1998; Wisor et al. 2001). Modafinil's mode of action is debated, but it also selectively inhibits dopamine reuptake (Mignot et al. 1994; Nishino and Kotorii 2010). All of these compounds are ineffective in dopamine transporter knockout mice, suggesting a primary mediation of wake promotion via the dopaminergic systems (Wisor et al. 2001). Dopamine reuptake blockers reduce total sleep time and slow-wave sleep (Nishino et al. 1998). Dopamine-specific reuptake blockers have little effect on REM sleep compared with adrenergic or serotonergic compounds (Nishino et al. 1997), and the selective dopamine reuptake inhibitors have little or no effect on cataplexy (Kanbayashi et al. 2000).

Evidence on Efficacy

The American Academy of Sleep Medicine (AASM) recommends the use of amphetamine-like stimulants, modafinil, and armodafinil for the treatment of narcolepsy (Wise et al. 2007). Amphetamine-like stimulants have a long history of effective use in clinical practice (Nishino and Mignot 2011b), but limited information is available on their benefit/risk ratio. This lack of information possibly reflects limited research funding for medications available in generic form rather than the clinical utility of these medications.

In contrast, 14 studies of modafinil, including four level-1 studies and two level-2 studies, are available. The approved recommended dosage of modafinil is 200 mg once daily, but higher doses and split-dose regimens have been investigated. Three level-1 studies indicated that use of a split-dose strategy provides better control of EDS than a single daily dose. One study demonstrated that adding a dose of modafinil 200 mg at 12:00 P.M. following a 400-mg dose at 7:00 A.M. improved scores on a maintenance of wakefulness test (MWT) done later in the day relative to scores after a 400-mg morning dose alone. A level-1 study by Black and Houghton (2006) compared combinations of active and placebo preparations of modafinil and sodium oxybate. Subjects receiving both active modafinil and sodium oxybate showed the most improvement, and suggesting an additive effect of the two compounds. One level-4 open-label study showed modafinil was effective in improving sleepiness and was generally well tolerated in 13 children (mean age 11 years) with narcolepsy or idiopathic hypersomnia. A level-1 study of 196 subjects assessed armodafinil for treatment of EDS in patients with narcolepsy. Subjects receiving armodafinil experienced significant improvements in sleepiness as measured by MWT mean sleep latency and on the Clinical Global Impression of Change scale (Morgenthaler et al. 2007).

Adverse Effects and Their Management

Amphetamines and amphetamine-like compounds have been effectively used in the management of EDS in narcolepsy since 1935 but are currently considered second-line therapy due to abuse potential (Nishino and Mignot 2011b). They should be prescribed at the minimum effective dose, with a preference for long-acting/extended-release agents. High doses may induce psychosis and long-term cardiac complications.

Modafinil is often considered to be first-line therapy for EDS in NT1 and is also approved for use in other disorders with hypersomnolence, such as shift work disorder and residual EDS in obstructive sleep apnea. Armodafinil is twice as potent as modafinil in a steady state (Nishino and Okuro 2008) and is typically dosed once daily in the morning, whereas modafinil is often more effective with twice-daily dosing. Currently, neither is approved by the FDA for idiopathic hypersomnia, although they are often prescribed off-label in these patients. The mechanism of action of armodafinil is presumably through dopamine transporter blockade (Nishino and Okuro 2008).

The lower abuse potential of modafinil in comparison with the other stimulant medications, notably the short-acting formulations, is likely due to the lack of a rapid-onset increase in dopamine release. One rare but important side effect risk with modafinil is a hypersensitivity reaction, including Stevens-Johnson syndrome. In addition, clinicians must inform patients that modafinil/armodafinil may reduce the efficacy of hormonal contraception; therefore, alternative means of contraception are required while using these drugs.

GAMMA-HYDROXYBUTYRIC ACID

Pharmacology

GHB is generally used in the salt form, such as sodium oxybate. Sodium oxybate is approved by the FDA as a prescription drug for narcolepsy. The exact mode of action of sodium oxybate on sleep and narcolepsy is unclear (Nishino 2010). It is a sedative anesthetic compound known to increase slow-wave sleep and, to a lesser extent, REM sleep, presumably through agonism at the GHB and $GABA_B$ receptors (Castelli et al. 2003). Sodium oxybate has a biphasic effect on dopamine transmission. It first reduces cell firing rates and dopamine release and then raises the brain content of dopamine (Castelli et al. 2003; Maitre 1997; Nishino and Mignot 1997). Other effects on levels or actions of opioids and glutamatergic and acetylcholine transmission have been reported (Castelli et al. 2003). Most studies to date suggest that the sedative-hypnotic effect of sodium oxybate is mediated via $GABA_B$ agonist activity (Castelli et al. 2003; Queva et al. 2003). Whether this effect also mediates the anticataplectic effects after long-term administration is unknown. Human or animal studies using other $GABA_B$ agonists would be needed to answer these questions.

Evidence on Efficacy

Sodium oxybate addresses multiple narcolepsy symptoms, including EDS, disrupted nocturnal sleep, cataplexy, and sleep attacks, thereby improving patients' overall daytime function (Alshaikh et al. 2012). Full therapeutic benefits may take weeks to months to fully manifest. The AASM recommends the use of sodium oxybate, and this recommendation is based on three level-1 and two level-4 studies (Wise et al. 2007). Three level-1 studies support the efficacy of sodium oxybate in treating cataplexy. One of these studies also supported its efficacy in treating EDS and disrupted sleep but found no significant improvement in hypnagogic hallucinations or sleep paralysis. Two additional level-1 studies supported its efficacy in treating EDS (Morgenthaler et al. 2007). In contrast, a level-4 study supported the efficacy of sodium oxybate in improving EDS, nighttime awakenings, sleep paralysis, and hypnagogic hallucinations (Mamelak et al. 2004).

Adverse Effects and Their Management

In the United States, due to its potential for abuse and possible adverse effects with heavy sedation and respiratory depression, sodium oxybate is dispensed from a central pharmacy and requires patient and provider enrollment in the pharmaceutical company's management program as mandated by the FDA. Other side effects include the possibility of weight loss due to appetite loss, nausea, and psychiatric side effects (Schneider and Mignot 2017). A slower titration schedule with lower starting dose may alleviate some of these side effects, particularly nausea. The high sodium load in the currently available drug preparation potentially presents a risk in patients with congestive heart failure, hypertension, or renal failure and warrants a strict low-salt diet. Intake of water or crackers with each dose can be recommended to mask any unpleasant taste.

ANTICATAPLECTIC AGENTS

Amphetamine-like stimulants and modafinil have little effect on cataplexy, and additional anticataplectics are needed for many NT1 patients (Nishino and Mignot 1997). The emotion-triggered, REM sleep–related atonia of cataplexy has been managed with REM sleep–suppressing antidepressants since the 1970s (Nishino 2010; Nishino and Kotorii 2010). Early use of tricyclic antidepressants (TCAs) established the immediate efficacy of antidepressants in reducing cataplexy. Unfortunately, the use of these compounds is limited by significant anticholinergic side effects, the high risk of overdose, and the lack of FDA approval. Recently, non-TCA and more selective monoamine reuptake inhibitors, such as noradrenergic and serotonergic/noradrenergic reuptake inhibitors, have been used with more success. Antidepressants are also effective for other REM sleep phenomena. As mentioned, sodium oxybate is also used for the treatment of cataplexy, but reports are conflicting on its effectiveness for other REM sleep phenomena, such as sleep paralysis and sleep-related hallucinations.

Pharmacology

Most TCA compounds are known to act on the monoaminergic systems (see Table 6–2). The compounds effective for EDS mostly target the presynaptic enhancement of dopaminergic neurotransmission (dopamine release and reuptake inhibition) (Nishino 2010; Nishino and Kotorii 2010), whereas anticataplectics are mostly mediated by enhancement of noradrenergic neurotransmission (Nishino et al. 1998). Animal data suggest that stimulants and anticataplectics are effective for both EDS and cataplexy regardless of hypocretin receptor dysfunction and ligand deficiency (Babcock et al. 1976; Nishino and Mignot 1997) and are likely to act on downstream pathways of hypocretin neurotransmission.

Among selective monoamine reuptake inhibitors, pure serotonergic antidepressants (selective serotonin reuptake inhibitors [SSRIs]) are less useful in the management of cataplexy. Extended-release venlafaxine, a serotonin-norepinephrine reuptake inhibitor (SNRI), is very effective and therefore is commonly used for first-line therapy. Atomoxetine, which is primarily a norepinephrine reuptake inhibitor (NRI), is also used in the treatment of cataplexy and EDS, particularly in children. REM-suppressing effects of these compounds may also be helpful in treating sleep paralysis and hypnagogic/hypnopompic hallucinations.

Evidence on Efficacy

The AASM recommends using selective monoamine reuptake inhibitors for the treatment of cataplexy, hypnagogic hallucinations, and sleep paralysis (Wise et al. 2007). Medications recommended for treatment of cataplexy have been expanded to include SSRIs, venlafaxine, and the NRI reboxetine. Evidence was limited regarding the treatment of cataplexy in the prior practice parameters, which may reflect limited sources of research funding for medications. In a review by the AASM in 2007 (Wise et al. 2007), only one level-4 study (Larrosa et al. 2001) involving treatment of cataplexy with a medication other than sodium oxybate was identified. Reboxetine, a selective NRI unavailable in the United States, has shown to reduce cataplexy in 12 subjects with narcolepsy with cataplexy. The recommendation for fluoxetine, an SSRI, was based on a level-2 and a level-5 study supporting its efficacy for treatment of cataplexy. The antidepressant venlafaxine, which inhibits serotonin and norepinephrine reuptake, may also reduce cataplexy (Morgenthaler et al. 2007).

Adverse Effects and Their Management

Use of TCAs in the treatment of cataplexy is hampered by several problems. The first is the relatively poor side effect profile of most tricyclic compounds. Side effects are mostly due to the drugs' anticholinergic properties and lead to dry mouth and associated dental problems, tachycardia, urinary retention, constipation, and blurred vision. Additional side effects are weight gain, sexual dysfunction (impotence or delayed orgasm), tremors, sedation from antihistaminic effects, and occasionally orthostatic hypotension due to the α_1-adrenergic blockade of some compounds. Nighttime sleep may also become more disturbed (Raynal 1976; Thorpy and Goswami 1990). A slow titration schedule can mitigate some of these side effects. However, non-TCA antidepressants should be considered if side effects persist. Selective monoamine reuptake inhibitors (SSRIs, SNRIs) have fewer anticholinergic properties and are better tolerated. Another disadvantage of these medications is the significant rebound of cataplexy that can occur when therapy is abruptly interrupted.

NONPHARMACOLOGICAL TREATMENTS

Nonpharmacological treatments with behavioral modification are often reported to be useful additions to the clinical management of patients with narcolepsy (Mullington and Broughton 1993; Roehrs et al. 1986; Rogers 1984; Thorpy and Goswami 1990). Regular napping usually relieves sleepiness for 1–2 hours and is the treatment of choice for some patients (Roehrs et al. 1986) but often has negative social and professional consequences. Exercising to avoid obesity, keeping a regular sleep-wake schedule, and having a supportive social environment such as through patient group organizations and support groups are also helpful. In almost all cases, however, pharmacological treatment is needed; 94% of patients reported using medications in a survey by a patient group organization (American Narcolepsy Association 1992).

EMERGING PHARMACOTHERAPIES

Current pharmacological treatments for narcolepsy are symptomatic and are not satisfactory to many patients due to undesirable side effects. Furthermore, most patients need to take two different classes of compounds to manage both EDS and cataplexy, and this brings various complications (Schneider and Mignot 2017). For these reasons, people have awaited a treatment that is more directly pathophysiologically oriented.

Hypocretin-Based Therapies

Hypocretin/Orexin peptides or their mimetics would theoretically be the most promising agents. However, large molecular peptides do not penetrate the brain efficiently, and oral administration is not applicable for neuropeptides. Thus, nonpeptide agonists need to be developed (Nepovimova et al. 2019). Possible hypocretin replacement therapies include intranasal hypocretin administration (Deadwyler et al. 2007), small molecule synthetic hypocretin receptor agonists (Irukayama-Tomobe et al. 2017; Nagahara et al. 2015), hypocretin gene therapy (Liu et al. 2016; Mieda et al. 2004), and hypocretin cell transplantation (Arias-Carrion and Murillo-Rodriguez 2014). Among these, nonpeptide small molecular hypocretin receptor agonists are considered to be the most promising. Although the identification of receptor agonists is generally complex and difficult, two potent nonpeptide hypocretin receptor 2–selective agonists, YNT-185 and TAK-925, were recently synthesized and proven effective in mouse models of narcolepsy. Of note, clinical trials of TAK-925 have recently been launched, and results are awaited. If ligand replacement therapy is demonstrated to be effective for hypocretin-deficient patients with narcolepsy, hypocretin cell transplant or gene therapy technology could also be applicable in the future.

Immune-Based Therapies

Immune-based treatments such as intravenous immunoglobulin (Dauvilliers et al. 2009), plasmapheresis (Chen et al. 2005), corticosteroids (Hecht et al. 2003), and alemtuzumab (Donjacour and Lammers 2012) have been tried to prevent the development of disease by preventing autoimmune attacks on hypocretin neurons. Unfortunately, most of these reports showed no effects, and intravenous immunoglobulin administration had mixed results (Dauvilliers et al. 2009; Knudsen et al. 2010, 2012; Valko et al. 2008).

Other Stimulants

Clarithromycin and flumazenil have been reported to improve subjective sleepiness in patients with NT2. These compounds are possible negative allosteric modulators of the $GABA_A$ receptor and may reduce GABA signaling. However, the exact mechanisms for improved sleepiness with clarithromycin and flumazenil are unknown (Rye et al. 2012; Trotti et al. 2015).

Conclusion

Narcolepsy is a chronic sleep disorder that is characterized by EDS, sleep fragmentation, and dissociated manifestations of REM sleep, including cataplexy, hypnagogic hallucinations, and sleep paralysis. In ICSD-3, narcolepsy was classified into NT1 (with cataplexy or hypocretin deficiency) and NT2 (without cataplexy and hypocretin deficiency). NT1 is most commonly caused by the loss of hypocretin-producing cells in the hypothalamus, and detection of low CSF hypocretin-1 can be used to diagnose the condition. NT1 is associated with *HLA-DQB1*06:02*, and this tight association suggests that the cause of most of the NT1 cases may be autoimmune destruction of these cells. Whereas most NT1 cases are caused by hypocretin cell loss, some cases with cataplexy and most cases without cataplexy (NT2) have normal CSF hypocretin-1 levels. This may reflect either disease heterogeneity or a partial loss of hypocretin neurons without significant CSF hypocretin-1 decrements. The hypocretin system sends strong excitatory projections onto monoaminergic cells. Current treatments are symptomatically based and act downstream of the hypocretin abnormality. Presynaptic stimulation of dopaminergic transmission and adrenergic reuptake inhibition mediate the wake-promoting effect of stimulants and anticataplectic effects of antidepressants, respectively. Sodium oxybate, a sedative compound, may act via $GABA_B$ receptors or specific GHB receptors.

Autoimmune treatments for NT1 using immunosuppressants have been attempted but have had mixed results. In contrast, much progress has been made in hypocretin replacement therapies for NT1; findings in animal models suggest that hypocretin replacement therapy with small molecular nonpeptide hypocretin receptor agonists is a new, promising therapeutic option and may improve both EDS and cataplexy. If ligand replacement therapy is demonstrated to be effective for patients with NT1, hypocretin cell transplant or gene therapy technology may also be applicable in the future.

KEY CLINICAL POINTS

- Narcolepsy is a syndrome that is characterized by EDS, sleep fragmentation, cataplexy, and other REM sleep phenomena caused by hypocretin deficiency due to the destruction of the hypocretin-producing neurons in the hypothalamus, presumably by autoimmune mechanisms.

- In the third edition of the *International Classification of Sleep Disorders* (ICSD-3), narcolepsy is classified based on the pathophysiology of the disease as NT1 (with cataplexy or hypocretin deficiency) or NT2 (without cataplexy and hypocretin deficiency).

- A large majority of patients with narcolepsy receive benefits from current pharmacological treatments. Three main categories of drugs include stimulants for excessive daytime sleepiness, antidepressants for REM sleep–related symptoms, and sodium oxybate for both symptoms. However, these treatments are all symptomatic, and no curative treatments currently exist.

- Although clinical data are still lacking, hypocretin replacement therapy such as small molecule synthetic hypocretin receptor agonists may be efficient for both cataplexy and sleepiness.

- Immune-based treatments would presumably play a pivotal role in preventing autoimmune destruction, especially if given at an early stage of the disease, but more work is needed in this area.

References

Ahmed SS, Schur PH, MacDonald NE, et al: Narcolepsy, 2009 A(H1N1) pandemic influenza, and pandemic influenza vaccinations: what is known and unknown about the neurological disorder, the role for autoimmunity, and vaccine adjuvants. J Autoimmun 50:1–11, 2014 24559657

Aldrich MS: The clinical spectrum of narcolepsy and idiopathic hypersomnia. Neurology 46(2):393–401, 1996 8614501

Alshaikh MK, Tricco AC, Tashkandi M, et al: Sodium oxybate for narcolepsy with cataplexy: systematic review and meta-analysis. J Clin Sleep Med 8(4):451–458, 2012 22893778

Ambati A, Poiret T, Svahn BM, et al: Increased beta-haemolytic group A streptococcal M6 serotype and streptodornase B-specific cellular immune responses in Swedish narcolepsy cases. J Intern Med 278(3):264–276, 2015 25683265

American Academy of Sleep Medicine: International Classification of Sleep Disorders, 3rd Edition. Rochester, MN, American Sleep Disorders Association, 2014

American Narcolepsy Association: Stimulant medication survey. The Eye Opener, January 1992:1–3, 1992

Aran A, Lin L, Nevsimalova S, et al: Elevated anti-streptococcal antibodies in patients with recent narcolepsy onset. Sleep 32(8):979–983, 2009 19725248

Arand D, Bonnet M, Hurwitz T, et al: The clinical use of the MSLT and MWT. Sleep 28(1):123–144, 2005 15700728

Arias-Carrion O, Murillo-Rodriguez E: Effects of hypocretin/orexin cell transplantation on narcoleptic-like sleep behavior in rats. PLoS One 9(4):e95342, 2014 24736646

Babcock DA, Narver EL, Mitler MM, et al: Cataplexy in dogs II: effects of imipramine, clomipramine and fluoxetine on cataplexy in dogs. Sleep Res 5:154, 1976

Bassetti C, Aldrich MS: Idiopathic hypersomnia. A series of 42 patients. Brain 120(Pt 8):1423–1435, 1997 9278632

Black J, Houghton WC: Sodium oxybate improves excessive daytime sleepiness in narcolepsy. Sleep 29(7):939–946, 2006 16895262

Black JE, Brooks SN, Nishino S: Narcolepsy and syndromes of primary excessive daytime somnolence. Semin Neurol 24(3):271–282, 2004 15449220

Castelli MP, Ferraro L, Mocci I, et al: Selective gamma-hydroxybutyric acid receptor ligands increase extracellular glutamate in the hippocampus, but fail to activate G protein and to produce the sedative/hypnotic effect of gamma-hydroxybutyric acid. J Neurochem 87(3):722–732, 2003 14535954

Chemelli RM, Willie JT, Sinton CM, et al: Narcolepsy in orexin knockout mice: molecular genetics of sleep regulation. Cell 98(4):437–451, 1999 10481909

Chen W, Black J, Call P, Mignot E: Late-onset narcolepsy presenting as rapidly progressing muscle weakness: response to plasmapheresis. Ann Neurol 58(3):489–490, 2005 16130098

Dauvilliers Y, Montplaisir J, Molinari N, et al: Age at onset of narcolepsy in two large populations of patients in France and Quebec. Neurology 57(11):2029–2033, 2001 11739821

Dauvilliers Y, Arnulf I, Mignot E: Narcolepsy with cataplexy. Lancet 369(9560):499–511, 2007 17292770

Dauvilliers Y, Abril B, Mas E, et al: Normalization of hypocretin-1 in narcolepsy after intravenous immunoglobulin treatment. Neurology 73(16):1333–1334, 2009 19841387

Dauvilliers Y, Arnulf I, Lecendreux M, et al: Increased risk of narcolepsy in children and adults after pandemic H1N1 vaccination in France. Brain 136(pt 8):2486–2496, 2013 23884811

de Lecea L, Kilduff TS, Peyron C, et al: The hypocretins: hypothalamus-specific peptides with neuroexcitatory activity. Proc Natl Acad Sci USA 95(1):322–327, 1998 9419374

Deadwyler SA, Porrino L, Siegel JM, et al: Systemic and nasal delivery of orexin-A (hypocretin-1) reduces the effects of sleep deprivation on cognitive performance in nonhuman primates. J Neurosci 27(52):14239–14247, 2007 18160631

Donjacour CE, Lammers GJ: A remarkable effect of alemtuzumab in a patient suffering from narcolepsy with cataplexy. J Sleep Res 21(4):479–480, 2012 22142323

Duffy J, Weintraub E, Vellozzi C, et al: Narcolepsy and influenza A (H1N1) pandemic 2009 vaccination in the United States. Neurology 83(20):1823–1830, 2014 25320099

Frauscher B, Ehrmann L, Mitterling T, et al: Delayed diagnosis, range of severity, and multiple sleep comorbidities: a clinical and polysomnographic analysis of 100 patients of the Innsbruck narcolepsy cohort. J Clin Sleep Med 9(8):805–812, 2013 23946711

Han F, Lin L, Warby SC, et al: Narcolepsy onset is seasonal and increased following the 2009 H1N1 pandemic in China. Ann Neurol 70(3):410–417, 2011 21866560

Hecht M, Lin L, Kushida CA, et al: Report of a case of immunosuppression with prednisone in an 8-year-old boy with an acute onset of hypocretin-deficiency narcolepsy. Sleep 26(7):809–810, 2003 14655912

Irukayama-Tomobe Y, Ogawa Y, Tominaga H, et al: Nonpeptide orexin type-2 receptor agonist ameliorates narcolepsy-cataplexy symptoms in mouse models. Proc Natl Acad Sci USA 114(22):5731–5736, 2017 28507129

Johns MW: A new method for measuring daytime sleepiness: the Epworth Sleepiness Scale. Sleep 14(6):540–545, 1991 1798888

Kanbayashi T, Honda K, Kodama T, et al: Implication of dopaminergic mechanisms in the wake-promoting effects of amphetamine: a study of D- and L-derivatives in canine narcolepsy. Neuroscience 99(4):651–659, 2000 10974428

Kanbayashi T, Shimohata T, Nakashima I, et al: Symptomatic narcolepsy in patients with neuromyelitis optica and multiple sclerosis: new neurochemical and immunological implications. Arch Neurol 66(12):1563–1566, 2009 20008665

Knudsen S, Mikkelsen JD, Bang B, et al: Intravenous immunoglobulin treatment and screening for hypocretin neuron-specific autoantibodies in recent onset childhood narcolepsy with cataplexy. Neuropediatrics 41(5):217–222, 2010 21210337

Knudsen S, Biering-Sørensen B, Kornum BR, et al: Early IVIg treatment has no effect on post-H1N1 narcolepsy phenotype or hypocretin deficiency. Neurology 79(1):102–103, 2012 22722630

Koepsell TD, Longstreth WT, Ton TG: Medical exposures in youth and the frequency of narcolepsy with cataplexy: a population-based case-control study in genetically predisposed people. J Sleep Res 19(1 pt 1):80–86, 2010 19732319

Lammers GJ, Arends J, Declerck AC, et al: Gamma-hydroxybutyrate and narcolepsy: a double-blind placebo-controlled study. Sleep 16(3):216–220, 1993 8506453

Larrosa O, de la Llave Y, Bario S, et al: Stimulant and anticataplectic effects of reboxetine in patients with narcolepsy: a pilot study. Sleep 24(3):282–285, 2001 11322710

Lin L, Faraco J, Li R, et al: The sleep disorder canine narcolepsy is caused by a mutation in the hypocretin (orexin) receptor 2 gene. Cell 98(3):365–376, 1999 10458611

Liu M, Blanco-Centurion C, Konadhode RR, et al: Orexin gene transfer into the amygdala suppresses both spontaneous and emotion-induced cataplexy in orexin-knockout mice. Eur J Neurosci 43(5):681–688, 2016 26741960

Longstreth WT Jr, Koepsell TD, Ton TG, et al: The epidemiology of narcolepsy. Sleep 30(1):13–26, 2007 17310860

Luo G, Ambati A, Lin L, et al: Autoimmunity to hypocretin and molecular mimicry to flu in type 1 narcolepsy. Proc Natl Acad Sci USA 115(52):E12323–E12332, 2018 30541895

Mahlios J, De la Herrán-Arita AK, Mignot E: The autoimmune basis of narcolepsy. Curr Opin Neurobiol 23(5):767–773, 2013 23725858

Maitre M: The gamma-hydroxybutyrate signalling system in brain: organization and functional implications. Prog Neurobiol 51(3):337–361, 1997 9089792

Mamelak M, Black J, Montplaisir J, et al: A pilot study on the effects of sodium oxybate on sleep architecture and daytime alertness in narcolepsy. Sleep 27(7):1327–1334, 2004 15586785

Mieda M, Willie JT, Hara J, et al: Orexin peptides prevent cataplexy and improve wakefulness in an orexin neuron-ablated model of narcolepsy in mice. Proc Natl Acad Sci USA 101(13):4649–4654, 2004 15070772

Mignot E, Nishino S, Guilleminault C, et al: Modafinil binds to the dopamine uptake carrier site with low affinity. Sleep 17(5):436–437, 1994 7991954

Mignot E, Hayduk R, Black J, et al: HLA DQB1*0602 is associated with cataplexy in 509 narcoleptic patients. Sleep 20(11):1012–1020, 1997 9456467

Mitler MM: Evaluation of treatment with stimulants in narcolepsy. Sleep 17(8 suppl):S103–S106, 1994 7701190

Montplaisir J, Petit D, Quinn MJ, et al: Risk of narcolepsy associated with inactivated adjuvanted (AS03) A/H1N1 (2009) pandemic influenza vaccine in Quebec. PLoS One 9(9):e108489, 2014 25264897

Morgenthaler TI, Kapur VK, Brown T, et al: Practice parameters for the treatment of narcolepsy and other hypersomnias of central origin. Sleep 30(12):1705–1711, 2007 18246980

Mullington J, Broughton R: Scheduled naps in the management of daytime sleepiness in narcolepsy-cataplexy. Sleep 16(5):444–456, 1993 8378686

Nagahara T, Saitoh T, Kutsumura N, et al: Design and synthesis of non-peptide, selective orexin receptor 2 agonists. J Med Chem 58(20):7931–7937, 2015 26267383

Nepovimova E, Janockova J, Misik J, et al: Orexin supplementation in narcolepsy treatment: a review. Med Res Rev 39(3):961–975, 2019 30426515

Nishino S: Modes of action of drugs related to narcolepsy: pharmacology of wake-promoting compounds and anticataplectics, in Narcolepsy: A Clinical Guide. Edited by Goswami M, Pandi-Perumal SR, Thorpy MJ. New York, Springer, 2010, pp 267–286

Nishino S, Kanbayashi T: Symptomatic narcolepsy, cataplexy and hypersomnia, and their implications in the hypothalamic hypocretin/orexin system. Sleep Med Rev 9(4):269–310, 2005 16006155

Nishino S, Kotorii N: Overview of management of narcolepsy, in Narcolepsy: A Clinical Guide. Edited by Goswami M, Pandi-Perumal SR, Thorpy MJ. New York, Springer, 2010, pp 251–265

Nishino S, Mignot E: Pharmacological aspects of human and canine narcolepsy. Prog Neurobiol 52(1):27–78, 1997 9185233

Nishino S, Mignot E: Narcolepsy and cataplexy. Handb Clin Neurol 99:783–814, 2011a 21056228

Nishino S, Mignot E: Wake-promoting medications: basic mechanisms and pharmacology, in Principles and Practice of Sleep Medicine, 5th Edition. Edited by Kryger MH, Roth T, Dement WC. St. Louis, MO, Elsevier Saunders, 2011b, pp 510–526

Nishino S, Okuro M: Armodafinil for excessive daytime sleepiness. Drugs Today (Barc) 44(6):395–414, 2008 18596995

Nishino S, Mao J, Sampathkumaran R, et al: Adrenergic, but not dopaminergic, uptake inhibition reduces REM sleep and cataplexy concomitantly. Sleep Res 26:445, 1997

Nishino S, Mao J, Sampathkumaran R, et al: Increased dopaminergic transmission mediates the wake-promoting effects of CNS stimulants. Sleep Res 1(1):49–61, 1998 11382857

Nishino S, Ripley B, Overeem S, et al: Low cerebrospinal fluid hypocretin (orexin) and altered energy homeostasis in human narcolepsy. Ann Neurol 50(3):381–388, 2001 11558795

Nishino S, Okuro M, Kotorii N, et al: Hypocretin/orexin and narcolepsy: new basic and clinical insights. Acta Physiol (Oxf) 198(3):209–222, 2010 19555382

O'Flanagan D, Barret AS, Foley M, et al: Investigation of an association between onset of narcolepsy and vaccination with pandemic influenza vaccine, Ireland April 2009–December 2010. Euro Surveill 19(17):15–25, 2014 24821121

Overeem S, van Nues SJ, van der Zande WL, et al: The clinical features of cataplexy: a questionnaire study in narcolepsy patients with and without hypocretin-1 deficiency. Sleep Med 12(1):12–18, 2011 21145280

Partinen M, Saarenpää-Heikkilä O, Ilveskoski I, et al: Increased incidence and clinical picture of childhood narcolepsy following the 2009 H1N1 pandemic vaccination campaign in Finland. PLoS One 7(3):e33723, 2012 22470463

Peyron C, Faraco J, Rogers W, et al: A mutation in a case of early onset narcolepsy and a generalized absence of hypocretin peptides in human narcoleptic brains. Nat Med 6(9):991–997, 2000 10973318

Queva C, Bremner-Danielsen M, Edlund A, et al: Effects of GABA agonists on body temperature regulation in $GABA_{B(1)}^{-/-}$ mice. Br J Pharmacol 140(2):315–322, 2003 12970075

Raynal D: Polygraphic aspects of narcolepsy, in Narcolepsy. Edited by Guilemminault C, Passouant P, Dement W. New York, Spectrum, 1976, pp 669–684

Rocca FL, Pizza F, Ricci E, Plazzi G: Narcolepsy during childhood: an update. Neuropediatrics 46(3):181–198, 2015 25961600

Roehrs T, Zorick F, Wittig R, et al: Alerting effects of naps in patients with narcolepsy. Sleep 9(1 pt 2):194–199, 1986 3704442

Rogers AE: Problems and coping strategies identified by narcoleptic patients. J Neurosurg Nurs 16(6):326–334, 1984 6568258

Roth T, Dauvilliers Y, Mignot E, et al: Disrupted nighttime sleep in narcolepsy. J Clin Sleep Med 9(9):955–965, 2013 23997709

Rye DB, Bliwise DL, Parker K, et al: Modulation of vigilance in the primary hypersomnias by endogenous enhancement of $GABA_A$ receptors. Sci Transl Med 4(161):161ra151, 2012 23175709

Sakurai T, Amemiya A, Ishii M, et al: Orexins and orexin receptors: a family of hypothalamic neuropeptides and G protein-coupled receptors that regulate feeding behavior. Cell 92(4):573–585, 1998 9491897

Saper CB, Scammell TE, Lu J: Hypothalamic regulation of sleep and circadian rhythms. Nature 437(7063):1257–1263, 2005 16251950

Saper CB, Fuller PM, Pedersen NP, et al: Sleep state switching. Neuron 68(6):1023–1042, 2010 21172606

Sarkanen T, Alakuijala A, Julkunen I, et al: Narcolepsy associated with Pandemrix vaccine. Curr Neurol Neurosci Rep 18(7):43, 2018 29855798

Schneider L, Mignot E: Diagnosis and management of narcolepsy. Semin Neurol 37(4):446–460, 2017 28837992

Scrima L, Hartman PG, Johnson FH Jr, et al: Efficacy of gamma-hydroxybutyrate versus placebo in treating narcolepsy-cataplexy: double-blind subjective measures. Biol Psychiatry 26(4):331–343, 1989 2669980

Serra L, Montagna P, Mignot E, et al: Cataplexy features in childhood narcolepsy. Mov Disord 23(6):858–865, 2008 18307264

Sorensen GL, Knudsen S, Jennum P: Sleep transitions in hypocretin-deficient narcolepsy. Sleep (Basel) 36(8):1173–1177, 2013 23904677

Taddei RN, Werth E, Poryazova R, et al: Diagnostic delay in narcolepsy type 1: combining the patients' and the doctors' perspectives. J Sleep Res 25(6):709–715, 2016 27149919

Thorpy MJ, Goswami M: Treatment of narcolepsy, in Handbook of Sleep Disorders. Edited by Thorpy MJ. New York, Marcel Dekker, 1990 pp 235–258

Toyoda H, Miyagawa T, Koike A, et al: A polymorphism in CCR1/CCR3 is associated with narcolepsy. Brain Behav Immun 49:148–155, 2015 25986216

Trotti LM, Saini P, Bliwise DL, et al: Clarithromycin in gamma-aminobutyric acid–related hypersomnolence: a randomized, crossover trial. Ann Neurol 78(3):454–465, 2015 26094838

Valko PO, Khatami R, Baumann CR, et al: No persistent effect of intravenous immunoglobulins in patients with narcolepsy with cataplexy. J Neurol 255(12):1900–1903, 2008 18825431

Winstone AM, Stellitano L, Verity C, et al: Clinical features of narcolepsy in children vaccinated with AS03 adjuvanted pandemic A/H1N1 2009 influenza vaccine in England. Dev Med Child Neurol 56(11):1117–1123, 2014 25041214

Wise M, Arand D, Auger R, et al: Treatment of narcolepsy and other hypersomnia of central origin. Sleep 30(12):1712–1727, 2007 18246981

Wisor JP, Nishino S, Sora I, et al: Dopaminergic role in stimulant-induced wakefulness. J Neurosci 21(5):1787–1794, 2001 11222668

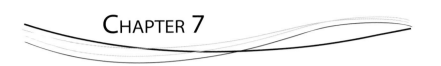

CHAPTER 7

Idiopathic Hypersomnia

Caroline Maness, M.D.

Lynn Marie Trotti, M.D., M.Sc.

Idiopathic hypersomnia (IH) is a chronic, potentially debilitating neurological condition that manifests as excessive sleepiness during waking hours and can be accompanied by pathologically prolonged sleep. The term *idiopathic hypersomnia* was first employed by Bedrich Roth in the 1970s (Roth 1976). In a large case series of his own patients, Roth described a subset who reported excessive daytime sleepiness (EDS) similar to that seen in narcolepsy but lacked the other prototypical features of narcolepsy. He described a monosymptomatic variant and a polysymptomatic variant of the disease: the monosymptomatic phenotype was characterized by EDS alone, whereas patients with the polysymptomatic form also reported abnormally long sleep durations and difficulties awakening (Roth 1976; Roth et al. 1972). Although Roth's lexicon is no longer used in describing the subtypes of IH, his early descriptions are echoed when a clinical and laboratory picture is built to support a diagnosis of IH.

Diagnostic Criteria

According to the third edition of the *International Classification of Sleep Disorders* (ICSD-3; American Academy of Sleep Medicine 2014), a diagnosis of IH should be considered in patients reporting at least 3 months of daily EDS as defined by "[an] irrepressible need to sleep or daytime lapses into sleep" without episodes of cataplexy (American Academy of Sleep Medicine 2014). Subsequent polysomnography/multiple sleep latency test (MSLT) should reveal no more than one sleep-onset REM period (SOREMP; REM within 15 minutes of sleep onset) on MSLT and the preceding night's polysomnogram combined. In addition, the mean sleep latency (MSL) on a daytime MSLT must be ≤8 minutes, or the pa-

TABLE 7–1. ICSD-3 diagnostic criteria for idiopathic hypersomnia

All criteria below must be met:

1. Patient must report daily episodes of an irrepressible need for sleep for ≥3 months.

2. Patient must not report cataplexy.

3. Patient must demonstrate fewer than two SOREMPs between MSLT and overnight polysomnography combined.

4. At least one of the following must be present:

    A. Mean sleep latency on MSLT must be ≤8 minutes.

    B. Patient must demonstrate ≥660 minutes of TST on either 24-hour polysomnography or on 7-day wrist actigraphy with ad-lib sleep (accompanied by a sleep log).

5. Insufficient sleep syndrome must be ruled out. If needed, wrist actigraphy can be performed to confirm patient is spending adequate time in bed.

6. Subjective and objective sleepiness must not be better attributable to other medical or psychiatric conditions or the use of drugs/medication.

Note.   ICSD-3=*International Classification of Sleep Disorders,* 3rd Edition; MSLT= multiple sleep latency test; SOREMP=sleep-onset REM period; TST=total sleep time.

Source.   American Academy of Sleep Medicine 2014.

tient must demonstrate a total sleep time (TST) ≥660 minutes on either extended 24-hour polysomnography or wrist actigraphy (American Academy of Sleep Medicine 2014). The full ICSD-3 diagnostic criteria are presented in Table 7–1.

Pathophysiology

As the term *idiopathic* implies, the precise pathophysiology of IH remains unclear. Given the various phenotypic presentations (Vernet and Arnulf 2009a), it is possible that the diagnosis captures a heterogeneous group of diseases. In contrast to patients with narcolepsy type 1 (NT1), levels of hypocretin in cerebrospinal fluid (CSF) are normal in patients with IH (Mignot et al. 2002). In addition, the *HLA-DQB1*06:02* genotype associated with NT1 is not thought to contribute to the development of IH, because the allele occurs with equal frequency in subjects with IH and in healthy control subjects (Vernet et al. 2010). Three studies have evaluated CSF histamine levels in patients with IH compared with control subjects; two found histamine to be decreased in the CSF of patients with IH, whereas the third showed no difference (Sowa 2016).

In vitro analysis of CSF reveals abnormal enhancement of $GABA_A$ receptor function by CSF in patients with IH compared with healthy control subjects (Rye et al. 2012). Furthermore, this abnormal enhancement is negated by the addition of GABA receptor antagonists in vitro, and improvements in vigilance parameters are observed in vivo when patients receive a $GABA_A$ antagonist intravenously (Rye et al. 2012). Taken together, these findings suggest that excessive endogenous activation of the GABAergic system may be responsible for the EDS and difficulty with sleep-wake transitions that are seen in some cases of IH. One subsequent study, however, was unable to reproduce this finding of excess $GABA_A$ receptor potentiation (Dauvilliers et al. 2016), although experimental techniques and study cohorts varied substantially between the two research centers.

It has also been hypothesized that IH is a disorder of patients' endogenous circadian rhythm, because recent studies have demonstrated a prolonged circadian period length in those with IH compared with control subjects (25.47 hours vs. 24.53 hours; $P<0.001$) (Materna et al. 2018). Given multiple hypothesized mechanisms at play, further research is imperative to clarify the causative pathology, or pathologies, in IH.

Epidemiology

PREVALENCE AND DEMOGRAPHIC CONSIDERATIONS

The exact prevalence of IH is unknown; estimates in the literature range from 0.002% to 0.010% (Sowa 2016). This may be an underestimation of the true prevalence of IH, because a population study indicates that 1.6% of the population sleeps >9 hours per night and has associated distress or impaired functioning due to excessive sleep (Ohayon et al. 2013).

Case series of patients with IH tend to be small, so information about sex predilection is limited; available data report a range from no sex difference to a female-to-male ratio of 1.8:1 (Bassetti and Aldrich 1997; Sowa 2016). Based on a systematic review, the mean age at onset is 21.9 years (interquartile range 19.9 [20.5–22.4]); however, diagnostic delays are common (Bassetti and Aldrich 1997; Sowa 2016).

RISK FACTORS

Case series have reported factors such as head trauma, viral illness, and general anesthesia to precede symptoms in some cases, but no definitive link has been confirmed (Billiard and Šonka 2016).

GENETICS

A culprit gene has not yet been identified in association with IH, although approximately one-third of patients report a positive family history of EDS or long sleep time (LST), suggesting a heritable component to the disease (Billiard and Šonka 2016). A recent genome-wide association study in a Japanese cohort of 408 patients with essential hypersomnia and 2,247 healthy control subjects revealed a single-nucleotide polymorphism (rs10988217) associated with essential hypersomnia (OR 2.63, $P=7.5 \times 10^{-9}$) (Miyagawa et al. 2018). The implication of this finding for patients captured by the ICSD-3 definition of IH is unclear, however, because the diagnosis "essential hypersomnia" includes patients with IH without long sleep time and those with narcolepsy without cataplexy (narcolepsy type 2 [NT2]).

Clinical Presentation

EDS that is not accompanied by cataplexy or other signs of REM dysregulation is the core diagnostic indicator of IH (American Academy of Sleep Medicine 2014). EDS may or may not be accompanied by abnormally long nighttime sleep durations, defined as >11 hours per night (American Academy of Sleep Medicine 2014). One subset of patients with IH even chiefly complains of prolonged nighttime sleep and is less bothered by daytime sleepiness (Vernet and Arnulf 2009a). LST is such a prominent feature of the disease that the prior iteration of the ICSD (American Academy of Sleep Medicine 2005) stipulated that diagnoses of IH be differentiated into IH with and without LST; however, this is no longer required based on ICSD-3 criteria (American Academy of Sleep Medicine 2014). Despite the change in nomenclature, the subtype of IH with LST must be taken into consideration when planning diagnostic testing, because MSL in these patients is significantly longer compared with those with IH without LST (9.6±0.7 minutes vs. 5.6±0.3 minutes), and most patients with IH with LST will not meet criteria for IH by MSLT (Vernet and Arnulf 2009a). In order to capture the LST variant, 24-hour polysomnography or 7-day actigraphy should be ordered, because patients with LST will generally demonstrate a significantly longer TST than those without (747±82 minutes vs. 635±82 minutes) (Vernet and Arnulf 2009a). Of note, in the United States, insurance will often not cover 24-hour polysomnography, so actigraphy may be the only option for diagnostic testing.

Unlike narcolepsy, patients with IH are also less likely to benefit from daytime napping and often experience great difficulty awakening from naps (Šonka et al. 2015; Trotti 2017; Vernet et al. 2010). Additionally, hypnagogic/hypnopompic hallucinations and sleep paralysis, which are considered part of the "narcolepsy tetrad," are only reported in about one-fourth of patients with IH (Vernet and Arnulf 2009a).

Severe sleep inertia, or "sleep drunkenness" (prolonged difficulty waking up with repeated returns to sleep, irritability, automatic behavior, and confusion), is reported in about 50% of patients with IH (Trotti 2017). This symptom supports a diagnosis of IH, although it is not required (American Academy of Sleep Medicine 2014). Some patients report sleep drunkenness to be the most disabling aspect of the disease, because they have difficulty awakening sufficiently to take wake-promoting agents.

In addition to EDS and sleep inertia, the symptom profile of IH often includes cognitive issues: patients with IH more commonly report memory problems, attention problems, and tendency to misplace objects than do healthy control subjects (79% vs. 43%, 55% vs. 18%, and 55% vs. 18%, respectively; $P < 0.01$ for all comparisons) (Vernet et al. 2010). Autonomic dysfunction also appears to be common in patients with IH, with as many as half of patients reporting orthostatic intolerance or Raynaud-like symptoms (Bassetti and Aldrich 1997).

The natural history of IH is heterogeneous, with spontaneous remission occurring in a minority of cases (reportedly 14%–33%) (Anderson et al. 2007; Bassetti and Aldrich 1997; Kim et al. 2016) and lifelong symptoms in others.

Diagnostic Testing

Diagnosing IH requires an adequate clinical history followed by polysomnography/MSLT to objectively document EDS. However, as mentioned, conventional polysomnography/MSLT may not be adequately sensitive to diagnose patients who have profound sleepiness but a normal MSL on MSLT. In these cases, 24-hour polysomnography or wrist actigraphy for ≥7 days, accompanied by a sleep log, is used to evaluate TST in a 24-hour period (≥660 minutes is diagnostic for IH) (American Academy of Sleep Medicine 2014). In certain situations, patients may have an MSL >8 minutes and a TST <660 minutes but otherwise have a clinical presentation consistent with IH. In these cases, clinical judgment can be used to decide if a diagnosis of IH is still appropriate, assuming other mimicking conditions have been excluded (American Academy of Sleep Medicine 2014).

Unlike NT1, serum genetic testing and CSF hypocretin testing will not aid in diagnosis. CSF studies conducted in vitro on patients with IH have shown that their CSF yields enhanced activity at $GABA_A$ receptors compared with control subjects (Rye et al. 2012); however, CSF testing is not part of the routine workup for IH.

Brain imaging via CT or MRI will not aid in confirming a diagnosis of IH but may be useful to rule out a causative brain lesion in a patient presenting with additional neurological signs or symptoms. For example, reports appear in the literature of patients developing EDS in conjunction with brain tumors or demyelinating disease, most often in the context of hypothalamic or thalamic lesions (Nishino and Kanbayashi 2005). However, in some of these cases, measurable CSF hypocretin is low, thus meeting criteria for NT1 as opposed to IH (Nishino and Kanbayashi 2005).

No patient questionnaires explicitly diagnose IH. The Epworth Sleepiness Scale is often used to assess degree of sleepiness in patients and treatment response in IH. One case series reported treatment-naive patients with IH to have an average Epworth Sleepiness Scale score of 16.3±3.3, which is similar to the average scores seen in narcolepsy.

Differential Diagnosis

Given that EDS is associated with various medical conditions, the differential diagnosis is broad when a patient presents to the clinic for sleepiness. A thorough history and polysomnogram can help greatly to rule out EDS caused by obstructive sleep apnea (see Chapters 8–11) or severe periodic leg movements (see Chapter 17). However, it can often be difficult, especially in patients with equivocal sleep studies and several comorbidities, to determine the primary pathology. Differential diagnostic considerations for EDS are detailed in the following sections.

NARCOLEPSY TYPE 1

NT1 is characterized by the "narcolepsy tetrad": EDS, cataplexy, sleep paralysis, and hypnagogic or hypnopompic hallucinations (see Chapter 6). Any reports of cataplexy suggest narcolepsy rather than IH. Sleep paralysis and sleep hallucinations, however, cannot be used clinically to differentiate the two disorders because they can occur in IH, albeit less frequently than in NT1 (Khan and Trotti 2015). Patients with NT1 tend to find short naps to be refreshing, whereas those with IH take long, unrefreshing naps (Šonka et al. 2015). In addition to disparate symptom profiles, polysomnography/MSLT distinguishes NT1 from IH: patients who have two or more SOREMPs on overnight polysomnography combined with the daytime MSLT and an MSL of ≤8 minutes should be di-

TABLE 7–2. Clinical features: idiopathic hypersomnia, narcolepsy type 1, and narcolepsy type 2

Clinical feature	Idiopathic hypersomnia	NT1	NT2
Excessive daytime sleepiness	+	+	+
Sleep paralysis	± (28%)[a]	± (40–58%)[b]	± (39%)[c]
Sleep hallucinations	± (24%)[a]	± (62%)[c]	± (44%)[c]
Cataplexy	—	+	—
Long sleep time	± (53%)[a]	± (18%)[d]	± (18%)[d]
Severe sleep inertia	Often present[b,e]	Rarely present[e]	May be present[f]
Cerebrospinal fluid hypocretin	Normal	<110 pg/mL	Normal
Nocturnal sleep disruption	Rarely present[e]	Often present[e]	May be present[e]
HLA-DQB1*06 positive	± (24%)[a]	+	± (15%)[c]

Note. NT1=narcolepsy type 1; NT2=narcolepsy type 2.
Source. Data from [a]Vernet and Arnulf 2009a; [b]Bassetti and Aldrich 1997; [c]Ruoff et al. 2018; [d]Vernet and Arnulf 2009b; [e]Šonka et al. 2015; [f]Bassetti et al. 2003.

agnosed with narcolepsy (American Academy of Sleep Medicine 2014). Sleep quality also helps differentiate the two, because patients with NT1 tend to have decreased sleep efficiency and trend toward more fragmented sleep compared with those with IH (Leu-Semenescu et al. 2016). See Table 7–2 for a comparison of features among IH, NT1, and NT2.

NARCOLEPSY TYPE 2

Unlike NT1 and IH, NT2 and IH can be difficult to distinguish based on clinical phenotype (see Chapter 6). Both IH and NT2 lack cataplexy. Presence or absence of sleep paralysis and sleep hallucinations is also less helpful in distinguishing NT2 from IH because both are present in similar frequencies in the two diseases (sleep paralysis: NT2 35% vs. IH 20%; sleep hallucinations: NT2 42% vs. IH 25%) (Khan and Trotti 2015). LST and sleep drunkenness, although classically described features of IH, can also be seen in NT2 (Vernet and Arnulf 2009b). The distinction currently relies solely on number of SOREMPS on MSLT (two or more SOREMPs indicates NT2). However, many variables affect REM sleep, and up to 4% of the general population has an MSLT result fulfilling criteria for narcolepsy. In addition, the low test-retest reliability of the MSLT further obscures the boundary between IH and NT2 (Ruoff et al. 2018; Trotti et al. 2013).

INSUFFICIENT SLEEP SYNDROME VERSUS IDIOPATHIC HYPERSOMNIA

Prolonged insufficient sleep durations can result in EDS similar to that reported in IH, and MSLT can even show short sleep latencies as a result. In these situations, a thorough clinical history is imperative to characterize actual time in bed. In select cases, sleep logs and actigraphy may be needed to rule out this possibility. If these data indicate insufficient sleep, the patient should be advised to change his or her sleep schedule to allow for at least 8 hours of sleep each night and be reassessed for EDS after several weeks of adequate sleep time.

KLEINE-LEVIN SYNDROME VERSUS IDIOPATHIC HYPERSOMNIA

Kleine-Levin syndrome (KLS) is a rare disorder of recurrent episodic hypersomnia that often presents during adolescence. The first episode of hypersomnia is often sudden, and patients will sleep as much as 18 hours per day (Arnulf et al. 2005). This severe sleepiness is accompanied by cognitive, behavioral, or psychological issues during waking hours. Episodes last between 2 days and 5 weeks and occur at least every 18 months (American Academy of Sleep Medicine 2014). The main differentiating factor between KLS and IH is the episodic nature of KLS. Patients with KLS should have reasonably normal sleep duration, alertness, and cognition between episodes, whereas patients with IH report unremitting hypersomnia.

HYPERSOMNIA ASSOCIATED WITH A PSYCHIATRIC DISORDER

Hypersomnolence may be present in up to 75% of young adults with major depressive disorder and was integral to the DSM-IV diagnosis of atypical depression (American Psychiatric Association 1994; Kaplan and Harvey 2009; Parker et al. 2006). To further muddy the clinical picture, patients known to have IH tend to report higher levels of anxiety and depression compared with healthy control subjects (Vernet et al. 2010). Diagnostic testing may not be as helpful as once thought in differentiating IH from hypersomnolence related to depression, because a recent study demonstrated that patients with hypersomnolence and co-occurring depression do not exhibit a reduced sleep efficiency as suggested by ICSD-3 (Plante et al. 2017). ICSD-3 explicitly avoids assigning causality in the diagnosis of hypersomnia *associated with* a mood disorder by choosing this wording over hypersomnia *due to* a mood disorder—acknowledging that cause and effect in this case are difficult to assign (American Academy of Sleep Medicine 2014). It is ultimately up to the acumen of the treating physician to parse out whether a patient's hypersomnolence is due primarily to a psychiatric disorder or if the patient simply has IH along with a comorbid mood disturbance.

HYPERSOMNIA DUE TO A MEDICAL DISORDER

Excessive sleepiness is known to accompany several medical and neurological conditions. For example, many patients with Parkinson's disease, dementia with Lewy bodies, or myotonic dystrophy report EDS (Chahine et al. 2017; Laberge et al. 2013). In these cases, timing of symptom onset is key; hypersomnolence presenting after a diagnosis of Parkinson's disease or myotonic dystrophy suggests secondary hypersomnia, but if hypersomnolence is the initial symptom, an appropriate etiological workup should be conducted with the emergence of any subsequent neurological symptoms.

EDS has also been associated with other medical conditions and metabolic derangements, such as hypothyroidism, genetic disorders, or infectious/postinfectious syndrome (Sowa 2016). As part of a workup for IH, patients should undergo basic laboratory testing to rule out anemia, iron deficiency, thyroid disorders, and vitamin B_{12} deficiency.

Iatrogenic causes of EDS should also be taken into consideration when evaluating a patient for potential IH. Many antidepressants and anticonvulsants can have sedating effects. Patients' medication lists should also be reviewed for antihistamines, antipsychotics, opiates, and antihypertensives that could be contributing to sleepiness.

Treatment

At this time, no disease-modifying or curative therapies are available for idiopathic hypersomnia. Available treatments are aimed at symptom reduction and often are needed indefinitely, except in rare cases of spontaneous remission. Unfortunately, even with treatment, patients with IH report poorer quality of life compared with the general population (Ozaki et al. 2012).

Regardless of primary pathology, depressive symptoms should be addressed with pharmacological and nonpharmacological options because they may contribute to burden of disease (Barateau et al. 2017; Neikrug et al. 2017).

BEHAVIORAL MODIFICATIONS

Up to 96.1% of patients with IH report using nonpharmacological strategies to manage symptoms; however, survey data have shown that patients with IH do not respond as favorably to behavioral modifications as do patients with narcolepsy (Neikrug et al. 2017). Although patients with narcolepsy find daytime napping somewhat effective in managing symptoms of their disease (scored by patients as 5 out of 10, where 0 represented "not at all effective" and 10 indicated "most effective"), patients with IH report practically no benefit from daytime napping, ranking it, on average, at 2.7 of out 10 (Neikrug et al. 2017). Other strategies employed by patients include scheduled nighttime sleep, exercise, use of caffeine, use of nicotine, and temperature manipulations. Among all methods, caffeine use was thought to be the most helpful, ranking 3.3 out of 10 in effectiveness (Neikrug et al. 2017). Caffeine gum may also be helpful in combatting the sleep inertia that often accompanies IH; a small study of healthy control subjects indicated that chewing caffeine gum shortly after awakening improved performance on a psychomotor vigilance task (Newman et al. 2013).

No studies explicitly speak to the role of dietary modifications in IH. One small study in patients with narcolepsy showed that a low-carbohydrate, ketogenic diet improved symptoms of sleepiness (Husain et al. 2004), but one must use caution in extrapolating this information to IH, given the different pathophysiologies.

Safety counseling is an important component of nonpharmacological management. Patients with IH, both treated and treatment naïve, have an increased risk of car accidents (OR 2.04, 95% CI 1.05–3.95, $P=0.002$) (Pizza et al. 2015). As such, patients should be reminded to avoid driving or operating heavy machinery while drowsy. Unfortunately, subjective sleepiness as rated by the Epworth Sleepiness Scale has not been shown to be a helpful indicator to assess risk of motor vehicle accident (Pizza et al. 2015). The maintenance of wakefulness test (MWT), however, has shown promise in assessing driving safety, because pathologically short sleep latencies predicted lapses in alertness during a driving simulation (Philip et al. 2013).

WAKE-PROMOTING AGENTS AND CNS STIMULANTS

To date, no medications are FDA approved for the treatment of IH. Few randomized controlled trials (RCTs) have assessed the efficacy of various therapies in IH, so most of the data come from small retrospective chart reviews and observational studies. As a result, many medications approved for the treatment of EDS in narcolepsy are used off-label for the treatment of IH. Although released prior to publication of the current existing RCTs, the 2007 practice parameters from the American Academy of Sleep Medicine recommended considering modafinil, methylphenidate, amphetamine, methamphetamine, or dextroamphetamine for the treatment of EDS in IH (Morgenthaler et al. 2007).

Modafinil

Modafinil is a nonstimulant wake-promoting agent that is considered standard therapy in narcolepsy and used off-label in IH. Its full mechanism of action is unclear, but it is known to increase extracellular dopamine concentration by inhibiting its presynaptic reuptake transporter. The two RCTs studying the use of modafinil in IH used 200 mg or 400 mg in two doses around 8 A.M. and 12 P.M. (Mayer et al. 2015; Philip et al. 2014). Patients are often initiated on modafinil 100 mg daily in two divided doses and then titrated up to 400 mg total daily. Armodafinil is the longer-acting R enantiomer of modafinil, which is a racemic compound. No studies have explicitly investigated the use of armodafinil in IH, but it is often used, because presumably it would have similar efficacy to modafinil. Armodafinil can be given as a 150-mg or 250-mg dose in the morning (Saini and Rye 2017).

The first RCT to specifically assess treatment outcomes in IH was a 2014 crossover trial looking at the effect of modafinil versus placebo on driving safety and MWT in patients with IH and narcolepsy (Philip et al. 2014). Patients treated with modafinil had significantly increased mean sleep latencies on MWT and fewer lapses of alertness during driving simulations compared with those receiving placebo. A subsequent RCT of 31 patients demonstrated a 6-point decrease (95% CI 2.92–7.67) in Epworth Sleepiness Scale score in patients treated with modafinil compared with a 1.5-point decrease (95% CI 0.089–3.80) in patients in the placebo arm (Mayer et al. 2015). Modafinil has been the most commonly used first-line drug for IH since its introduction to the marketplace in 1998 (Ali et al. 2009).

Modafinil is often preferred for first-line use over stimulants due to its lower abuse potential and milder side effect profile. Side effects of modafinil include headache, nausea, and anxiety, which often remit with continued use (Ali et al. 2009). Although not a side effect per se, one retrospective review indicated the most common reason for discontinuation of modafinil was the high cost of the medication (Ali et al. 2009). Also of note, modafinil decreases the efficacy of oral contraceptives, which must be taken into consideration in women of childbearing age.

Methylphenidate

Methylphenidate is a stimulant medication also commonly used in IH. It principally works by blocking the reuptake of both dopamine and norepinephrine. Although no RCTs are available to support its use, it is often used as second-line therapy in IH. A retrospective review indicated the average daily dosage of methylphenidate in IH patients is 50.6 mg (±27.3) divided into three or four doses (Ali et al. 2009).

Methylphenidate can be an effective monotherapy for IH and possibly more effective than modafinil, because a recent retrospective study showed more patients chose to continue this agent as monotherapy compared with modafinil (51% vs. 32%) (Ali et al. 2009). Dosing of methylphenidate is often limited by side effects, which include restlessness, palpitations, and insomnia (Ali et al. 2009). Taken together, stimulant medications put patients at increased risk for psychosis, polysubstance abuse (including stimulant abuse), weight loss, and tachyarrhythmias, especially at higher doses (Auger et al. 2005). Patients should be monitored for weight loss, hypertension, emergent anxiety/psychosis, and new arrhythmias while taking stimulants.

Dextroamphetamine, Methamphetamine, Amphetamine/Dextroamphetamine

Dextroamphetamine, methamphetamine, and amphetamine/dextroamphetamine preparations are occasionally used in the treatment of IH, although no RCTs have tested the efficacy of their use. These drugs exert their CNS effects via three mechanisms: increasing synaptic release of dopamine and norepinephrine, inhibiting dopamine and norepinephrine reuptake, and inhibiting monoamine oxidase. Although these are more potent stimulants than methylphenidate, they are used with caution given their serious side effect profile.

Bupropion

Bupropion is an antidepressant that works by inhibiting synaptic reuptake of norepinephrine and dopamine. No studies have specifically evaluated its use in IH, but in a pooled analysis of six RCTs comparing bupropion and selective serotonin reuptake inhibitors (SSRIs) in patients with depression and excessive sleepiness, patients who achieved symptomatic remission from depression with bupropion were less likely to have residual sleepiness than those treated with SSRIs (Cooper et al. 2014). These results suggest bupropion may have a role in the treatment of patients with hypersomnia and concomitant mood disorders. Solriamfetol is another dopamine and norepinephrine reuptake inhibitor approved by the FDA for the treatment of EDS in narcolepsy. This agent could potentially benefit patients with IH.

EMERGING THERAPIES

Many patients with IH respond to traditional wake-promoting agents, with as many as 65% achieving complete response and another 26% achieving a partial response (Ali et al. 2009). However, a subset of patients do not exhibit an adequate response despite multiple traditional agents or are unable to tolerate these therapies due to side effects. In these cases, novel or repurposed alternate therapies are needed to control symptoms.

Pitolisant

Pitolisant is a new histaminergic wake-promoting agent recently approved in the United States for the treatment of narcolepsy. Pitolisant is an inverse agonist of the histamine H_3 receptor and works by increasing histamine release in the cortex and hypothalamus (Leu-Semenescu et al. 2014). It is dosed once daily in the morning, with dose ranges of 5–50 mg. In a retrospective chart review on the efficacy of pitolisant for IH, the average maximum daily dosage achieved was 40 mg/day (Leu-Semenescu et al. 2014). This review also reported a mean 1.9-point decrease (±2.6) in Epworth Sleepiness Scale score compared with pretreatment baseline in patients treated with pitolisant. The most common side effects of treatment seem to be abdominal pain, increased appetite, and headache. The only side effects severe enough to cause patients to stop taking the drug despite clear benefit were rare cases of major anxiety, severe depression, and nightmares. No addiction or abuse was observed.

Sodium Oxybate

Sodium oxybate is a medication that has been used in the treatment of EDS and cataplexy associated with narcolepsy for more than a decade. It is dosed twice nightly and increases slow-wave sleep (Leu-Semenescu et al. 2016). A recent retrospective chart review evaluated the efficacy of sodium oxybate in IH and found that it reduced EDS to the same extent in patients with IH as in those with narcolepsy (decline in Epworth score of >3 points compared with pretreatment status) and also decreased sleep inertia in 71% of patients with IH (Leu-Semenescu et al. 2016). However, its side effect profile is limiting; patients with IH given sodium oxybate experienced more severe nausea, headache, and dizziness than did patients with narcolepsy who received it (Leu-Semenescu et al. 2016). Sodium oxybate also must be prescribed with caution, must be stored in a secure location, and may not be mixed with alcohol or other sedatives. The medication carries a black box warning due to concern for misuse/abuse, obtundation, and severe respiratory depression, especially when used in combination with other CNS depressants. Providers must also be cognizant of the risk of emergent depression and suicidality in patients taking sodium oxybate. All prescribers and patients receiving sodium oxybate must enroll in a risk evaluation and mitigation strategy program to ensure safe prescribing practices.

GABA$_A$ Receptor Antagonists

Extrapolating from the discovery that the CSF of patients with EDS yielded unexpected excess activation at the GABA$_A$ receptor (Rye et al. 2012), medications known to act as negative allosteric GABA$_A$ receptor modulators have been trialed in these patients to combat sleepiness. One such modulator is the antibiotic clarithromycin, which has been shown in a randomized crossover trial to significantly reduce subjective sleepiness (Trotti et al. 2015). Flumazenil is another GABA$_A$ receptor modulator that may have therapeutic potential. In vitro studies of the CSF of patients with IH have shown that the increased potentiation at GABA$_A$ receptors is reversed with the addition of flumazenil (Rye et al. 2012). A subsequent large, retrospective chart review indicated that either transdermal or sublingually dosed flumazenil yielded symptomatic benefit in a majority of patients who had previously been considered to have treatment-refractory IH (Trotti et al. 2016). Unfortunately, flumazenil administration is complicated due to issues of drug delivery. Given extensive hepatic first-pass metabolism, oral dosing is not feasible, and thus the drug must be compounded for long-term use as either a sublingual lozenge or transcutaneous cream (Trotti et al. 2016). Patients and physicians must also exercise caution with extended flumazenil use because it has historically only been used short term for the reversal of anesthesia, and its long-term sequelae are unknown. Intravenous flumazenil carries a known risk of seizures; however, this risk is thought to be greatest in patients with long-term use of benzodiazepines (Trotti et al. 2016). No seizures were reported in the cohort of patients with IH who were trialed on compounded preparations of the medication (Trotti et al. 2016).

Conclusion

IH is a potentially debilitating, often lifelong disease characterized by EDS, prolonged nighttime sleep, and often-profound difficulties awakening. Much is still unknown about the pathophysiology of the disease, but given the diverse phenotypes, it is likely that multiple culprit etiologies are being captured in the diagnosis. In lieu of clear pathophysiology, the mainstay of current treatment involves wake-promoting medications, which often do not adequately control symptoms. Future avenues of research should focus on clarifying the pathophysiological mechanism(s) at play so that more targeted and effective therapies can be developed.

KEY CLINICAL POINTS

- Idiopathic hypersomnia (IH) is thought to be rare based on limited available prevalence data, although symptoms of excessive sleepiness and long sleep durations are not uncommon in population studies.

- The pathophysiology of IH is unknown, although some emerging cerebrospinal fluid studies suggest pathology of the histaminergic, GABAergic, or prolonged circadian rhythm.

- Diagnosis of IH requires evaluation by a sleep physician, overnight polysomnography, and either 24-hour polysomnography, multiple sleep latency testing, or wrist actigraphy.

- To diagnose IH, excessive sleepiness caused by insufficient sleep syndrome, medical conditions, and psychiatric conditions must be excluded. Other conditions of excessive sleepiness, such as narcolepsy and Kleine-Levin syndrome, must also be considered.

- Modafinil is generally used as first-line treatment in IH based on two randomized controlled trials demonstrating its efficacy. Stimulant medications may also be used in IH, although data supporting their use are limited.

- Pitolisant, a histaminergic drug, has been shown in a retrospective chart review to be effective in combating sleepiness in IH, although it is not yet approved for use in the United States.

- $GABA_A$ receptor modulators flumazenil and clarithromycin have shown promise in alleviating sleepiness in patients with poor response to traditional wake-promoting agents.

References

Ali M, Auger RR, Slocumb NL, et al: Idiopathic hypersomnia: clinical features and response to treatment. J Clin Sleep Med 5(6):562–568, 2009 20465024

American Academy of Sleep Medicine: International Classification of Sleep Disorders, 2nd Edition. Darien, IL, American Academy of Sleep Medicine, 2005

American Academy of Sleep Medicine: International Classification of Sleep Disorders, 3rd Edition. Darien, IL, American Academy of Sleep Medicine, 2014

American Psychiatric Association: Diagnostic and Statistical Manual of Mental Disorders, 4th Edition. Washington, DC, American Psychiatric Association, 1994

Anderson KN, Pilsworth S, Sharples LD, et al: Idiopathic hypersomnia: a study of 77 cases. Sleep 30(10):1274–1281, 2007 17969461

Arnulf I, Zeitzer JM, File J, et al: Kleine-Levin syndrome: a systematic review of 186 cases in the literature. Brain 128(12):2763–2776, 2005 16230322

Auger RR, Goodman SH, Silber MH, et al: Risks of high-dose stimulants in the treatment of disorders of excessive somnolence: a case-control study. Sleep 28(6):667–672, 2005 16477952

Barateau L, Lopez R, Franchi JA, et al: Hypersomnolence, hypersomnia, and mood disorders. Curr Psychiatry Rep 19(2):13, 2017 28243864

Bassetti C, Aldrich MS: Idiopathic hypersomnia. A series of 42 patients. Brain 120(8):1423–1435, 1997 9278632

Bassetti C, Gugger M, Bischof M, et al: The narcoleptic borderland: a multimodal diagnostic approach including cerebrospinal fluid levels of hypocretin-1 (orexin A). Sleep Med 4(1):7–12, 2003

Billiard M, Šonka K: Idiopathic hypersomnia. Sleep Med Rev 29(Oct):23–33, 2016 26599679

Chahine LM, Amara AW, Videnovic A: A systematic review of the literature on disorders of sleep and wakefulness in Parkinson's disease from 2005 to 2015. Sleep Med Rev 35(Oct):33–50, 2017 27863901

Cooper JA, Tucker VL, Papakostas GI: Resolution of sleepiness and fatigue: a comparison of bupropion and selective serotonin reuptake inhibitors in subjects with major depressive disorder achieving remission at doses approved in the European Union. J Psychopharmacol 28(2):118–124, 2014 24352716

Dauvilliers Y, Evangelista E, Lopez R, et al: Absence of gamma-aminobutyric acid—a receptor potentiation in central hypersomnolence disorders. Ann Neurol 80(2):259–268, 2016 27315195

Husain AM, Yancy WS Jr, Carwile ST, et al: Diet therapy for narcolepsy. Neurology 62(12):2300–2302, 2004 15210901

Kaplan KA, Harvey AG: Hypersomnia across mood disorders: a review and synthesis. Sleep Med Rev 13(4):275–285, 2009 19269201

Khan Z, Trotti LM: Central disorders of hypersomnolence: focus on the narcolepsies and idiopathic hypersomnia. Chest 148(1):262–273, 2015 26149554

Kim T, Lee JH, Lee CS, et al: Different fates of excessive daytime sleepiness: survival analysis for remission. Acta Neurol Scand 134(1):35–41, 2016 26392230

Laberge L, Gagnon C, Dauvilliers Y: Daytime sleepiness and myotonic dystrophy. Curr Neurol Neurosci Rep 13(4):340, 2013 23430686

Leu-Semenescu S, Nittur N, Golmard J-L, et al: Effects of pitolisant, a histamine H3 inverse agonist, in drug-resistant idiopathic and symptomatic hypersomnia: a chart review. Sleep Med 15(6):681–687, 2014 24854887

Leu-Semenescu S, Louis P, Arnulf I: Benefits and risk of sodium oxybate in idiopathic hypersomnia versus narcolepsy type 1: a chart review. Sleep Med 17(suppl C):38–44, 2016 26847972

Materna L, Halfter H, Heidbreder A, et al: Idiopathic hypersomnia patients revealed longer circadian period length in peripheral skin fibroblasts. Front Neurol 9:424, 2018 29930532

Mayer G, Benes H, Young P, et al: Modafinil in the treatment of idiopathic hypersomnia without long sleep time—a randomized, double-blind, placebo-controlled study. J Sleep Res 24(1):74–81, 2015 25196321

Mignot E, Lammers GJ, Ripley B, et al: The role of cerebrospinal fluid hypocretin measurement in the diagnosis of narcolepsy and other hypersomnias. Arch Neurol 59(10):1553–1562, 2002 12374492

Miyagawa T, Khor S-S, Toyoda H, et al: A variant at 9q34.11 is associated with *HLA-DQB1*06:02* negative essential hypersomnia. J Hum Genet 63(12):1259–1267, 2018 30266950

Morgenthaler TI, Kapur VK, Brown T, et al: Practice parameters for the treatment of narcolepsy and other hypersomnias of central origin. Sleep 30(12):1705–1711, 2007 18246980

Neikrug AB, Crawford MR, Ong JC: Behavioral sleep medicine services for hypersomnia disorders: a survey study. Behav Sleep Med 15(2):158–171, 2017 26788889

Newman RA, Kamimori GH, Wesensten NJ, et al: Caffeine gum minimizes sleep inertia. Percept Mot Skills 116(1):280–293, 2013 23829154

Nishino S, Kanbayashi T: Symptomatic narcolepsy, cataplexy and hypersomnia, and their implications in the hypothalamic hypocretin/orexin system. Sleep Med Rev 9(4):269–310, 2005 16006155

Ohayon MM, Reynolds CF III, Dauvilliers Y: Excessive sleep duration and quality of life. Ann Neurol 73(6):785–794, 2013 23846792

Ozaki A, Inoue Y, Hayashida K, et al: Quality of life in patients with narcolepsy with cataplexy, narcolepsy without cataplexy, and idiopathic hypersomnia without long sleep time: comparison between patients on psychostimulants, drug-naïve patients and the general Japanese population. Sleep Med 13(2):200–206, 2012 22137109

Parker G, Malhi G, Hadzi-Pavlovic D, et al: Sleeping in? The impact of age and depressive sub-type on hypersomnia. J Affect Disord 90(1):73–76, 2006 16325918

Philip P, Chaufton C, Taillard J, et al: Maintenance of wakefulness test scores and driving performance in sleep disorder patients and controls. Int J Psychophysiol 89(2):195–202, 2013 23727627

Philip P, Chaufton C, Taillard J, et al: Modafinil improves real driving performance in patients with hypersomnia: a randomized double-blind placebo-controlled crossover clinical trial. Sleep (Basel) 37(3):483–487, 2014 24587570

Pizza F, Jaussent I, Lopez R, et al: Car crashes and central disorders of hypersomnolence: a French study. PLoS One 10(6):e0129386, 2015 26052938

Plante DT, Cook JD, Goldstein MR: Objective measures of sleep duration and continuity in major depressive disorder with comorbid hypersomnolence: a primary investigation with contiguous systematic review and meta-analysis. J Sleep Res 26(3):255–265, 2017 28145043

Roth B: Narcolepsy and hypersomnia: review and classification of 642 personally observed cases. Neurochirurgie Psychiatrie 119(1):31–41, 1976

Roth B, Nevsimalova S, Rechtschaffen A: Hypersomnia with "sleep drunkenness." Arch Gen Psychiatry 26(5):456–462, 1972 5019884

Ruoff C, Pizza F, Trotti LM, et al: The MSLT is repeatable in narcolepsy type 1 but not narcolepsy type 2: a retrospective patient study. J Clin Sleep Med 14(1):65–74, 2018 29198301

Rye DB, Bliwise DL, Parker K, et al: Modulation of vigilance in the primary hypersomnias by endogenous enhancement of GABAA receptors. Sci Transl Med 4(161):161ra151, 2012 23175709

Saini P, Rye DB: Hypersomnia: evaluation, treatment, and social and economic aspects. Sleep Med Clin 12(1):47–60, 2017 28159097

Šonka K, Šusta M, Billiard M: Narcolepsy with and without cataplexy, idiopathic hypersomnia with and without long sleep time: a cluster analysis. Sleep Med 16(2):225–231, 2015 25576137

Sowa NA: Idiopathic hypersomnia and hypersomnolence disorder: a systematic review of the literature. Psychosomatics 57(2):152–164, 2016 26895727

Trotti LM: Waking up is the hardest thing I do all day: sleep inertia and sleep drunkenness. Sleep Med Rev 35(October):76–84, 2017 27692973

Trotti LM, Staab BA, Rye DB: Test-retest reliability of the multiple sleep latency test in narcolepsy without cataplexy and idiopathic hypersomnia. J Clin Sleep Med 9(8):789–795, 2013 23946709

Trotti LM, Saini P, Bliwise DL, et al: Clarithromycin in γ-aminobutyric acid-related hypersomnolence: a randomized, crossover trial. Ann Neurol 78(3):454–465, 2015 26094838

Trotti LM, Saini P, Koola C, et al: Flumazenil for the treatment of refractory hypersomnolence: clinical experience with 153 patients. J Clin Sleep Med 12(10):1389–1394, 2016 27568889

Vernet C, Arnulf I: Idiopathic hypersomnia with and without long sleep time: a controlled series of 75 patients. Sleep 32(6):753–759, 2009a 19544751

Vernet C, Arnulf I: Narcolepsy with long sleep time: a specific entity? Sleep 32(9):1229–1235, 2009b 19750928

Vernet C, Leu-Semenescu S, Buzare M-A, et al: Subjective symptoms in idiopathic hypersomnia: beyond excessive sleepiness. J Sleep Res 19(4):525–534, 2010 20408941

CHAPTER 8

Adult Obstructive Sleep Apnea

Chester Wu, M.D.

Christian Guilleminault, M.D.

Initially described in 1976 (Guilleminault et al. 1976), obstructive sleep apnea (OSA) is the repetitive narrowing and collapse of the pharyngeal airway during sleep. OSA results in decreased airflow (hypopneas) or cessation of airflow (apneas), and subsequent sleep disruption (arousals) and disturbances in gas exchange (hypoxemia and hypercapnia). The following chapter reviews the epidemiology, pathophysiology, risk factors for, presentation of, and diagnosis and treatment of OSA.

Definition

The current definition of OSA requires the combination of at least 5 partial (hypopneas) or complete (apneas) obstructive breathing events per hour of sleep with the presence of signs or symptoms of impaired breathing, sleep disruption, or medical complications, or the presence of at least 15 breathing events per hour regardless of associated consequences. This measurement of average number of breathing events per hour is called the apnea-hypopnea index (AHI) and is the most widely used metric to assess OSA severity. The severity of OSA ranges from mild (AHI of 5–15 events per hour) to moderate and severe (AHI of 15–30 and >30 events per hour, respectively).

The Concept of the Apnea-Hypopnea Index

The AHI is a metric intended to measure and communicate in a shared language the severity of sleep-disordered breathing, including OSA. The AHI includes breathing events that are associated with either oxygen desaturation (hypoxia) or sleep fragmentation (number of cortical arousals). The respective importance of these two consequences of obstructive breathing events continues to be a matter of debate. Depending on the setting, such as different health care payers or diagnostic procedures (home sleep apnea testing vs. in-lab polysomnogram that includes electroencephalography), the AHI may not include breathing events causing cortical arousals or O_2 desaturation events not reaching a 4% decrement in O_2 saturation. Furthermore, the AHI may vary from night to night as affected by sleep stages achieved or body position. Therefore, the notion of the "AHI" should not be understood as an absolute marker of disease severity.

Extending the definition of OSA beyond the limitations of the AHI, other physiological aspects such as autonomic activation (subcortical) and electroencephalographic (cortical) instability (cyclic alternating patterns) have been shown to be associated with subtle obstructive breathing events. The concept of upper airway resistance syndrome was created to describe the phenomenon of these subtle breathing events that still result in daytime symptoms in the absence of hypoxia (Guilleminault and Khramtsov 2001; Guilleminault et al. 1993; Lopes and Guilleminault 2006). On the other end of the spectrum, the importance of hypoxia may not be limited to the number of oxygen desaturations (oxygen desaturation index) but also include their severity (lowest oxygen saturation reached) and duration (time spent during sleep below a 90% or 88% oxygen saturation cutoff). These aspects continue to be a matter of active research and suggest that OSA should be seen as a spectrum of disease with multiple dimensions and various presentations that evolve with age and disease progression.

Epidemiology

OSA is the most prevalent sleep breathing disorder. Originally thought to affect 1%–5% of the population, more recent studies have suggested much higher prevalence rates as awareness of sleep-disordered breathing has grown, the rate of obesity has increased, the recommended techniques to monitor breathing events have changed, and criteria for OSA have been redefined.

It is estimated that 33.9% of men and 17.4% of women between the ages of 30 and 70 years meet mild OSA criteria, with an AHI cutoff of >5 events per hour and hypopneas associated with a 4% oxygen desaturation (Peppard et al. 2013). However, the proportion of patients who also have excessive daytime sleepiness (EDS), indicated by an Epworth Sleepiness Scale score >10, is lower, decreasing the prevalence to 14.3% and 5.0% in men and women, respectively. A more recent study that used the 2012 American Academy of Sleep Medicine (AASM) definition for hypopneas (30% decrease in nasal pressure flow associated with either a 3-second electroencephalographic activity change or a 3% oxygen desaturation) in a sample of the Swiss population ages 40–85 years found that 83.8% of men and 60.8% of women have an AHI of >5 events per hour (at least mild OSA), and 49.7% of men and 23.4% of women have an AHI of >15 (at least moderate OSA). The mean BMI in this population sample was 25.6 kg/m^2 (Heinzer et al. 2015).

Pathophysiology

Classically, the two main contributors to OSA were thought to be upper airway anatomy (luminal cross-sectional area and collapsibility) and upper airway muscle function. However, investigators have more recently suggested that OSA is more heterogeneous and that other physiological traits may contribute to the risk of developing OSA. Therefore, OSA can be conceptualized as having different phenotypes. These other physiological traits include the propensity for awakening from sleep during airway narrowing (arousal threshold) and the stability of the ventilatory control system (loop gain).

UPPER AIRWAY ANATOMY

Studies employing various imaging techniques consistently demonstrate that the airway is smaller in patients with OSA than in healthy control subjects. Upper airway space is influenced by bony craniofacial anatomy and soft tissue structures that are developed in late fetal life and early childhood.

Early studies demonstrated that abnormalities of maxillary and mandibular position and size (particularly shorter mandibular length and mandibular retroposition) and lower hyoid bone position are correlated with increased risk of sleep apnea (Jamieson et al. 1986). These variations effectively reduce the boundaries or increase the length of the airway, respectively. Patients with abnormal development of the maxillary bones (indicated by a narrow palate) also have reduced upper airway space.

Soft tissue in the upper airway may also reduce its lumen size. Patients with OSA also tend to have an invasion of adipocytes in this area, which results in a larger tongue with a higher percentage of fat, thicker lateral pharyngeal walls, and a thicker and enlarged soft palate (Edwards et al. 2017). Tonsillar and adenoid hypertrophy can also increase the risk of upper airway obstruction by impinging on luminal space.

UPPER AIRWAY INTEGRITY AND GENIOGLOSSUS RESPONSIVENESS AND EFFECTIVENESS

In addition to structural anatomy, structural integrity or collapsibility of the airway is also vital to the pathophysiology of sleep apnea. Studies demonstrate that the propensity for the upper airway to collapse during sleep positively correlates with likelihood and severity of sleep apnea (Isono et al. 1997).

The largest and most significant upper airway dilator is the genioglossus muscle, which has been thoroughly investigated for its relation to OSA. Genioglossus activity is reduced at sleep onset and particularly in REM in both healthy individuals and those with sleep apnea. The genioglossus muscle and other upper airway muscles must not only respond to airway collapse but also effectively maintain airway patency.

Evidence is mixed regarding genioglossus muscle responsiveness in patients with OSA versus healthy control subjects. However, studies suggest that genioglossus muscle contraction in the latter is more effective in maintaining airway patency than that in the former (Edwards et al. 2017).

AROUSAL THRESHOLD

The propensity to awaken as a result of airway narrowing was historically assumed to be a protective mechanism in sleep. Indeed, studies have demonstrated that patients with severe sleep apnea tend to have a higher respiratory arousal threshold (i.e., are less likely to awaken with airway narrowing). However, an excessively low respiratory arousal threshold has also been proposed as a cause of OSA, particularly in patients with milder disease (Eckert and Younes 2014). Several possible explanations for this have been proposed.

One theory is that frequent arousals decrease the progression to slow-wave sleep, which is associated with improved breathing stability. Another potential explanation is that the protective mechanism of pharyngeal muscle activation, which is driven by pressure swings and changes in blood gases, is undermined if the patient awakens before this mechanism can be triggered. Upper airway muscle reflexes to increase tone in response to upper airway resistance may also be blunted by repeated, frequent arousals. Lastly, an excessive number of arousals from sleep may result in a ventilatory overcorrection of carbon dioxide, which can perpetuate ventilatory control instability in sleep.

Studies have demonstrated that arousal threshold strongly relates to markers of sleep apnea severity, including AHI, nadir oxygen, and the percentage of all respiratory events that are hypopneas; these factors could be used as a screening tool to identify patients with low arousal thresholds (Edwards et al. 2014a).

VENTILATORY CONTROL (LOOP GAIN)

Another proposed phenotype of OSA is that of an overly sensitive ventilatory control system (high loop gain) that results in overcorrection of carbon dioxide to a given ventilatory disturbance. Ventilatory control is influenced by innate sensitivity to hypercapnia and hypoxemia (to a lesser degree), the difference between inspired and arterial blood gas levels for carbon dioxide or oxygen, a timing factor of the circulation time between the lungs and chemoreceptors, and lung volume. High loop gain is thought to be a potential culprit, particularly in those with only a mild predisposition to upper airway collapse instead of a highly collapsible airway.

POSITION

Sleeping position often influences sleep apnea severity, with some studies demonstrating that the respiratory disturbance index can be as much as 40%–50% lower when patients sleep in a lateral position compared with supine (Oksenberg et al. 1997). Overall, 50% of patients have supine-predominant OSA (i.e., AHI at least twice as high in supine position), and 15% have supine-isolated OSA (i.e., AHI <5 in nonsupine position and at least twice as high in supine position) (Joosten et al. 2014).

OTHER CONTRIBUTING MECHANISMS

Some other factors proposed to contribute to the risk of OSA include lung volume, surface tension, and fluid or vascular shifts. Studies have suggested that increased lung volume reduces airway collapsibility (Squier et al. 2010), possibly by directly stretching or dilating the airway. Surface tension or "stickiness" of the airway may lead to more folds in the upper airway and subsequently increase collapsibility. Lastly, rostral fluid shifts, particularly in patients with disorders predisposing to fluid retention, such as heart failure and end-stage renal disease, may potentiate OSA. Fluid shift from the legs at night to the tissues of the neck increases neck circumference, upper airway tissue volume, and pressure, collectively increasing the risk for OSA (Yumino et al. 2010).

Sleep stage influences the previously described pathophysiological factors. Normal REM sleep causes atonia, including of the upper airway muscles, which increases their collapsibility. Additionally, loop gain is more sensitive in non-REM sleep, decreases in sensitivity during deeper sleep, and is lowest in REM sleep (Deacon-Diaz and Malhotra 2018).

AGE-DEPENDENT PATHOPHYSIOLOGY

Studies have demonstrated not only that OSA is a consequence of the interaction of many of these physiological factors but also that age influences all of these variables. Upper airway anatomy and collapsibility seem to be the primary pathophysiology for OSA in older patients, whereas abnormal ventilatory control is more common in younger patients (Edwards et al. 2014b). That said, upper airway anatomy in young children may lead to less obvious airway collapse that is not formally recognized (Guilleminault and Huang 2018).

Risk Factors and Comorbidities

Established risk factors for OSA include sex, age, ethnicity, obesity, craniofacial anatomy, and upper airway soft tissue abnormalities. Other proposed risk factors include smoking, nasal congestion, substance use, and comorbid medical and psychiatric conditions (Young et al. 2004).

SEX AND HORMONES

OSA is more common in men than in women, with an approximately two- to threefold higher risk for men. Potential explanations include hormonal effects on upper airway muscles and collapsibility, sex differences in fat distribution and anatomy, and different occupational and social exposures. The theory of hormones contributing to risk of OSA is supported by the increased prevalence of OSA in post- compared with premenopausal women, particularly if they are not receiving hormone replacement therapy.

AGE

Risk factors leading to OSA may be present at birth and can impact anatomical development of the upper airway, resulting in abnormal breathing during sleep in children (see Chapter 9). The prevalence of OSA increases with age, starting in young adulthood and increasing until approximately age 65, at which time it either plateaus or begins to decrease in prevalence. A conclusive explanation for this phenomenon has not been found, although one potential explanation is increased mortality associated with OSA.

ETHNICITY

Population-based studies have primarily been conducted in the United States, Europe, and Asia. In the United States, studies suggest that African Americans have a higher risk of severe sleep apnea compared with white subjects, even when adjusted for BMI (Ancoli-Israel et al. 1995). Studies have found that the correlation between BMI and sleep apnea severity is weaker in Asian men than in white men. Even when age and BMI are comparable, Asian men have significantly more severe OSA than do white men (Li et al. 2000). The prevailing theory for these observations in ethnicity and OSA is suspected to be ethnic variations in craniofacial anatomy.

OBESITY

The positive correlation between increased OSA prevalence and severity with obesity is well established. Several mechanisms explaining this relationship are alterations in upper airway structure (especially increased volume and mass) or function (collapsibility), disturbance of ventilatory control, and exacerbation of OSA via obesity-related reduction in functional residual lung capacity.

CRANIOFACIAL AND UPPER AIRWAY STRUCTURE

As mentioned, anatomical abnormalities of the upper airway, including dysmorphisms of mandibular and maxillary size and position, narrowed nasal cavities, and tonsillar and adenoid hypertrophy, increase the risk of OSA. Many of these abnormalities can be identified at birth and during childhood.

NASAL CONGESTION

Epidemiological and experimental studies have demonstrated that nasal congestion is positively correlated with OSA. One study has suggested that the odds ratio for an AHI of ≥ 5 in chronic nasal congestion versus no nasal congestion is 1.8 (Young et al. 1997).

SMOKING

The relationship between smoking and sleep apnea has been controversial, with some studies finding up to a threefold risk of sleep apnea in current smokers (Wetter et al. 1994). Meanwhile, other studies have found an inverse relationship between smoking and sleep apnea severity (Newman et al. 2001). It has been proposed that smoking not only induces airway inflammation but also causes sleep instability due to nicotine withdrawal at night.

ALCOHOL

It is hypothesized that alcohol induces upper airway muscle hypotonia, impacting reflex responses, and depresses the CNS arousal response. Studies have suggested that acute alcohol ingestion before sleep worsens snoring, increases frequency and duration of obstructive respiratory events, and results in more precipitous oxygen desaturation (Issa and Sullivan 1982).

MEDICATIONS

Benzodiazepines, hypnotics, and opiates likely exacerbate OSA. Studies have demonstrated that chronic high-dosage hypnotic use increases the likelihood of a subsequent diagnosis of sleep-related breathing disorders (Li et al. 2000). This may be due to inhibition of the CNS, decreased ventilation response to hypoxia, or decreased muscle tone in the upper airway muscles caused by these medications.

COMORBID MEDICAL CONDITIONS

The prevalence of OSA is increased in patients with other disorders, including diabetes, chronic lung disease, hypertension, coronary artery disease, congestive heart failure, end-stage renal disease, myocardial infarction, stroke, chronic lung disease, depression, anxiety, and PTSD. These correlations are likely due to a combination of shared risk factors rather than causal. Other syndromes have a direct impact on the upper airway anatomy, such as acromegaly and trisomy 21, or affect orofacial growth, such as in cartilage diseases (e.g., Ehlers-Danlos syndrome, Marfan syndrome, neuromuscular disease, or premature septal deviation).

Clinical Presentation and Physical Examination

SYMPTOMS

The combination on polysomnography of OSA and daytime sleepiness is referred to as *obstructive sleep apnea syndrome*. Although daytime sleepiness is the most common complaint, OSA is a heterogeneous disorder with many symptoms. Other commonly reported symptoms in patients with OSA include snoring, gasping and choking at night, witnessed apneic episodes, insomnia, restless sleep, bruxism, frequent nocturia, waking up feeling unrefreshed, morning headaches, waking up with a dry mouth, cognitive deficits or "brain fog" during the day, poor concentration, memory decline, erectile dysfunction, and changes in mood such as depression and irritability.

Although snoring is highly prevalent and sensitive for OSA, it is not specific. Nocturnal gasping and choking in adults has been found to be the single most reliable symptom to indicate sleep apnea, with a likelihood ratio of 3.3 (Myers et al. 2013). However, with the multitude of potential pathological causes of OSA and comorbid conditions, no single symptom or sign can sufficiently predict a diagnosis. In general, symptoms and sequelae of OSA increase as OSA severity increases.

CLINICAL SIGNS AND PHYSICAL EXAMINATION

Several of the most prominent risk factors of OSA are readily apparent after a thorough evaluation including age, sex, ethnicity, obesity status, medical and psychiatric comorbidities, current medications, and alcohol and tobacco use. Physical examination helps practitioners stratify a patient's risk for OSA, determine precipitating causes of the patient's OSA, and guide treatment planning.

Craniofacial Structure

Maxillary and mandibular deficiency and posterior positioning have been associated with an increased risk for OSA (Lowe et al. 1986). Mandibular retropositioning (retrognathia) is defined as a >0.5 cm retroposition of the most inferior contour of the chin (the "gnathion") relative to the deepest point of the superior aspect of the nasal bone (the "nasion"). Additionally, a "long face" and inferior-placed hyoid bone are associated with sleep apnea.

Nose

The evaluation of the nose for sleep apnea involves evaluation for septal deviation, nasal collapse, turbinate hypertrophy, and nasal polyps that can affect nasal airflow (Shah et al. 2016).

Oropharynx

The presence of a narrow hard palate and a posterior buccal crossbite (upper molars sitting inside the lower molars) collectively suggest maxillary constriction that may increase airflow resistance and risk of sleep apnea. Other oropharyngeal findings that increase the risk of sleep apnea include an elongated uvula and soft palate, lateral peritonsillar narrowing, tonsillar hypertrophy, macroglossia, dental overbite with the upper teeth covering the lower third of the lower teeth, and dental overjet as defined by a >3-mm anterior-posterior distance between the upper and lower incisors.

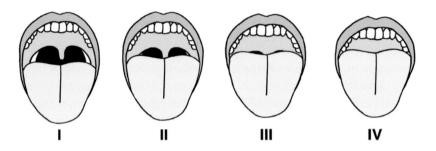

FIGURE 8-1. Modified Mallampati classification.

Classification based on modified Mallampati. Class I: Soft palate, uvula, fauces (opening between the pharynx and the tongue), faucial pillars (anterior and posterior arches that form the tonsillar fossae laterally) visible; Class II: Soft palate, major part of uvula, fauces visible; Class III: Soft palate, base of uvula visible; Class IV: Only hard palate visible.

The modified Mallampati classification system, originally developed as a predictor of airway intubation difficulty, is also regularly assessed in patients with concern for OSA (Figure 8–1). A Mallampati class of three or four is pathologically small.

Neck

A neck circumference that measures >43 cm (17 in) in men and >40.5 cm (16 in) in women while sitting upright at the superior border of the cricothyroid membrane is associated with increased risk of sleep apnea.

Diagnostic Procedures, Tests, and Questionnaires

The AASM clinical guidelines task force strongly recommends use of either polysomnography or home sleep apnea testing in conjunction with a comprehensive sleep evaluation and adequate follow-up to diagnose OSA and evaluate pathology severity. However, some screening tools and assessments can be used in clinical practice to select individuals with a high pretest probability.

SCREENING TOOLS

Many clinical questionnaires have been developed with the intent of identifying patients with OSA or to correlate with severity of OSA. However, although sensitivity of the questionnaires tends to be reasonably high, specificity tends to be low, resulting in false positives (Kapur et al. 2017).

Epworth Sleepiness Scale

The Epworth Sleepiness Scale is an eight-item questionnaire generally accepted as the standard for assessing subjective daytime sleepiness. Patients report their likelihood of falling asleep during the day in various situations. It has also been tested as a tool for predicting OSA, but its performance against polysomnography in identifying patients with OSA has been limited. For an AHI of ≥5, sensitivity ranges from 0.27 to 0.72 and specificity from 0.50 to 0.76, with an accuracy between 51% and 59%. The result is a high number of false negatives. The AASM task force has deemed that the overall quality of evidence for the Epworth Sleepiness Scale to predict OSA is low (Kapur et al. 2017).

STOP-BANG Questionnaire

The STOP-BANG is a screening tool that combines patient Yes/No responses to symptoms of OSA with an assessment of clinical risk factors. It comprises **S**noring, **T**iredness, **O**bserved apneas, blood **P**ressure, **B**MI, **A**ge, **N**eck circumference, and **G**ender (sex). The STOP-BANG's sensitivity is 0.93 for an AHI of ≥5, but specificity is low at 0.36, with an accuracy of 52%–53%. The AASM task force has deemed that the overall quality of evidence for the STOP-BANG to predict OSA is moderate (Kapur et al. 2017).

Other Prediction Tools

Other commonly used screening tools for OSA include the Berlin questionnaire, Sleep Apnea Clinical Score, Multivariable Apnea Prediction instrument, and the Kushida Index in adults. Despite these many tools developed to aid in the diagnosis of OSA, the AASM task force has made an umbrella recommendation against the singular use of any of these tools to make the diagnosis. Furthermore, due to the potential risk for and ramifications of false-negative and false-positive results, it has been concluded that the use of these clinical tools as the sole means to diagnose OSA causes more potential harm than potential benefit (Kapur et al. 2017).

HOME SLEEP APNEA TESTING

In patients who have had a clinical evaluation and have a high likelihood of moderate to severe uncomplicated (meaning without comorbidities) OSA, home sleep apnea testing can be used to establish a diagnosis. Most home sleep studies evaluate nasal pressure, chest and abdominal respiratory inductance plethysmography to assess respiratory effort, and oximetry. The WatchPAT, another home sleep apnea testing device, monitors only peripheral arterial tone, pulse oximetry, heart rate, and actigraphy (measure of movements, or accelerometry).

The advantages of home tests are the convenience of doing them at home, lower cost, and improved access for patients. However, the disadvantages are multiple and include the absence of a technologist to adjust any sensor misplacement, which results in higher rates of failure; varied sensor technology; inability to accurately distinguish obstructive and central events or monitor body position with certain home devices; and the lack of sleep staging. The lack of staging causes a propensity to underestimate the AHI, resulting in more false-negative results for two reasons. First, the AHI can only be calculated as the number of events over total machine recording time instead of actual sleep time. Second, hypopneas associated with electroencephalographic arousals in the absence of oxygen desaturation, as well as respiratory effort–related arousals, cannot be detected. This may be especially important in younger, nonobese, and premenopausal subjects who tend to have more arousal-associated hypopneas than oxygen desaturation arousals. Overall technical failure rate of home sleep apnea testing devices ranges from 3% to 18% (Flemons et al. 2003).

POLYSOMNOGRAPHY

Despite the increasing prevalence of home testing, an overnight, in-lab, supervised polysomnographic study remains the gold standard to diagnose OSA. Polysomnography is indicated in the event of a negative, inconclusive, or technically inadequate home apnea test (Kapur et al. 2017). Additional indications are the presence of significant medical comorbidities that increase the risk of non-obstructive sleep-disordered breathing; the concern for other, nonrespiratory sleep disorders; or if environmental or personal factors preclude use of home testing (Kapur et al. 2017).

In addition to nasal pressure, chest and abdominal respiratory inductance plethysmography, and oximetry evaluated by home sleep apnea tests, polysomnography can provide many other variables. The AASM formally recommends all polysomnograms include electroencephalograms, electrooculograms, submental electromyogram activity, a thermistor to detect airflow (specifically, mouth breathing that nasal pressure cannot detect) in addition to a nasal pressure transducer, respiratory effort and oxygen saturation, body position, electrocardiograms, and leg electromyograms. Additionally, polysomnograms can assess thoracic and abdominal respiratory muscle electromyographic activity, snoring via a microphone, end-tidal and transcutaneous carbon dioxide, and abnormal movements and behaviors through video recording and upper-extremity electromyogram. Esophageal manometry can also be used to monitor changes in inspiratory and expiratory effort.

Diagnostic Criteria

The current *International Classification of Sleep Disorders* definition for OSA in adults is (American Academy of Sleep Medicine 2014):

1. Five or more predominantly obstructive respiratory events (i.e., obstructive and mixed apneas, hypopneas, or respiratory effort–related arousals) per hour of sleep (for polysomnography) or recording time (for home sleep apnea tests) in a patient with one or more of the following:

   - Sleepiness, nonrestorative sleep, fatigue, or insomnia symptoms
   - Waking up with breath holding, gasping, or choking
   - Habitual snoring, breathing interruptions, or both noted by a bed partner or other observer
   - Hypertension, mood disorder, cognitive dysfunction, coronary artery disease, stroke, congestive heart failure, atrial fibrillation, frequent cardiac arrhythmias, or type 2 diabetes mellitus

   OR

2. Fifteen or more predominantly obstructive respiratory events (apneas, hypopneas, or respiratory effort–related arousals) per hour of sleep (for polysomnography) or recording time (for home sleep apnea tests), regardless of the presence of associated symptoms or comorbidities.

Differential Diagnosis

BENIGN SNORING

The differential diagnosis of OSA depends on the patient's presenting complaint. Although snoring is almost unanimously present in OSA, with studies reporting that up to 97% of patients with OSA snore, the positive value of snoring to predict OSA may be much lower. One meta-analysis demonstrated that snoring has a positive predictive value of 18%–20% for an AHI of ≥5 based on polysomnography and that patients with mild snoring and a BMI <26 are unlikely to have more than mild OSA (Myers et al. 2013). However, other studies have demonstrated that in treatment-seeking patients, the positive predictive value of snoring can be as high as 84.7% to predict an AHI of ≥5 using polysomnography (Romero et al. 2010). Nevertheless, benign snoring without OSA should be considered.

OTHER CAUSES OF HYPERSOMNIA

EDS, which is very prominent in OSA, can also be caused by other sleep or medical and psychiatric disorders. Sleep disorders that cause excessive sleepiness include insufficient sleep, circadian rhythm disorders (see Chapters 12 and 13), periodic limb movement disorder (Chapter 17), narcolepsy (Chapter 6), and idiopathic hypersomnia (Chapter 7), as well as other sleep-related behavior disorders such as sleep-related hypoventilation and central sleep apnea (Chapters 10 and 11, respectively). Medical and psychiatric conditions, such as neurodegenerative disorders (notably dementia with Lewy bodies), anemia, hypothyroidism, renal disease, adrenal insufficiency, depression, anxiety, or substance abuse, and use of sedating medications should also be considered in patients with EDS.

OTHER MIMICS

The differential diagnosis for gasping and choking at night, witnessed apneas, and disrupted sleep include central sleep apnea (see Chapter 11), gastroesophageal reflux disease, asthma, chronic obstructive pulmonary disease, congestive heart failure, and panic disorder.

Adverse Consequences

The adverse effects that OSA has on cardiovascular risk and metabolic syndrome/insulin resistance are well established. Patients with OSA are at increased risk of hypertension, pulmonary artery hypertension, coronary artery disease, cardiac arrhythmias, heart failure, stroke, diabetes, obesity, cognitive impairment and dementia, preeclampsia, impotence, and increased overall mortality.

Other adverse effects of OSA include impaired daytime function and quality of life; increased risk of psychiatric conditions, such as depressive and anxiety disorders; and increased health care costs. Additionally, patients and clinicians must be conscientious of the increased risk of motor vehicle accidents in patients with OSA. Diagnosed patients should be educated regarding the increased risk of motor vehicle accidents due to drowsy driving in untreated OSA. This is especially important for patients with high-risk occupations, such as commercial drivers, pilots, and medical staff, because OSA has been shown to increase the risk of motor vehicle accidents two- to threefold (Strohl et al. 2013). Fortunately, proper treatment of OSA is associated with a significant reduction in this risk (Tregear et al. 2010).

Treatment

The purpose of OSA treatment is to relieve obstruction and maintain airway patency during sleep, which translates to the elimination of apneas, hypopneas, arousals, oxygen desaturation, and carbon dioxide changes. In addition to improving sleep quality and daytime symptoms, the impact of OSA therapy lies in recuperating the effects that OSA has on quality of life, cognition, cardiovascular risk, metabolic syndrome, mental health, mortality, and health care cost. Treatment options for OSA have rapidly expanded since it was first described. Although positive airway pressure (PAP) therapy remains the gold standard and most prevalent treatment for OSA, many alternative therapies are now commonly available to patients.

BEHAVIORAL MODIFICATION AND NONINVASIVE THERAPIES

Weight Loss and Exercise

It is essential to educate overweight patients with OSA about the positive correlation between obesity and OSA. Studies have demonstrated that a 10% weight loss from stable weight can reduce the AHI by 26% (Peppard et al. 2000). Weight loss can also help improve many of the medical conditions shared between OSA and obesity, including hypertension, cardiovascular morbidity, and reduced quality of life.

Positional Therapy

OSA severity and the risk of upper airway collapse during sleep are strongly influenced by body position, particularly supine position compared with nonsupine (lateral recumbent or prone) positions (Penzel et al. 2001). Many commercial products ranging from alarms to positional belts and specialized pillows have been developed to promote nonsupine sleep. However, sleep position change is generally recommended as an adjunctive therapy for OSA (Epstein et al. 2009).

Myofunctional Therapy

Myofunctional therapy involves various oropharyngeal and tongue exercises with the intent to strengthen oropharynx muscles, including the genioglossus. Studies have suggested that myofunctional therapy can significantly reduce AHI and snoring in adults with OSA, making it a viable adjunctive therapy for OSA (Camacho et al. 2015).

Alcohol and Exacerbating Medication Avoidance

As mentioned, acute alcohol ingestion can worsen snoring, increase obstructive respiratory events, and result in more precipitous oxygen desaturation. Therefore, patients with OSA should be instructed to avoid alcohol. If feasible, medications that inhibit the CNS and dampen respiratory effort, such as benzodiazepines and opiates, should also be avoided in patients with OSA.

Other Noninvasive Therapies

Medications treating the underlying conditions that contribute to OSA, such as nasal steroids for chronic rhinitis or thyroid hormones to treat hypothyroidism, are recommended (Lin et al. 2012).

POSITIVE AIRWAY PRESSURE THERAPY

Since being introduced in 1981, continuous positive airway pressure (CPAP) has been established as the gold standard, "one-size-fits-all" treatment of OSA. PAP therapy delivers pressurized air into the airway to relieve obstruction during sleep. Although CPAP delivers the same pressure regardless of the respiratory cycle, other modalities such as bilevel PAP or adaptive servo ventilation can deliver different inspiratory PAP, expiratory PAP, and pressure support. These other modalities are more commonly used in patients with complex sleep-disordered breathing resulting in hypoventilation or central sleep apnea.

Although PAP therapy is highly effective, its impact relies on patient adherence, which can be challenging. Some studies suggest that nonadherence rates range from 46% to 83% (Weaver and Grunstein 2008). Although no consensus threshold to define nonadherence has been found, the average nightly usage of CPAP in most studies is 4 hours. At this threshold, many studies demonstrate significant improvement of daytime symptoms, quality of life, neurocognitive function, and cardiovascular health. Therefore, it is recommended that patients use PAP therapy at a minimum for 4 hours per night, but ideally 6 hours or longer. One concern associated with PAP treatment is the physical pressure exerted on the face, particularly with full face masks, that may impact maxillary bone growth in preadolescents and adolescents. In adults, full face mask anteroposterior pressure on the mandible may also lead to increased obstructive events.

ORAL APPLIANCE THERAPY

Oral appliances enlarge the upper airway and may also decrease its collapsibility. The most common oral appliances are the mandibular advancement devices, which are designed to hold the lower jaw in an anterior position during sleep to prevent upper airway collapse. Some may also result in the anterior advancement of the tongue, but dedicated tongue-retaining devices have also been developed to hold the tongue in an anterior position and thus maintain airway patency. Potential adverse effects of oral appliances include temporomandibular joint pain, mouth dryness, tooth pain, gum irritation, sialorrhea, and headaches. Long-term usage may result in substantial dental changes of occlusion and bite. That said, oral appliances are a reasonable alternative to PAP therapy for patients with mild to moderate OSA. Oral appliances are not recommended as a first-line therapy for patients with severe OSA, more significant reductions in oxygen saturation, or significant cardiovascular disease (Cao et al. 2017). Systematic bite evaluation should be performed annually, with regular follow-up by an orthodontist.

SURGERIES

Surgery of the upper airway is indicated as an adjunctive therapy with PAP or an oral appliance when anatomy is compromising the airway or reducing primary treatment efficacy or tolerance. Surgery is also a second-line therapy if other interventions have failed or were intolerable to the patient. Although many procedures may improve OSA, the specific surgery is predicated on a thorough interview and physical examination. Nasopharyngoscopy, imaging, or drug-induced sleep endoscopy may also assist the evaluation.

Nasal Surgery

Nasal breathing may be improved with surgeries to correct structural abnormalities such as deviated nasal septum, turbinate hypertrophy, nasal valve collapse, or nasal polyps. Improving nasal breathing has been shown to improve CPAP tolerance. However, nasal surgery alone has not been demonstrated to cure or improve OSA (Cao et al. 2017).

Oropharyngeal and Palatal Surgery

Other surgeries with the primary goal of relieving oropharyngeal obstruction include tonsillectomy, uvulopalatopharyngoplasty (UPPP), tongue reduction, genioglossus advancement, and maxillomandibular advancement. Tonsillectomy may significantly improve the AHI in some patients with significant tonsillar hypertrophy (grade 3–4) and may even be curative, but this has not been consistently demonstrated. Tonsillar hypertrophy can also adversely affect CPAP therapy. Tonsillectomy in these patients reduces CPAP pressure requirements and improves adherence (Chandrashekariah et al. 2008).

UPPP traditionally involves the removal of the uvula, parts of the soft palate, tonsils, and the tonsillar pillars. It is not recommended as a primary intervention for OSA (Aurora et al. 2010), because success rates can be highly variable between 16% and 83% (Cao et al. 2017). Furthermore, initial improvement of OSA from UPPP progressively decays over time (Boot et al. 2000), and UPPP can cause more difficulties with CPAP adherence due to worsened mouth leak.

Maxillomandibular Advancement

Maxillomandibular advancement moves the entire lower facial skeleton and attached soft tissues anteriorly to widen the posterior upper airway space. Studies have demonstrated that this procedure is an effective treatment for OSA (Zaghi et al. 2016). It is indicated for the treatment of severe OSA in patients who cannot tolerate or are unwilling to try PAP therapy or oral appliances (Aurora et al. 2010).

Palatal Expansion

Rapid maxillary expansion is an orthodontic procedure to widen the upper airway and was initially used to treat OSA in children. However, skull maturation and suture ossification limit the use of rapid maxillary expansion in adolescents and adults. The philosophy of maxillary expansion has been adapted for adults using a combination of surgery and orthodontic techniques. Studies in adults demonstrate significant improvement in OSA using palatal expansion (Li et al. 2019).

Upper Airway Stimulation

Distal, intermittent hypoglossal nerve stimulation has been approved by the FDA and shown to significantly improve OSA (Strollo et al. 2014). A neurostimulator implanted in the chest directly stimulates the distal branches of the hypoglossal nerve from the end of expiration to the end of inspiration, causing an anterior protrusion of the tongue that subsequently relieves upper airway obstruction during sleep. Hypoglossal nerve stimulation is an option for patients without significant obesity who have at least moderate to severe OSA that is not supine isolated. It is indicated in those who are unable to tolerate PAP therapy and are not deemed good candidates for, or have failed, other therapies. Upper airway stimulation has demonstrated substantial and sustained improvement in AHI after several years of treatment (Woodson et al. 2018).

Patients are selected based on the absence of complete concentric collapse (mostly anterior-posterior collapse) at the velopharynx (soft palate) on drug-induced sleep endoscopy. Potential disadvantages include the need for invasive surgery, future contraindication to chest and neck MRI, the need to replace the battery at regular intervals, and discomfort from electrical stimulation.

OXYGEN

Given the several potential pathophysiological causes of OSA, the use of oxygen has been tried but is not currently recommended for the treatment of OSA. Supplemental oxygen can be used as an adjunct to treat hypoxemia, but use of oxygen alone may reduce respiratory drive (relative hypoventilation), thereby prolonging apneas and worsening nocturnal hypercapnia (Epstein et al. 2009).

PHARMACOTHERAPY

Many pharmacotherapies such as antidepressants (desipramine, protriptyline), acetylcholinesterase inhibitors, and estrogen supplementation have been tried but have shown mixed results. In a recent, randomized, placebo-controlled crossover trial, a combination of atomoxetine (noradrenergic) and oxybutynin (antimuscarinic) showed a 63% reduction in AHI compared with placebo in a group of patients with a mean BMI of 34.8 (Taranto-Montemurro et al. 2019). Because none of these drugs alone produced such results, it is assumed that they may have a synergistic effect on the upper airway dilator muscles. More trials are needed to confirm the efficacy and safety of pharmacotherapies targeting upper airway muscle strength and collapsibility during sleep, loop gain, and arousal threshold.

Conclusion

The prevalence and awareness of OSA may continue to increase as physicians and patients further recognize its impact on patient health, as the obesity epidemic continues, and as we increasingly recognize the various phenotypes of OSA. We are hopeful that the ability to accurately diagnose OSA will improve as our understanding of the phenotypes and pathophysiology of OSA increases. Although PAP therapy remains the gold standard, "one-size-fits-all" treatment, alternatives are constantly being developed. In the future, physicians may be able to categorize patients with OSA and curate optimal, patient-specific treatment for their condition.

KEY CLINICAL POINTS

- Common symptoms of obstructive sleep apnea (OSA) include daytime sleepiness, snoring, gasping and choking at night, witnessed apneic episodes, insomnia, restless sleep, morning headaches, and cognitive deficits.

- Risk factors for OSA include male sex (and postmenopausal females), middle to older age, obesity, craniofacial abnormalities, nasal congestion, alcohol use, and medications that depress CNS function.

- Clinic screening tools are insufficient to diagnose OSA. A home sleep apnea test and, preferably, in-laboratory polysomnography are the only approved modalities for diagnosis.

- Adverse effects of OSA include increased cardiovascular risk, metabolic syndrome, impaired cognition, increased risk of psychiatric disorders, motor vehicle accidents, and overall increased mortality and health care cost.

- Patients with OSA should be educated about increased driving risk and noninvasive interventions for treatment (e.g., weight loss and exercise, sleep position, myofunctional therapy, and avoidance of alcohol/exacerbating medications).

- Positive airway pressure therapy remains the gold standard treatment for OSA, but alternatives include oral appliances for patients with mild to moderate disease and surgery as an adjunct or second-line treatment in the event of first-line treatment failure or intolerance.

References

American Academy of Sleep Medicine: International Classification of Sleep Disorders, 3rd Edition. Darien, IL, American Academy of Sleep Medicine, 2014

Ancoli-Israel S, Klauber MR, Stepnowsky C, et al: Sleep-disordered breathing in African-American elderly. Am J Respir Crit Care Med 152(6 pt 1):1946–1949, 1995 8520760

Aurora RN, Casey KR, Kristo D, et al: Practice parameters for the surgical modifications of the upper airway for obstructive sleep apnea in adults. Sleep 33(10):1408–1413, 2010 21061864

Boot H, van Wegen R, Poublon RML, et al: Long-term results of uvulopalatopharyngoplasty for obstructive sleep apnea syndrome. Laryngoscope 110(3 pt 1):469–475, 2000 10718440

Camacho M, Certal V, Abdullatif J, et al: Myofunctional therapy to treat obstructive sleep apnea: a systematic review and meta-analysis. Sleep (Basel) 38(5):669–675, 2015 25348130

Cao MT, Sternbach JM, Guilleminault C: Continuous positive airway pressure therapy in obstuctive sleep apnea: benefits and alternatives. Expert Rev Respir Med 11(4):259–272, 2017 28287009

Chandrashekariah R, Shaman Z, Auckley D: Impact of upper airway surgery on CPAP compliance in difficult-to-manage obstructive sleep apnea. Arch Otolaryngol Head Neck Surg 134(9):926–930, 2008 18794435

Deacon-Diaz N, Malhotra A: Inherent vs. induced loop gain abnormalities in obstructive sleep apnea. Front Neurol 9(Nov):896, 2018 30450076

Eckert DJ, Younes MK: Arousal from sleep: implications for obstructive sleep apnea pathogenesis and treatment. J Appl Physiol 116(3):302–313, 2014

Edwards BA, Eckert DJ, McSharry DG, et al: Clinical predictors of the respiratory arousal threshold in patients with obstructive sleep apnea. Am J Respir Crit Care Med 190(11):1293–1300, 2014a 25321848

Edwards BA, Wellman A, Sands SA, et al: Obstructive sleep apnea in older adults is a distinctly different physiological phenotype. Sleep (Basel) 37(7):1227–1236, 2014b 25061251

Edwards BA, Eckert DJ, Jordan AS: Obstructive sleep apnoea pathogenesis from mild to severe: is it all the same? Respirology 22(1):33–42, 2017 27699919

Epstein LJ, Kristo D, Strollo PJ Jr, et al: Clinical guideline for the evaluation, management and long-term care of obstructive sleep apnea in adults. J Clin Sleep Med 5(3):263–276, 2009 19960649

Flemons WW, Littner MR, Rowley JA, et al: Home diagnosis of sleep apnea: a systematic review of the literature. An evidence review cosponsored by the American Academy of Sleep Medicine, the American College of Chest Physicians, and the American Thoracic Society. Chest 124(4):1543–1579, 2003 14555592

Guilleminault C, Huang Y: From oral facial dysfunction to dysmorphism and the onset of pediatric OSA. Sleep Med Rev 40:203–214, 2018

Guilleminault C, Khramtsov A: Upper airway resistance syndrome in children: a clinical review. Semin Pediatr Neurol 8(4):207–215, 2001 11768783

Guilleminault C, Tilkian A, Dement WC: The sleep apnea syndromes. Annu Rev Med 27:465–484, 1976 180875

Guilleminault C, Stoohs R, Clerk A, et al: A cause of excessive daytime sleepiness. The upper airway resistance syndrome. Chest 104(3):781–787, 1993 8365289

Heinzer R, Vat S, Marques-Vidal P, et al: Prevalence of sleep-disordered breathing in the general population: the HypnoLaus study. Lancet Respir Med 3(4):310–318, 2015 25682233

Isono S, Remmers JE, Tanaka A, et al: Anatomy of pharynx in patients with obstructive sleep apnea and in normal subjects. J Appl Physiol 82(4):1319–1326, 1997

Issa FG, Sullivan CE: Alcohol, snoring and sleep apnea. J Neurol Neurosurg Psychiatry 45(4):353–359, 1982 7077345

Jamieson A, Guilleminault C, Partinen M, et al: Obstructive sleep apneic patients have craniomandibular abnormalities. Sleep 9(4):469–477, 1986 3809860

Joosten SA, O'Driscoll DM, Berger PJ, et al: Supine position related obstructive sleep apnea in adults: pathogenesis and treatment. Sleep Med Rev 18(1):7–17, 2014 23669094

Kapur VK, Auckley DH, Chowdhuri S, et al: Clinical practice guideline for diagnostic testing for adult obstructive sleep apnea: an American Academy of Sleep Medicine clinical practice guideline. J Clin Sleep Med 13(3):479–504, 2017 28162150

Li KK, Kushida C, Powell NB, et al: Obstructive sleep apnea syndrome: a comparison between Far-East Asian and white men. Laryngoscope 110(10 pt 1):1689–1693, 2000 11037826

Li K, Quo S, Guilleminault C: Endoscopically assisted surgical expansion (EASE) for the treatment of obstructive sleep apnea. Sleep Med 60:53–59, 2019 30393018

Lin CM, Huang YS, Guilleminault C: Pharmacotherapy of obstructive sleep apnea. Expert Opin Pharmacother 13(6):841–857, 2012 22424320

Lopes MC, Guilleminault C: Chronic snoring and sleep in children: a demonstration of sleep disruption. Pediatrics 118(3):e741–e746, 2006 16950965

Lowe AA, Santamaria JD, Fleetham JA, et al: Facial morphology and obstructive sleep apnea. Am J Orthod Dentofacial Orthop 90(6):484–491, 1986 3098087

Myers KA, Mrkobrada M, Simel DL: Does this patient have obstructive sleep apnea? The rational clinical examination systematic review. JAMA 310(7):731–741, 2013 23989984

Newman AB, Nieto FJ, Guidry U, et al: Relation of sleep-disordered breathing to cardiovascular disease risk factors: the Sleep Heart Health Study. Am J Epidemiol 154(1):50–59, 2001 11434366

Oksenberg A, Silverberg DS, Arons E, et al: Positional vs nonpositional obstructive sleep apnea patients: anthropomorphic, nocturnal polysomnographic, and multiple sleep latency test data. Chest 112(3):629–639, 1997 9315794

Penzel T, Möller M, Becker HF, et al: Effect of sleep position and sleep stage on the collapsibility of the upper airways in patients with sleep apnea. Sleep 24(1):90–95, 2001 11204057

Peppard PE, Young T, Palta M, et al: Longitudinal study of moderate weight change and sleep-disordered breathing. JAMA 284(23):3015–3021, 2000 11122588

Peppard PE, Young T, Barnet JH, et al: Increased prevalence of sleep-disordered breathing in adults. Am J Epidemiol 177(9):1006–1014, 2013 23589584

Romero E, Krakow B, Haynes P, et al: Nocturia and snoring: predictive symptoms for obstructive sleep apnea. Sleep Breath 14(4):337–343, 2010 19865841

Shah JA, George A, Chauhan N, et al: Obstructive sleep apnea: role of an otorhinolaryngologist. Indian J Otolaryngol Head Neck Surg 68(1):71–74, 2016 27066415

Squier SB, Patil SP, Schneider H, et al: Effect of end-expiratory lung volume on upper airway collapsibility in sleeping men and women. J Appl Physiol 109(4):977–985, 2010

Strohl KP, Brown DB, Collop N, et al: An official American Thoracic Society Clinical Practice Guideline: sleep apnea, sleepiness, and driving risk in noncommercial drivers. An update of a 1994 statement. Am J Respir Crit Care Med 187(11):1259–1266, 2013 23725615

Strollo PJ Jr, Soose RJ, Maurer JT, et al: Upper-airway stimulation for obstructive sleep apnea. N Engl J Med 370(2):139–149, 2014 24401051

Taranto-Montemurro L, Messineo L, Sands SA, et al: The combination of atomoxetine and oxybutynin greatly reduces obstructive sleep apnea severity: a randomized, placebo-controlled, double-blind crossover trial. Am J Respir Crit Care Med 199(10):1267–1276, 2019 30395486

Tregear S, Reston J, Schoelles K, et al: Continuous positive airway pressure reduces risk of motor vehicle crash among drivers with obstructive sleep apnea: systematic review and meta-analysis. Sleep 33(10):1373–1380, 2010 21061860

Weaver TE, Grunstein RR: Adherence to continuous positive airway pressure therapy: the challenge to effective treatment. Proc Am Thorac Soc 5(2):173–178, 2008 18250209

Wetter DW, Young TB, Bidwell TR, et al: Smoking as a risk factor for sleep-disordered breathing. Arch Intern Med 154(19):2219–2224, 1994 7944843

Woodson BT, Strohl KP, Soose RJ, et al: Upper airway stimulation for obstructive sleep apnea: 5-year outcomes. Otolaryngol Head Neck Surg 159(1):194–202, 2018

Young T, Finn L, Kim H, et al: Nasal obstruction as a risk factor for sleep-disordered breathing. J Allergy Clin Immunol 99(2):S757–S762, 1997 9042068

Young T, Skatrud J, Peppard PE: Risk factors for obstructive sleep apnea in adults. JAMA 291(16):2013–2016, 2004 15113821

Yumino D, Redolfi S, Ruttanaumpawan P, et al: Nocturnal rostral fluid shift: a unifying concept for the pathogenesis of obstructive and central sleep apnea in men with heart failure. Circulation 121(14):1598–1605, 2010 20351237

Zaghi S, Holty J-EC, Certal V, et al: Maxillomandibular advancement for treatment of obstructive sleep apnea: a meta-analysis. JAMA Otolaryngol Head Neck Surg 142(1):58–66, 2016 26606321

CHAPTER 9

Pediatric Obstructive Sleep Apnea

Payal Kenia Gu, M.D.

Shannon S. Sullivan, M.D.

Of all disorders classified in the *International Classification of Sleep Disorders*, 3rd Edition (ICSD-3), published by the American Academy of Sleep Medicine (AASM; 2014), only pediatric obstructive sleep apnea (OSA) retains a specialized diagnostic category for pediatrics. This reflects the varied and quite unique aspects of the clinical syndrome, which are distinct from the adult phenotype (see Chapter 8). Pediatric OSA involves intermittent complete (apneas) or partial (hypopneas) obstruction of the upper airway or prolonged periods of increased resistance to airflow and partial obstruction that disrupt normal ventilation in sleep.

A more inclusive and accurate term is pediatric sleep-disordered breathing (SDB), because in many cases, especially in the absence of obesity or certain congenital disorders, the pediatric phenotype may not include obstructive apneas but rather hypopneas, hypoventilation, or other abnormal breathing patterns that affect sleep quality. Compared with adults, children often do not have classical cortical arousals associated with these breathing abnormalities but may instead manifest frequent nocturnal movement or autonomic activation in sleep. Such phenomena have been hypothesized to be linked to the preponderance of slow-wave sleep seen in children, one of the features of which is a higher arousal threshold (Figure 9–1).

The concept of upper airway resistance–associated sleep disturbance, including both scoreable cortical arousals (termed *upper airway resistance syndrome*) and evidence of sleep instability (measured on electroencephalography by an elevated frequency of cyclic alternating pattern activity), has been described in children (Guilleminault and Khramtsov 2001; Lopes and Guilleminault 2006). In such cases, increased resistance to air-

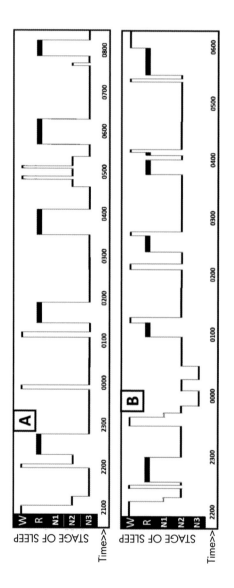

FIGURE 9–1.   Hypnograms demonstrating various stages of sleep cycled through in one night in a child (A) and an adult (B).

A, Over the course of the night, sleep in children is characterized by a preponderance of slow-wave sleep. **B,** This is in stark comparison to adult sleep, where slow-wave sleep represents a much smaller proportion of total sleep time, predominantly seen in the first few hours of the night.

flow through the upper airway precipitates cortical arousals and disturbance in sleep, with symptomatic consequences, and so is included in the spectrum of SDB. Additionally, children who do have apneas may have a greater degree of oxygen desaturation/hypoxemia than adults, thought to be due to lower functional residual capacity as well as higher metabolic rate (Berry et al. 2018).

Diagnostic Criteria

Pediatric OSA is defined for children ages 1–18 years when both clinical and polysomnographic criteria are met. Compared with earlier versions, the diagnostic criteria have been simplified, with symptoms consolidated into a single criterion. At least one nocturnal symptom (snoring, labored/obstructed breathing) or daytime consequence (sleepiness, hyperactivity, behavioral or learning problems) must be present. Polysomnographic criteria per the AASM require either an apnea/hypopnea index (AHI) of at least 1 or hypercapnia for at least 25% of total sleep time that is associated with evidence of obstructed breathing (snoring, nasal flow limitation, or paradoxical chest motion) (Berry et al. 2018). Of note, no exact criteria have been agreed upon for the diagnosis of OSA in infants younger than 1 year.

Epidemiology

The prevalence of pediatric OSA was estimated more than a decade ago by Lumeng and Chervin (2008) in a meta-analysis of epidemiological studies completed worldwide. The prevalence of parent-reported snoring in children was 7.45%. OSA prevalence ranged from 1% to 4%. Peak ages of presentation occurs in preschoolers and young school-age children age 2–8 years, although a second peak has been described in adolescence.

Certain risk factors have been associated with pediatric OSA. These include obesity, history of prematurity, adenotonsillar hypertrophy, craniofacial features, and environmental tobacco smoke (Dayyat et al. 2009; Dudley and Patel 2016; Kaditis et al. 2008). Although in prepubertal children the prevalence is thought to be equal between sexes, evidence suggests a higher prevalence in adolescent boys (Lumeng and Chervin 2008). Several studies have found a higher rate of pediatric OSA in African American children, although not all racial and ethnic groups have been well studied (Ruiter et al. 2010). Risk for OSA is often familial (Friberg et al. 2009). In the Cleveland Family Study, SDB was identified

TABLE 9–1.   Chronic conditions associated with sleep-disordered breathing

Craniofacial abnormalities (e.g., Pierre Robin sequence, Treacher Collins syndrome, cleft lip/palate)

Neuromuscular disorders (e.g., Duchenne muscular dystrophy)

Achondroplasia

Down syndrome

Mucopolysaccharidoses

Prader-Willi syndrome

Cerebral palsy

Chiari malformation

in children of families with OSA three to four times more often than in children of control families (Redline et al. 1999). In that study, comorbid asthma and allergies were also independent risk factors for SDB. Children diagnosed with other forms of chronic diseases listed in Table 9–1 are predisposed to SDB and warrant systematic screening for OSA (Kaditis et al. 2012).

Pathophysiology

Breathing during sleep is a complex interplay of multiple factors, including the tone of muscles of the upper airway, chest, and rib cage and the diaphragm and its interplay with the chest wall; the brain stem as the central mediator; and the central and peripheral chemoreceptors allowing for central control, as well as vagal afferents and other neuromodulation of breathing. The maturation of these components markedly differentiates sleep-related breathing in infants from that of older children. Similarly, physiology is altered in children compared with adults. The upper airway has been argued to be more resistant to total collapse in children than in adults. Ventilatory responsiveness to chemoreception also diminishes with age (Carroll and Donnelly 2014). These factors help explain why thresholds for normal apnea/hypopnea frequency are much lower for children than adults.

As compared with wakefulness, muscles maintaining the stability of the airway during sleep have less tone and result in a smaller and more collapsible airway. Neurons regulating activation of the airway fire differently during sleep as compared with wakefulness, with relative downregulation of activity noted during sleep (Carroll and Donnelly 2014).

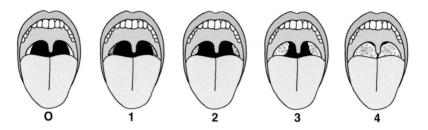

FIGURE 9–2. Grading of tonsillar hypertrophy.

This graphic demonstrates the numeric grading scale used to quantify the relative size of the palatine tonsils based on visual appearance within the oropharynx (Friedman et al. 1999). Grade 0=no tonsillar tissue (removed); Grade 1=tonsils barely visible behind anterior pillars; Grade 2=tonsils visible beyond anterior pillars; Grade 3=tonsils extend three-quarters (75%) of the distance to midline; Grade 4=tonsils touch and completely obstruct airway.

Intercostal muscles, which contribute to thoracic cage expansion, also have reduced tone and result in lower functional residual capacity. These are expected physiological changes during sleep. In addition to relatively different rib cage and diaphragmatic orientation in young children, factors that increase airway resistance (e.g., adenotonsillar hypertrophy or nasal obstruction) may aggravate this delicate physiological balance to contribute to OSA and other variants of SDB.

The most common obstructive factor identified in prepubertal children with sleep apnea is adenotonsillar enlargement (Figure 9–2). Children diagnosed with OSA in the preschool years are frequently found to have enlargement of the tonsils and adenoids (Linder-Aronson and Leighton 1983). The adenoidal-nasopharyngeal area is narrowest at 4.5 years, followed by adenoidal growth between ages 7 and 10 years, with a gradual reduction in growth of this space by the age of 12 years. Association between adenoidal growth and OSA severity decreases in adolescence, whereas the impact of tonsillar growth remains significant from early childhood into late adolescence (Kang et al. 2013). Tonsillectomy is primarily performed in combination with adenoidectomy, and few data exist regarding the relative impact of removal of tonsillar versus adenoidal tissue.

However, the etiology of OSA is often multifactorial, as shown in several studies where children still had symptoms and persistent evidence of OSA after tonsillectomy and adenoidectomy (Guilleminault et al. 2007; Mitchell and Boss 2009; Tauman et al. 2006). Obesity increases risk of residual OSA after adenotonsillectomy (Mitchell and Boss 2009; Tauman et al. 2006). Skeletal and soft tissue changes also impact OSA by contributing to increased upper airway resistance. Some features include midface hypoplasia (or maxillary deficiency), retrognathia, narrow palate, or nasal obstruction. Nasal obstruction may manifest as turbinate hypertrophy, choanal atresia, nasal polyps, or septal deviation. Neuromuscular weakness and hypotonia are less frequently encountered but still represent an important predisposition to OSA and SDB in children. Commonly affected populations include children with muscular dystrophy. These children may have bulbar weakness, which further diminishes the tone of their airway beyond physiological changes expected during sleep. They may also have respiratory muscle weakness and thus added decline in functional residual capacity during sleep.

Clinical Presentation, Course, and Complications

Children with OSA often present with a history of habitual snoring. However, it is important to note that not all children with OSA will snore but, rather, will be described as restless sleepers, have frequent nocturnal awakenings, have parasomnias including sleepwalking and sleep talking (Guilleminault et al. 2003, 2005), or have nocturnal enuresis (Kovacevic et al. 2014). Although presenting symptoms classically involve a spectrum of nocturnal disturbances, daytime symptoms that warrant screening for SDB include daytime sleepiness, morning headaches, inattention, hyperactivity, and behavioral disturbances (Table 9–2) (Kaditis et al. 2016; Marcus et al. 2012). Studies demonstrating improvements in academic and neurocognitive performance (Chervin et al. 2006; Gozal 1998) as well as behavioral problems (Stewart et al. 2005) after treatment of OSA support these observed associations.

In the long term, untreated sleep apnea can be associated with risk for cor pulmonale, hypertension, and even growth failure in the very young (Guilleminault et al. 1976). A reversal of growth restriction is frequently observed after surgical management of adenotonsillar hypertrophy, independent of whether a preceding diagnosis of SDB has been made. Subsequent studies have shown significant postoperative increases in the substrates of growth hormone activity and improved height and weight (Kiris et al. 2010). Prospective longitudinal cohort studies are lacking, and no data have suggested that the syndrome spontaneously resolves with passage into adulthood. On this note, limitations regarding what is known of the natural history of OSA must be considered. In the Childhood Adenotonsillectomy Trial (Chervin et al. 2015), of the 94 children ages 5–9 years who had a baseline AHI of ≥5 and were randomized to

TABLE 9–2.   Symptoms associated with sleep-disordered breathing

Nocturnal symptoms	Daytime symptoms
Frequent awakenings	Aggressive behavior
Nocturnal enuresis (bedwetting)	Daytime sleepiness
Parasomnias (nightmares, night terrors, sleepwalking)	Hyperactivity
Restless sleep	Impaired memory/learning
Snoring	Inattention
Sweating in sleep	Irritability
Witnessed apneas (pauses in breathing)	Poor academic performance

watchful waiting for 7 months, 24% had spontaneous resolution of their OSA by polysomnographic criteria (AHI <2). In another study, 70 children ages 6–13 years with a prior diagnosis of primary snoring (i.e., without OSA) were reevaluated with polysomnography 4 years later. Of these, 37% now met criteria for OSA (obstructive AHI >1), 31% still met criteria for primary snoring, and 25% had resolution of snoring and normal polysomnogram results (Li et al. 2013).

Diagnostic Procedures, Tests, and Questionnaires

All children should be screened for snoring regularly by their primary physicians. When a positive history is obtained, further clinical query regarding symptoms (as described earlier) should follow. Alternative methods for screening based on symptomatology include the Pediatric Sleep Questionnaire, a 22-item closed-response question survey validated for use in patients ages 2–18 years. This questionnaire screens for symptoms such as snoring, daytime sleepiness, behavioral disturbance, and hyperactivity and generates a score ranging from 0 to 1.0 (0 = normal and 1.0=highest probability of OSA). A mean score of 0.33 or higher has been demonstrated to correlate with a diagnosis of OSA on polysomnography (Chervin et al. 2007). Ultimately, overnight, attended, in-lab polysomnography is accepted as the worldwide gold standard for objective diagnosis of OSA and other forms of obstructive SDB. If polysomnography is unavailable, alternative methods with less predictive value may be employed, such as nocturnal video recording, nocturnal oximetry, daytime nap polysomnogram, or ambulatory polysomnogram (Kaditis et al. 2016; Marcus et al. 2012). In-lab polysomnography includes continuous electroencephalography. This allows for measurement of brain wave activity at the level of the skull, which allows for sleep staging and identification of brain arousals associated with SDB. Among other monitoring parameters, in-lab monitoring provides audio and video input, along with monitoring of eye movements, chin and leg electromyogram, autonomic variables of heart rate and pulse oximetry, and respiratory monitoring via nasal cannula, mouth thermistor, and abdominal and thoracic bands.

As previously discussed, according to the ICSD-3, OSA is diagnosed in children who have an average of at least one respiratory event (apnea, mixed apnea, or hypopnea) per hour of sleep (AHI ≥1). This satisfies mild sleep apnea, although many clinicians will treat for clinical symptoms associated with a higher minimum AHI of 1.5–2. In children, an AHI between 5 and 10 is consistent with moderate sleep apnea, and >10 is consistent with severe sleep apnea. When discrete events of obstruction are not present, a diagnosis of OSA can still be made when evidence of obstructive hypoventilation is found with observation of both hypercapnia (arterial partial pressure of carbon dioxide [$PaCO_2$] >50 mm Hg) for at least 25% of total sleep time and upper airway resistance (e.g., snoring, nasal flow limitation, or paradoxical chest movement).

Differential Diagnosis

When obstructive SDB is not identified on polysomnogram but other clinical symptoms such as daytime sleepiness or difficulty focusing are present, other factors should be ruled out. For example, a closer look at a sleep log over several nights may reveal other helpful details. For the child who is staying up until 1 A.M. to complete homework nightly and waking up at 5:30 A.M. to make it to swimming practice, insufficient sleep syndrome would be suspected if no history of snoring, nocturia, or nighttime awakenings is present. In another case, a mother may complain that her adolescent son cannot fall asleep before 1 A.M. on school nights and struggles to get to school on time, yet he reports a similar bedtime on weekends and late morning awakening with no daytime difficulties on these days. With no nocturnal symptoms, his likely diagnosis may be delayed sleep phase syndrome (see Chapter 12).

In another scenario, a 10-year-old girl presents to the clinic with her mother. The parent reports the child was healthy and well until 3 months ago, when she started to fall asleep in unexpected circumstances for short naps during the day despite sleeping normal hours at night without interruptions or snoring. She has had a 15-lb weight gain in the past

3 months. The mother recalls an unusual episode the other day where the child was telling a joke and began to slur her words as she was laughing. According to the parent, the child dropped the cup she was holding and claimed that she had lost control of her hand. Her mother distantly recalls a flu-like illness affecting multiple family members 9 months ago. The history and course are most likely suggestive of type 1 narcolepsy (see Chapter 6), an autoimmune disorder that leads to reduction of hypocretin/orexin production and disruption of normal sleep and wake states. Thus, a detailed history, including bedtime routine and weekday and weekend sleep logs, is equally as important as the findings from a polysomnogram to obtaining a correct diagnosis.

Treatment

Currently two guidelines exist regarding management of OSA in children: the 2012 clinical practice guidelines published by the American Academy of Pediatrics (AAP) and the 2015 task force report by the European Respiratory Society (ERS). The latter is more expansive and provides a greater array of treatment options, with the added scope of not only treating OSA but also addressing future risk for OSA.

ADENOTONSILLECTOMY

According to both guidelines, adenotonsillectomy is considered the first-line treatment for OSA when adenotonsillar hypertrophy is present. If risk factors for postoperative respiratory compromise are present (Table 9–3), the AAP recommends close postoperative monitoring as well as consideration for rescheduling if the child has an acute respiratory infection on the day of surgery.

However, adenotonsillectomy is not uniformly effective in resolving OSA syndrome and results in normalization of OSA (obstructive AHI <1–2 events per hour depending on study) in 30%–90% of children (Bhattacharjee et al. 2010; Marcus et al. 2013). Tonsillar tissue is visible on oral examination and can be scored by a tonsil grading scale (see Figure 9–2). Tonsillar hypertrophy is defined as grades 3 and 4 (as proposed by Friedman et al. 1999); however, tonsillectomy may be performed for grade 2 tonsils as well. A significant improvement in quality of life was noted in children with grade 2–4 tonsils with mild OSA (AHI 1–5) (Volsky et al. 2014). Adenoidal tissue is not visible on simple oral examination but should be systematically evaluated by a pediatric otorhinolaryngologist for possible surgical reduction with tonsillectomy or alone (if tonsils are not also enlarged).

TABLE 9–3. **Risk factors for postoperative respiratory complications in children with obstructive sleep apnea undergoing adenotonsillectomy**

Age younger than 3 years

Severe obstructive sleep apnea on polysomnography (defined as minimum oxygen saturation <80%, apnea-hypopnea index ≥24 per hour, or peak carbon dioxide ≥60 mm Hg*)

Cardiac complications of obstructive sleep apnea syndrome

Failure to thrive

Obesity

Craniofacial anomalies

Neuromuscular disorders

Current respiratory infection

*Peak transcutaneous or end-tidal carbon dioxide levels on polysomnography.

OTHER NONSURGICAL THERAPIES AND TREATMENT OF ALLERGIES

Alternative therapies for nonsurgical management as advised by the AAP are limited to anti-inflammatory therapy and weight loss. The ERS guidelines offer a more comprehensive approach, including alternative treatment modalities. Each of these alternative treatments is dependent upon the presence of specific risk factors. If allergic symptoms are present in a child with pediatric OSA, intranasal steroids or oral leukotriene inhibitor therapy (montelukast) for 6–12 weeks may be beneficial. Montelukast therapy is expected to treat adenoidal hypertrophy because adenoidal and tonsillar tissues in children with SDB have been shown to have increased leukotriene receptors (Goldbart et al. 2004; Scadding 2010). Finally, weight loss may be considered in children above the 95th percentile for BMI based on age and sex.

POSITIVE AIRWAY PRESSURE THERAPY

Noninvasive positive pressure therapy with continuous or bilevel positive airway pressure (PAP) therapy can be equally or more efficacious than adenotonsillectomy. However, outcomes are often significantly limited by discomfort or poor adherence (Marcus et al. 2006). Additionally, some evidence has indicated that prolonged nasal PAP therapy with a nasal mask is associated with long-term maxillary retrusion (Fauroux et al. 2005; Roberts et al. 2016).

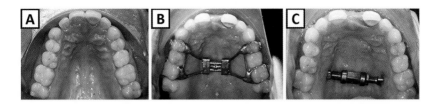

FIGURE 9–3. **Progressive transverse widening with rapid maxillary expansion.**

A, Maxilla before expansion. **B,** Maxilla with expander anchored upon teeth. **C,** The same maxilla with an expander anchored in the bony hard palate for further widening of the hard palate.

Source. Images courtesy of Dr. Stacey Quo.

RAPID MAXILLARY EXPANSION

Rapid maxillary expansion is considered for a child with maxillary constriction, which is found in children with a high-arched or narrow palate. This treatment involves placement of a palatal expander by an orthodontist (shown in Figure 9–3). The expander is attached to two or four teeth (usually molars or premolars) with an attached screw that can be manually rotated to expand the palatal space at the midpalatal suture (which is still cartilaginous in children). Progressive rotations of the screw place force on the suture and cause it to widen. The process expands the maxilla and the nasal cavity in the transverse diameter, improving maxillary constriction (Pirelli et al. 2015; Vale et al. 2017) and reducing nasal resistance. For older children, the expander may be attached to the bony hard palate rather than the teeth for a more effective expansion of the nasal cavity, also known as transpalatal distraction.

MYOFUNCTIONAL THERAPY

Reinforcement of the long-term impact of maxillary expansion has been seen with the associated practice of long-term myofunctional therapy, which involves regular practice of certain oropharyngeal exercises (Guilleminault et al. 2013). The mechanism is poorly understood, but the impact of these exercises has been seen in adults and children with OSA in the form reduced overall severity of sleep apnea (reduced AHI) and reduced snoring duration (Camacho et al. 2015). Although long-term follow-up on the stability of improvement from treatments is generally lacking, in select children, rapid maxillary expansion has been shown to maintain improvements at 12-year follow up (Pirelli et al. 2015).

COMBINED SEQUENTIAL APPROACH

In our practice, intervention with adenotonsillectomy is prioritized when clinically appropriate. Thereafter, a repeat polysomnogram 4–6 months after surgery is recommended. If residual sleep apnea persists along with clinical symptoms, all pertinent alternative therapies are employed to optimize the patient's risk factors. If the patient has some history of atopy, referral to an allergist is made. At the same time, referral to an orthodontist for rapid maxillary expansion may be considered alone or in combination with ongoing myofunctional therapy. Continuous PAP is also considered in select patients, in particular those with severe sleep-related respiratory abnormalities or severe daytime symptoms.

KEY CLINICAL POINTS

- The prevalence of pediatric obstructive sleep apnea (OSA) is 1%–4%. Family history of OSA, obesity, history of prematurity, adenotonsillar hypertrophy, and African American race, as well as some congenital, craniofacial, and chronic airway pediatric conditions are risk factors.

- Variables that increase upper airway resistance are most likely to aggravate risk for OSA, and reduction or resolution of these elements is implicit to treatment of pediatric OSA.

- Treatment modalities include primarily adenotonsillectomy but may also involve some combination of positive airway pressure therapy, anti-inflammatory therapy, maxillary expansion, and weight loss.

- Overnight polysomnography remains the gold standard for objective diagnosis of pediatric OSA and is important in reassessment of severity after treatment.

- Pediatric criteria for mild, moderate, and severe sleep apnea are different from adult criteria because a lower threshold is held for abnormal.

- When a diagnosis of mild sleep apnea is made in a child, the treatment plan should be made in parallel with the severity of ongoing symptoms.

References

American Academy of Sleep Medicine: International Classification of Sleep Disorders, 3rd Edition. Darien, IL, American Academy of Sleep Medicine, 2014

Berry RB, Brooks R, Gamaldo CE, et al: AASM Manual for the Scoring of Sleep and Associated Events: Rules, Terminology and Technical Specifications. Version 2.5. Darien, IL, American Academy of Sleep Medicine, 2018

Bhattacharjee R, Kheirandish-Gozal L, Spruyt K, et al: Adenotonsillectomy outcomes in treatment of obstructive sleep apnea in children: a multicenter retrospective study. Am J Respir Crit Care Med 182(5):676–683, 2010 20448096

Camacho M, Certal V, Abdullatif J, et al: Myofunctional therapy to treat obstructive sleep apnea: a systematic review and meta-analysis. Sleep (Basel) 38(5):669–675, 2015 25348130

Carroll JL, Donnelly DF: Respiratory physiology and pathophysiology during sleep, in Principles and Practice of Pediatric Sleep Medicine. Edited by Sheldon SH, Ferber R, Kryger MH, et al. London, Elsevier Saunders, 2014, pp 179–194

Chervin RD, Weatherly RA, Ruzicka DL, et al: Subjective sleepiness and polysomnographic correlates in children scheduled for adenotonsillectomy vs other surgical care. Sleep 29(4):495–503, 2006 16676783

Chervin RD, Weatherly RA, Garetz SL, et al: Pediatric sleep questionnaire: prediction of sleep apnea and outcomes. Arch Otolaryngol Head Neck Surg 133(3):216–222, 2007 17372077

Chervin RD, Ellenberg SS, Hou X, et al: Prognosis for spontaneous resolution of OSA in children. Chest 148(5):1204–1213, 2015 25811889

Dayyat E, Kheirandish-Gozal L, Sans Capdevila O, et al: Obstructive sleep apnea in children: relative contributions of body mass index and adenotonsillar hypertrophy. Chest 136(1):137–144, 2009 19225059

Dudley KA, Patel SR: Disparities and genetic risk factors in obstructive sleep apnea. Sleep Med 18:96–102, 2016 26428843

Fauroux B, Lavis JF, Nicot F, et al: Facial side effects during noninvasive positive pressure ventilation in children. Intensive Care Med 31(7):965–969, 2005 15924228

Friberg D, Sundquist J, Li X, et al: Sibling risk of pediatric obstructive sleep apnea syndrome and adenotonsillar hypertrophy. Sleep 32(8):1077–1083, 2009 19725259

Friedman M, Tanyeri H, La Rosa M, et al: Clinical predictors of obstructive sleep apnea. Laryngoscope 109:1901–1907, 1999 10591345

Goldbart AD, Goldman JL, Li RC, et al: Differential expression of cysteinyl leukotriene receptors 1 and 2 in tonsils of children with obstructive sleep apnea syndrome or recurrent infection. Chest 126(1):13–18, 2004 15249436

Gozal D: Sleep-disordered breathing and school performance in children. Pediatrics 102(3 Pt 1):616–620, 1998 9738185

Guilleminault C, Khramtsov A: Upper airway resistance syndrome in children: a clinical review. Semin Pediatr Neurol 8(4):207–215, 2001 11768783

Guilleminault C, Eldridge FL, Simmons FB, et al: Sleep apnea in eight children. Pediatrics 58(1):23–30, 1976 934781

Guilleminault C, Palombini L, Pelayo R, et al: Sleepwalking and sleep terrors in prepubertal children: what triggers them? Pediatrics 111(1): e17–e25, 2003

Guilleminault C, Lee JH, Chan A, et al: Non-REM-sleep instability in recurrent sleepwalking in pre-pubertal children. Sleep Med 6(6):515–521, 2005 15994122

Guilleminault C, Huang YS, Glamann C, et al: Adenotonsillectomy and obstructive sleep apnea in children: a prospective survey. Otolaryngol Head Neck Surg 136(2):169–175, 2007 17275534

Guilleminault C, Huang YS, Monteyrol PJ, et al: Critical role of myofascial reeducation in pediatric sleep-disordered breathing. Sleep Med 14(6):518–525, 2013 23522724

Kaditis AG, Alexopoulos EI, Hatzi F, et al: Adiposity in relation to age as predictor of severity of sleep apnea in children with snoring. Sleep Breath 12(1):25–31, 2008 17684780

Kaditis A, Kheirandish-Gozal L, Gozal D: Algorithm for the diagnosis and treatment of pediatric OSA: a proposal of two pediatric sleep centers. Sleep Med 13(3):217–227, 2012 22300748

Kaditis AG, Alonso Alvarez ML, Boudewyns A, et al: Obstructive sleep disordered breathing in 2- to 18-year-old children: diagnosis and management. Eur Respir J 47(1):69–94, 2016 26541535

Kang KT, Chou CH, Weng WC, et al: Associations between adenotonsillar hypertrophy, age, and obesity in children with obstructive sleep apnea. PLoS One 8(10):e78666, 2013 24205291

Kiris M, Muderris T, Celebi S, et al: Changes in serum IGF-1 and IGFBP-3 levels and growth in children following adenoidectomy, tonsillectomy or adenotonsillectomy. Int J Pediatr Otorhinolaryngol 74(5):528–531, 2010 20303184

Kovacevic L, Wolfe-Christensen C, Lu H, et al: Why does adenotonsillectomy not correct enuresis in all children with sleep disordered breathing? J Urol 191(5 suppl):1592–1596, 2014 24679871

Li AM, Zhu Y, Au CT, et al: Natural history of primary snoring in school-aged children: a 4-year follow-up study. Chest 143(3):729–735, 2013 23099418

Linder-Aronson S, Leighton BC: A longitudinal study of the development of the posterior nasopharyngeal wall between 3 and 16 years of age. Eur J Orthod 5(1):47–58, 1983 6572594

Lopes MC, Guilleminault C: Chronic snoring and sleep in children: a demonstration of sleep disruption. Pediatrics 118(3):e741–e746, 2006 16950965

Lumeng JC, Chervin RD: Epidemiology of pediatric obstructive sleep apnea. Proc Am Thorac Soc 5(2):242–252, 2008 18250218

Marcus CL, Rosen G, Ward SL, et al: Adherence to and effectiveness of positive airway pressure therapy in children with obstructive sleep apnea. Pediatrics 117(3):e442–e451, 2006 16510622

Marcus CL, Brooks LJ, Draper KA, et al: Diagnosis and management of childhood obstructive sleep apnea syndrome. Pediatrics 130(3):576–584, 2012 22926173

Marcus CL, Moore RH, Rosen CL, et al: A randomized trial of adenotonsillectomy for childhood sleep apnea. N Engl J Med 368(25):2366–2376, 2013 23692173

Mitchell RB, Boss EF: Pediatric obstructive sleep apnea in obese and normal-weight children: impact of adenotonsillectomy on quality-of-life and behavior. Dev Neuropsychol 34(5):650–661, 2009 20183725

Pirelli P, Saponara M, Guilleminault C: Rapid maxillary expansion (RME) for pediatric obstructive sleep apnea: a 12-year follow-up. Sleep Med 16(8):933–935, 2015 26141004

Redline S, Tishler PV, Schluchter M, et al: Risk factors for sleep-disordered breathing in children. Associations with obesity, race, and respiratory problems. Am J Respir Crit Care Med 159(5 Pt 1):1527–1532, 1999 10228121

Roberts SD, Kapadia H, Greenlee G, Chen ML: Midfacial and dental changes associated with nasal positive airway pressure in children with obstructive sleep apnea and craniofacial conditions. J Clin Sleep Med 12(4):469–475, 2016 26715402

Ruiter ME, DeCoster J, Jacobs L, Lichstein KL: Sleep disorders in African Americans and Caucasian Americans: a meta-analysis. Behav Sleep Med 8(4):246–259, 2010 20924837

Scadding G: Non-surgical treatment of adenoidal hypertrophy: the role of treating IgE-mediated inflammation. Pediatr Allergy Immunol 21(8):1095–1106, 2010 20609137

Stewart MG, Glaze DG, Friedman EM, et al: Quality of life and sleep study findings after adenotonsillectomy in children with obstructive sleep apnea. Arch Otolaryngol Head Neck Surg 131(4):308–314, 2005 15837898

Tauman R, Gulliver TE, Krishna J, et al: Persistence of obstructive sleep apnea syndrome in children after adenotonsillectomy. J Pediatr 149(6):803–808, 2006 17137896

Vale F, Albergaria M, Carrilho E, et al: Efficacy of rapid maxillary expansion in the treatment of obstructive sleep apnea syndrome: a systematic review with meta-analysis. J Evid Based Dent Pract 17(3):159–168, 2017 28865812

Volsky PG, Woughter MA, Beydoun HA, et al: Adenotonsillectomy vs observation for management of mild obstructive sleep apnea in children. Otolaryngol Head Neck Surg 150(1):126–132, 2014 24170659

CHAPTER 10

Sleep-Related Hypoventilation Syndromes

William Auyeung, M.D.
Michelle Cao, D.O.

Sleep-related hypoventilation refers to an impairment in ventilation during sleep that causes elevations in arterial partial pressure of carbon dioxide ($PaCO_2$) levels. The causes of sleep-related hypoventilation are numerous. The 3rd edition of the *International Classification of Sleep Disorders* placed sleep-related hypoventilation as a separate category from sleep-related hypoxemia (American Academy of Sleep Medicine 2014; Kryger et al. 2017). Disorders of sleep-related hypoventilation include congenital central alveolar hypoventilation syndrome (CCHS), late-onset central hypoventilation with hypothalamic dysfunction, idiopathic central alveolar hypoventilation, obesity hypoventilation syndrome, sleep-related alveolar hypoventilation due to a medication or substance, and sleep-related alveolar hypoventilation due to a medical disorder. Awake hypoventilation may or may not be present in these disorders except for obesity hypoventilation syndrome, which requires the demonstration of not only sleep-related but also daytime hypercapnia. Obstructive sleep apnea (OSA; see Chapter 8) may also be present in any of these conditions.

Monitoring of $PaCO_2$ during polysomnography is required to make the diagnosis and is most accurate with arterial blood gas measurement, although surrogates such as transcutaneous or end-tidal carbon dioxide monitors can be used with some caveats. Although not strictly required for adults, $PaCO_2$ monitoring is recommended by the American Academy of Sleep Medicine (AASM) practice guidelines for diagnostic polysomnography in all children (Berry et al. 2018). The *AASM Manual for the Scoring of Sleep and Associated Events* (Berry et al. 2018) defines hypoventilation in adults as an increase in $PaCO_2$ either 1) to a value >55 mm Hg for ≥10 minutes or 2) ≥10 mm Hg above an awake supine value to a value >50 mm Hg for ≥10 minutes. For children, sleep hypoventilation is defined simply as an increase in $PaCO_2$ to a value >50 mm Hg for >25% of total sleep time. However, insurance providers such as Medicare may require awake arterial blood gas testing to document a $PaCO_2$ >45 mm Hg to qualify the patient for a respiratory assist device.

Congenital Central Alveolar Hypoventilation Syndrome

CCHS is a rare autosomal dominant disorder due to mutations in the *PHOX2B* gene (Weese-Mayer et al. 2010). This syndrome is characterized by absent or minimal respiratory responses to hypoxia and hypercapnia despite normal lung and respiratory muscle function, resulting in hypoventilation during sleep but preserved conscious control of ventilation. Voluntary maneuvers such as coughing are preserved. The label of "Ondine's curse" is discouraged due to the negative connotations and nonspecific use in describing noncongenital disorders of central hypoventilation.

CCHS typically presents in the neonatal period as duskiness or cyanosis during sleep without distress, although this may be nonspecific. Milder cases of CCHS may manifest later in adulthood as delayed recovery from general anesthesia or respiratory illnesses or as unexplained seizures during sleep. CCHS is associated with neural crest tumors and defects in the autonomic nervous system. Ophthalmological and cardiac rhythm abnormalities have also been described. Patients with CCHS are cognitively normal unless hypoventilation is poorly managed.

Diagnosis of CCHS requires the presence of sleep-related hypoventilation and a mutation in the *PHOX2B* gene. Other conditions causing central hypoventilation or neuromuscular weakness must be excluded. Most *PHOX2B* mutations are de novo and involve a polyalanine repeat mutation (PARM). The presence of longer PARMs or a non-PARM results in worsened severity. Approximately 1,000 cases worldwide with confirmed *PHOX2B* mutations have been documented, but this is likely an underestimate.

Rapid-Onset Obesity With Hypothalamic Dysfunction, Hypoventilation, and Autonomic Dysregulation

Rapid-onset obesity with hypothalamic dysfunction, hypoventilation, and autonomic dysregulation (ROHHAD) is a rare syndrome of hypoventilation in children that is distinct from CCHS. It is also known as late-onset central hypoventilation syndrome with hypothalamic dysfunction. The discovery of *PHOX2B* mutations allowed CCHS to be distinguished from ROHHAD, although both share features of autonomic dysfunction and an increased risk for neural crest–derived tumors. A genetic basis for ROHHAD has not been identified, and the prevalence is unknown. The finding of lymphocytic infiltrates of the hypothalamus in some affected patients has led to the postulation of an autoimmune etiology (Kryger et al. 2017).

ROHHAD is diagnosed clinically based on a combination of obesity, neural crest tumors, emotional/behavioral disturbances, and hypothalamic dysfunction. *PHOX2B* mutations must be absent (American Academy of Sleep Medicine 2014). The classic description is of a previously normal child between 18 months and 7 years of age who develops hyperphagia with rapid weight gain, typically 20–40 lb over 6–12 months. Affected children also have absent responses to hypoxia and hypercapnia, although the onset of this may be insidious and occur years after the onset of obesity. Children may also have comorbid OSA, and in some cases the diagnosis of OSA may precede that of nocturnal hypoventilation (Reppucci et al. 2016). The associated hypothalamic dysfunction may present variably, for example, as diabetes insipidus, central hypothyroidism, adrenal insufficiency, or hypogonadism. The patient may also have developmental delays or behavioral disturbances, such as violent outbursts, reduced social reciprocity, or cognitive inflexibility.

Obesity Hypoventilation Syndrome

Obesity and hypoventilation with an awake $PaCO_2$ >45 mm Hg are the defining traits of obesity hypoventilation syndrome (OHS). *Obesity* is defined as a BMI >30 kg/m^2 for adults, or a BMI greater than the 95th percentile for age/sex in children. The diagnosis also requires the exclusion of hypoventilation related to another medical condition, substance, or medication. Nocturnal hypoxia is often present but is not part of the diagnostic criteria. Usage of "Pickwickian syndrome" is discouraged due to its misapplication to obese patients without OHS (American Academy of Sleep Medicine 2014). The prevalence in the general population is conservatively estimated to be 0.6%, but the true prevalence remains unknown (Mokhlesi 2010; Olson and Zwillich 2005). Up to 20% of obese patients with OSA have OHS. Conversely, 90% of patients with OHS have comorbid OSA.

The exact pathophysiology is unclear but likely involves a combination of impaired respiratory mechanics related to physical loading of the chest wall, increased dead space fraction of breaths, increased tissue carbon dioxide production, and impaired ventilatory responses to hypoxia and hypercapnia (Olson and Zwillich 2005). Elevated serum bicarbonate levels >27 mEq/L are typically seen and have been proposed as a screening tool, but this measure is not diagnostic by itself (Balachandran et al. 2014). Patients may have awake hypoxia as well. OHS has also been associated with diabetes, hypertension, and heart failure. Affected patients appear to be at higher risk of pulmonary hypertension and both left- and right-sided congestive heart failure compared with BMI-matched control subjects (Berg et al. 2001).

Other Causes of Sleep-Related Hypoventilation

Sleep-related hypoventilation can also be precipitated by substances that either inhibit ventilatory drive ("won't breathe") or impair respiratory mechanics ("can't breathe").

TOXIC AND IATROGENIC CAUSES

Substances that affect ventilatory drive may directly involve the respiratory centers responsible for the rhythmogenesis of breathing or any part of the neurological pathways responsible for responses to hypoxia and hypercapnia. Substances that inhibit ventilatory drive include ethanol, opiates, sedative-hypnotics, and anesthetic agents such as propofol, etomidate, and inhaled organofluorides (e.g., halothane) (American Academy of Sleep Medicine 2014). *Respiratory mechanics* refers to the combination of chest wall compliance, pulmonary parenchymal compliance, and respiratory muscle strength. Some medications may have effects on both ventilatory drive and respiratory mechanics, such as fentanyl, which at high doses inhibits respiratory drive via opioid receptors and impairs respiratory mechanics via increased chest wall rigidity.

NEUROMUSCULAR DISORDERS

Sleep-related hypoventilation may be caused by a medical condition instead of a substance. Mechanisms include impaired respiratory drive, abnormal gas exchange, or worsened respiratory mechanics as previously mentioned, which also includes neuromuscular weakness. Neuromuscular disorders are heterogeneous in onset and severity and include conditions such as neuropathies, motor neuron diseases (e.g., amyotrophic lateral sclerosis [ALS]), neuromuscular junction disorders (e.g., myasthenia gravis), and myopathies such as muscular or myotonic dystrophies. Neuromuscular patients generally have an intact respiratory drive but have low minute ventilation that is exacerbated during sleep due to low inspired tidal volumes from respiratory muscle weakness. Notably, respiratory failure is the primary cause of death in most patients with neuromuscular disease, such as ALS.

PULMONARY DISEASE AND OTHER CAUSES OF SLEEP-RELATED HYPOVENTILATION

Respiratory mechanics are also dependent on the size and compliance of the thoracic cavity. For example, severe kyphoscoliosis may cause reduced thoracic volume and thus reduced tidal volumes. Causes of abnormal gas exchange include abnormal airways, lung parenchyma, or lung perfusion. An example of this is chronic obstructive pulmonary disease (COPD), in which destruction of the capillary bed within the lungs leads to reduced efficiency of carbon dioxide removal for each breath. Other medical conditions may not have a specific mechanism but instead are related to global metabolism, such as severe hypothyroidism. Congenital causes of sleep-related hypoventilation should also be excluded.

Treatment

GENERAL PRINCIPLES

Treatment of sleep-related hypoventilation involves augmenting ventilation, managing comorbid conditions, and treating the underlying cause when possible. Offending substances such as opiates or sedatives should be down-titrated or discontinued when possible. Supplemental oxygen alone is not recommended because it can depress the hypoxic ventilatory drive to breathe and subsequently worsen hypoventilation. Continuous positive airway pressure (CPAP) devices are designed to treat upper airway obstruction (i.e., OSA) and generally should not be used to treat patients with hypoventilation or respiratory impairment. Noninvasive positive pressure ventilation (NIPPV) is recommended for hypoventilation syndromes and hypercapnic respiratory failure syndromes. NIPPV involves bilevel positive airway pressure (BPAP) delivered via nasal or full-face mask. The difference between the inspiratory positive airway pressure (PAP) and expiratory PAP is called "pressure support" and is needed to augment tidal volume.

Volume assured pressure support (VAPS), a specialized mode of NIPPV, delivers a clinician-specified tidal volume (6–10 mL/kg ideal body weight) by adjusting the pressure support over a series of breaths. VAPS modes are available on specific respiratory assist devices and portable home mechanical ventilators. Respiratory assist devices, such as BPAP with backup respiratory rate and VAPS, are designed to guarantee a minimum respiratory rate in order to control and optimize nocturnal ventilation. Separately, auto or adapt servo ventilation devices should not be used in patients with hypoventilation because servo ventilation algorithms are designed to reduce average minute ventilation below the patient's resting minute ventilation in order to stabilize periodic breathing, resulting in relative hypoventilation.

Portable home mechanical ventilators can be used in the outpatient setting where ventilation must be ensured to prevent progressive hypercapnic respiratory failure, such as in patients with CCHS or neuromuscular disease. The primary advantage of a portable ventilator is the internal battery, which allows for continued function in the home setting even in the event of a power failure as well as for ambulatory purposes such as when traveling. Respiratory assist devices are dependent on power from an electrical grid and are thus unsuitable for dedicated life-support applications. Portable home ventilators also provide the option of daytime NIPPV for patients who need diurnal ventilatory support (via mouthpiece ventilation or mask interface), whereas respiratory assist devices are designed for nocturnal use. Negative pressure body ventilators have fallen out of favor with advances in NIPPV support devices. The details of home mechanical ventilation initiation and support, such as logistics and provider responsibility, are not discussed here.

Although polysomnography can be used to document nocturnal hypercapnia and sleep-disordered breathing in patients with sleep-related hypoventilation, its most important value lies in the titration portion to optimize nocturnal ventilation. This involves adjustment of expiratory PAP to overcome any airway obstruction and, most importantly, adjustment of inspiratory pressures to augment tidal volumes, reduce hypercapnia, and optimize synchronization of patient and device. A low amount of expiratory pressure is needed to deliver ventilation by providing upper airway patency. High expiratory pressures can increase the work of breathing in specific conditions, such as neuromuscular disease or diaphragmatic impairment. In the specific case of neuromuscular disease, electromyographic monitoring of respiratory muscles such as the scalene and sternocleidomastoid muscles is performed to demonstrate reduction in the work of breathing during sleep while on NIPPV. These titration studies should be performed in an accredited sleep laboratory with experienced personnel trained in advanced titration protocols, with real-time monitoring of carbon dioxide.

TREATMENT OF SLEEP-RELATED HYPOVENTILATION DUE TO CCHS AND ROHHAD

Patients with CCHS and ROHHAD inevitably require dedicated ventilatory support during sleep and may also require daytime ventilatory support. Patients with CCHS do not respond to respiratory stimulants and cannot be trained to overcome their hypoventilation. Thus, mechanical ventilation via tracheostomy is recommended from the neonatal period through childhood. Older children with CCHS who only require nocturnal ventilation may be transitioned to nighttime noninvasive ventilation via nasal or face mask in conjunction with the option of diaphragmatic pacing. The severity of hypoventilation in ROHHAD can be variable at the time of diagnosis but progresses over time, with many needing long-term, continuous mechanical ventilation via tracheostomy (Ize-Ludlow et al. 2007). Sleep-related hypoventilation in ROHHAD does not improve with weight loss, unlike in OHS. Case reports exist of improvement in behavioral symptoms with cyclophosphamide immunosuppression, but the efficacy for treating hypoventilation has not been studied (Jacobson et al. 2016; Paz-Priel et al. 2011). Screening for neural crest–derived tumors is recommended for patients with either CCHS or ROHHAD. Long-term outcomes for these patients are not well studied.

TREATMENT OF SLEEP-RELATED HYPOVENTILATION DUE TO OBESITY HYPOVENTILATION SYNDROME

Patients with OHS may be successfully treated with either CPAP therapy or NIPPV via BPAP. It is unclear whether BPAP is superior to CPAP for improving daytime hypercapnia, sleep quality, or quality of life (Howard et al. 2017; Masa et al. 2015; Piper et al. 2008). Lifestyle modification with caloric restriction and exercise may modestly improve daytime hypercapnia but is overall less effective than noninvasive ventilation (Masa et al. 2015). Nevertheless, lifestyle modification is an important adjunct to any therapeutic plan. CPAP is considered the first-line treatment option for most patients with OHS. Patients should be followed closely to monitor improvements in gas exchange and oxygenation. For patients who continue to have nocturnal hypoxia, persistent hypoventilation, or daytime symptoms despite optimal CPAP therapy, noninvasive ventilation such as BPAP should be considered. Supplemental oxygen should not be used as the sole treatment modality for OHS because this may worsen hypercapnia (Hollier et al. 2014; Wijesinghe et al. 2011). Bariatric surgery may be an option for patients with OHS for whom lifestyle modification has been ineffective. Respiratory stimulants such as progestins (e.g., medroxyprogesterone) or carbonic anhydrase inhibitors (e.g., acetazolamide) have shown limited success in small case series but should not be considered as first-line therapy because they cannot treat comorbid OSA (Mokhlesi and Tulaimat 2007).

TREATMENT OF SLEEP-RELATED HYPOVENTILATION DUE TO NEUROMUSCULAR DISORDERS

NIPPV in patients with neuromuscular disease has been shown to provide a survival benefit as well as improved quality of life. Patients with ALS or Duchenne muscular dystrophy (DMD) treated with NIPPV have demonstrated prolonged survival at 2-year follow-up in small randomized studies. Historically, respiratory failure was the leading cause of death in patients with DMD, so the introduction of NIPPV was truly revolutionary and doubled their median survival (Vianello et al. 1994). However, prophylactic use of NIPPV in patients with DMD without symptoms or evidence of hypoventilation has not been shown to postpone the onset of respiratory failure (Mehta and Hill 2001). Patients with ALS who were placed on NIPPV have improved survival and quality of life compared with those receiving care without ventilatory support, and subanalysis revealed that patients with relatively preserved bulbar function experienced the greatest benefit from NIPPV, with an increase in median survival of 205 days (Bourke et al. 2006). One case series of patients with ALS has shown prolonged survival of patients receiving ventilation via tracheostomy compared with those receiving NIPPV, with some surviving beyond 10 years (Cazzolli and Oppenheimer 1996). However, with impressive technological advances in NIPPV and its ability to support a patient's ventilatory failure diurnally, tracheostomy is no longer the recommended route.

Titration of NIPPV in patients with neuromuscular disease should be performed in the sleep lab to achieve adequate minute ventilation and limit respiratory muscle fatigue. Otherwise, comprehensive management of these patients also involves attention to airway clearance strategies to prevent aspiration pneumonia, typically involving mechanical cough-assist devices. Patients with neuromuscular disease who develop respiratory infections may develop worsening hypoventilation that may exceed the support provided by their current NIPPV settings and therefore must be monitored carefully.

TREATMENT OF SLEEP-RELATED HYPOVENTILATION DUE TO CHRONIC OBSTRUCTIVE PULMONARY DISEASE

Treatment of hypoventilation due to COPD with nocturnal high-intensity NIPPV may be of benefit. High-intensity NIPPV refers to implementation of very high inspiratory PAP and low expiratory PAP, with a pressure support of ≥15 cm of water as well as the addition of a high backup respiratory rate, with the goal of guaranteeing minute ventilation and normalizing hypercapnia. Earlier studies of NIPPV in patients with stable COPD without high-intensity pressure support have shown contradictory effects on blood gas measurements, sleep quality, and sleep duration, although patients with greater hypercapnia and better tolerance of NIPPV may have derived more benefit (Mehta and Hill 2001). Use of high-intensity NIPPV in these patients tends to improve respiratory quality of life but not sleep quality (Dreher et al. 2010; Murphy et al. 2012; Weir et al. 2015). Randomized controlled trials are conflicting but suggest readmission rates are lowered and long-term survival is improved when patients with stable but severe COPD and daytime hypercapnia are treated with high-intensity NIPPV (Köhnlein et al. 2014; Murphy et al. 2017; Struik et al. 2014).

Conclusion

Timely implementation of NIPPV has resulted in improved survival and quality of life in patients with congenital disorders of hypoventilation and neuromuscular diseases. Although polysomnography can diagnose sleep-related hypoventilation and sleep-disordered breathing, including OSA, its value lies in the titration portion, which is used to determine the best settings for NIPPV to optimize nocturnal ventilatory support and reduce the work of breathing. This is especially true for patients with neuromuscular disease for whom optimization also involves offloading the work of breathing at night in order to improve daytime function. Otherwise, management of sleep-related hypoventilation should involve treating the underlying condition and any comorbid conditions, such as OSA.

KEY CLINICAL POINTS

- Polysomnography is recommended to detect nocturnal elevations in arterial carbon dioxide to make the diagnosis of sleep-related hypoventilation.

- The optimal settings for ventilatory support devices should be determined using the titration portion of a sleep study, rather than empirically.

- Bilevel and continuous positive airway pressure are both effective at improving daytime hypercapnia, sleep quality, and quality of life in patients with obesity hypoventilation syndrome.

- Noninvasive positive pressure ventilation (NIPPV) for patients with neuromuscular disease such as Duchenne muscular dystrophy and amyotrophic lateral sclerosis has been revolutionary in prolonging their survival, including the ability to provide daytime ventilation.

- High-intensity NIPPV may offer improved survival and reduced readmission rates for a subset of patients with stable severe chronic obstructive pulmonary disease with hypercapnia without obstructive sleep apnea.

- Respiratory assist devices are not meant for dedicated life-support applications; instead, a portable ventilator with an internal battery should be used, such as for patients with congenital central alveolar hypoventilation syndrome or severe neuromuscular disease.

- Supplemental oxygen alone is insufficient for treating hypoventilation and hypoxemia because it may worsen hypercapnia and should be used in conjunction with NIPPV.

References

American Academy of Sleep Medicine (ed): International Classification of Sleep Disorders, 3rd Edition. Darien, IL, American Academy of Sleep Medicine, 2014

Balachandran JS, Masa JF, Mokhlesi B: Obesity hypoventilation syndrome epidemiology and diagnosis. Sleep Med Clin 9(3):341–347, 2014 25360072

Berg G, Delaive K, Manfreda J, et al: The use of health-care resources in obesity-hypoventilation syndrome. Chest 120(2):377–383, 2001 11502632

Berry RB, Claude LA, Harding SM, et al (eds): The AASM Manual for the Scoring of Sleep and Associated Events, Version 2.5. Darien, IL, American Academy of Sleep Medicine, 2018

Bourke SC, Tomlinson M, Williams TL, et al: Effects of non-invasive ventilation on survival and quality of life in patients with amyotrophic lateral sclerosis: a randomised controlled trial. Lancet Neurol 5(2):140–147, 2006 16426990

Cazzolli PA, Oppenheimer EA: Home mechanical ventilation for amyotrophic lateral sclerosis: nasal compared to tracheostomy-intermittent positive pressure ventilation. J Neurol Sci 139(suppl):123–128, 1996 8899671

Dreher M, Storre JH, Schmoor C, et al: High-intensity versus low-intensity non-invasive ventilation in patients with stable hypercapnic COPD: a randomised crossover trial. Thorax 65(4):303–308, 2010 20388753

Hollier CA, Harmer AR, Maxwell LJ, et al: Moderate concentrations of supplemental oxygen worsen hypercapnia in obesity hypoventilation syndrome: a randomised crossover study. Thorax 69(4):346–353, 2014 24253834

Howard ME, Piper AJ, Stevens B, et al: A randomised controlled trial of CPAP versus non-invasive ventilation for initial treatment of obesity hypoventilation syndrome. Thorax 72(5):437–444, 2017

Ize-Ludlow D, Gray JA, Sperling MA, et al: Rapid-onset obesity with hypothalamic dysfunction, hypoventilation, and autonomic dysregulation presenting in childhood. Pediatrics 120(1):e179–e188, 2007 17606542

Jacobson LA, Rane S, McReynolds LJ, et al: Improved behavior and neuropsychological function in children with ROHHAD after high-dose cyclophosphamide. Pediatrics 138(1):e20151080, 2016 27313069

Köhnlein T, Windisch W, Köhler D, et al: Non-invasive positive pressure ventilation for the treatment of severe stable chronic obstructive pulmonary disease: a prospective, multicentre, randomised, controlled clinical trial. Lancet Respir Med 2(9):698–705, 2014 25066329

Kryger M, Roth T, Dement W (eds): Principles and Practice of Sleep Medicine, 6th Edition. Philadelphia, PA, Elsevier, 2017

Masa JF, Corral J, Alonso ML, et al: Efficacy of different treatment alternatives for obesity hypoventilation syndrome. Pickwick study. Am J Respir Crit Care Med 192(1):86–95, 2015 25915102

Mehta S, Hill NS: Noninvasive ventilation. Am J Respir Crit Care Med 163(2):540–577, 2001 11179136

Mokhlesi B: Obesity hypoventilation syndrome: a state-of-the-art review. Respir Care 55(10):1347–1362, discussion 1363–1365, 2010 20875161

Mokhlesi B, Tulaimat A: Recent advances in obesity hypoventilation syndrome. Chest 132(4):1322–1336, 2007 17934118

Murphy PB, Brignall K, Moxham J, et al: High pressure versus high intensity noninvasive ventilation in stable hypercapnic chronic obstructive pulmonary disease: a randomized crossover trial. Int J Chron Obstruct Pulmon Dis 7:811–818, 2012 23271905

Murphy PB, Rehal S, Arbane G, et al: Effect of home noninvasive ventilation with oxygen therapy vs oxygen therapy alone on hospital readmission or death after an acute COPD exacerbation: a randomized clinical trial. JAMA 317(21):2177–2186, 2017 28528348

Olson AL, Zwillich C: The obesity hypoventilation syndrome. Am J Med 118(9):948–956, 2005 16164877

Paz-Priel I, Cooke DW, Chen AR: Cyclophosphamide for rapid-onset obesity, hypothalamic dysfunction, hypoventilation, and autonomic dysregulation syndrome. J Pediatr 158(2):337–339, 2011 20727534

Piper AJ, Wang D, Yee BJ, et al: Randomised trial of CPAP vs bilevel support in the treatment of obesity hypoventilation syndrome without severe nocturnal desaturation. Thorax 63(5):395–401, 2008 18203817

Reppucci D, Hamilton J, Yeh EA, et al: ROHHAD syndrome and evolution of sleep disordered breathing. Orphanet J Rare Dis 11(1):106, 2016 27473663

Struik FM, Sprooten RT, Kerstjens HA, et al: Nocturnal non-invasive ventilation in COPD patients with prolonged hypercapnia after ventilatory support for acute respiratory failure: a randomised, controlled, parallel-group study. Thorax 69(9):826–834, 2014 24781217

Vianello A, Bevilacqua M, Salvador V, et al: Long-term nasal intermittent positive pressure ventilation in advanced Duchenne's muscular dystrophy. Chest 105(2):445–448, 1994 8306744

Weese-Mayer DE, Berry-Kravis EM, Ceccherini I, et al: An official ATS clinical
    policy statement: congenital central hypoventilation syndrome: genetic ba-
    sis, diagnosis, and management. Am J Respir Crit Care Med 181(6):626–644,
    2010 20208042
Weir M, Marchetti N, Czysz A, et al: High intensity non-invasive positive pressure
    ventilation (HINPPV) for stable hypercapnic chronic obstructive pulmonary
    disease (COPD) patients. Chronic Obstr Pulm Dis (Miami) 2(4):313–320, 2015
    28848853
Wijesinghe M, Williams M, Perrin K, et al: The effect of supplemental oxygen on
    hypercapnia in subjects with obesity-associated hypoventilation: a ran-
    domized, crossover, clinical study. Chest 139(5):1018–1024, 2011 20947648

CHAPTER 11

Central Sleep Apneas

Gaurav Singh, M.D., M.P.H.

As opposed to the upper airway obstruction that characterizes obstructive sleep apnea (OSA; see Chapter 8), the key feature of central sleep apnea (CSA) is a lack of drive to breathe while asleep. Therefore, repetitive periods of absent airflow during sleep in patients with CSA are due to a reduction or loss of respiratory effort despite a patent airway, rather than a loss of airway patency (i.e., upper airway obstruction), whereas respiratory effort is preserved among individuals with OSA. As part of the broader category of sleep-related breathing disorders, CSA encompasses various subtypes with different etiologies, pathophysiologies, and treatments. These are reviewed in this chapter.

Diagnostic Criteria

The *International Classification of Sleep Disorders*, 3rd Edition (ICSD-3; American Academy of Sleep Medicine 2014), lists diagnostic criteria for eight different CSA disorders: primary CSA, CSA with Cheyne-Stokes breathing (CSB), CSA due to a medical disorder without CSB, CSA due to a medication or substance, CSA due to high-altitude periodic breathing (HAPB), treatment-emergent (TE)-CSA, primary CSA of infancy, and primary CSA of prematurity.

UNDERLYING CENTRAL SLEEP APNEA DISORDERS, EXCLUDING INFANTS

Diagnostic criteria for underlying CSA conditions, excluding those of infants, are summarized in Table 11–1. Note that symptoms and polysomnographic features are nearly identical for the various CSA disorders,

TABLE 11–1. ICSD-3 criteria for underlying CSA conditions (excluding disorders in infants)

Type of CSA	Symptoms	PSG features	Etiology	Exclusions
Primary[a]	1. Sleepiness 2. Difficulty initiating or maintaining sleep, frequent nocturnal awakenings, or nonrestorative sleep 3. Awakening short of breath 4. Snoring 5. Witnessed apneas	1. CAHI ≥5 2. Total number of central apneas/hypopneas >50% of total number of apneas/hypopneas 3. Absence of CSB	Idiopathic (no daytime or nocturnal hypoventilation)	Not better explained by another current sleep disorder, medical or neurological disorder, medication use (e.g., opiates), or substance use disorder
CSB[b]	Same as primary CSA	Same as primary CSA, except pattern of breathing meets criteria for CSB during diagnostic or PAP titration PSG	Presence of atrial fibrillation/flutter, CHF, or a neurological disorder	Not better explained by another current sleep disorder, medication use (e.g., opiates), or substance use disorder
Medical disorder without CSB[a]	Same as primary CSA	Same as primary CSA	Occurs as consequence of a medical or neurological disorder	Not due to medication or substance use

TABLE 11–1. ICSD-3 criteria for underlying CSA conditions (excluding disorders in infants) *(continued)*

Type of CSA	Symptoms	PSG features	Etiology	Exclusions
Medication or substance[a]	Same as primary CSA	Same as primary CSA	Due to use of opioids or other respiratory depressant	Not better explained by another current cause
High-altitude periodic breathing[c]	Same as primary CSA, except includes awakening with morning headaches and snoring not included	If performed, demonstrates CAHI ≥5 primarily during non-REM sleep	Recent ascent to high altitude	Same as primary CSA

[a]Criteria from all columns are required for diagnosis.
[b]Criteria from *either* "Symptoms" *or* "Etiology," along with "PSG features" and "Exclusions," are required for diagnosis.
[c]PSG is not required for diagnosis if symptoms are clinically attributable to HAPB.
CAHI=central apnea–central hypopnea index; CHF=congestive heart failure; CSA=central sleep apnea; CSB=Cheyne-Stokes breathing; ICSD-3=
International Classification of Sleep Disorders, 3rd Edition; PAP=positive airway pressure; PSG=polysomnography.

aside from some key differences. Awakening with morning headaches is included as a symptom of CSA due to HAPB, whereas snoring is not. Symptoms are discussed further in the "Clinical Presentation, Course, and Complications" section later in this chapter. Polysomnography is not required for diagnosing HAPB if symptoms are clinically attributable to this condition. CSA with CSB requires a pattern of breathing on a diagnostic or positive airway pressure (PAP) titration polysomnogram that meets criteria for CSB, whereas the other CSA subtypes require absence of CSB (American Academy of Sleep Medicine 2014; Berry et al. 2018). This pattern and polysomnography criteria for CSA disorders are discussed further in the "Diagnostic Procedures and Testing" section.

TREATMENT-EMERGENT CSA

Diagnosis of TE-CSA requires *both* diagnostic polysomnography demonstrating five or more predominantly obstructive respiratory events (obstructive or mixed apneas, hypopneas, or respiratory effort related arousals) per hour of sleep *and* polysomnography while receiving PAP without a backup rate demonstrating resolution of obstructive events and emergence or persistence of central events. Specifically, diagnosis requires a central apnea–central hypopnea index (CAHI) of ≥5 events per hour, *and* 50% or more of the total number of apneas and hypopneas must be of central etiology. Finally, the CSA cannot be better explained by another CSA disorder (e.g., CSA with CSB or CSA due to a medication or substance) (American Academy of Sleep Medicine 2014).

CSA DISORDERS IN INFANTS

ICSD-3 also includes two CSA conditions seen in infants. Primary CSA of infancy occurs in infants with a conceptional age of ≥37 weeks at the time of symptom onset, whereas primary CSA of prematurity occurs in infants with a conceptional age <37 weeks at onset. Clinical features of both conditions include apneas or cyanosis witnessed by an observer or an episode of central apnea or desaturation noted by monitoring during sleep. A unique feature of the latter disorder is bradycardia detected by monitoring during sleep. Polysomnography or alternative monitoring demonstrates either recurrent prolonged central apneas (>20 seconds) or periodic breathing for ≥5% of total sleep time. Finally, either disorder cannot be better explained by another sleep disorder, medical or neurological disorder, or medication. CSA disorders in infants are not discussed further here but are reviewed in detail elsewhere (American Academy of Sleep Medicine 2014).

Pathophysiology

CSA is characterized by a reduction or loss of respiratory effort during sleep that results in repetitive periods of absent airflow. Different mechanisms may lead to cessation of ventilatory effort during sleep. A classification system of CSA based on carbon dioxide levels and degree of ventilation is discussed in the following sections. First, a brief review of normal respiratory physiology during sleep is presented to place CSA pathophysiology in context. Table 11–2 provides a summary of relevant CSA pathophysiology.

NORMAL RESPIRATORY PHYSIOLOGY DURING SLEEP

Behavioral control of respiration is lost during sleep, and breathing is regulated primarily by metabolic control, which is determined by pH, arterial partial pressure of oxygen (PaO_2), and arterial partial pressure of carbon dioxide ($PaCO_2$). Hypercapnia is a more potent stimulus of ventilation than hypoxemia, but ventilatory responses to either stimulus decline during progressive stages of sleep, with the most diminished responses occurring during REM sleep. PaO_2 decreases by 2–12 mm Hg and $PaCO_2$ increases by 2–8 mm Hg during sleep. The set point for response to $PaCO_2$, known as the *apneic threshold*, which is typically 1–2 mm Hg below eucapnic levels during wakefulness, also rises during sleep but normally remains 2–6 mm Hg below eucapnic sleep levels. Ventilation occurs at $PaCO_2$ levels above the apneic threshold but ceases when $PaCO_2$ falls below it, resulting in apnea. *Loop gain* refers to feedback mechanisms that stabilize ventilation and maintain $PaCO_2$ within a range suitable for normal breathing. Loop gain comprises controller gain (chemoresponsiveness and ventilatory response to changes in $PaCO_2$ and PaO_2) and plant gain (efficiency of carbon dioxide elimination by the lungs and respiratory muscles).

PATHOLOGICAL MECHANISMS OF CSA DURING SLEEP

CSA may result when this tightly regulated respiratory control system is perturbed due to high loop gain, which causes $PaCO_2$ levels to repeatedly oscillate above and below the apneic threshold. These fluctuations induce hyperventilation and apnea, respectively. Factors that contribute to high loop gain include increased chemoreceptor responsiveness to hy-

TABLE 11–2.   Pathophysiology of CSA disorders

Type of central sleep apnea	CO$_2$/Ventilation level	Primary mechanisms involved*	Awake PaCO$_2$ and HCO$_3$ levels	Most common sleep stages
Primary	Nonhypercapnic/Hyperventilation	↑ Chemoresponsiveness ↑ Ventilatory drive ↓ Arousal threshold ↓ HAT/PaCO$_2$ difference	Normal or ↓	N1/N2
CSB	Nonhypercapnic/Hyperventilation	↑ Chemoresponsiveness ↑ Ventilatory drive ↑ Circulation time (i.e., delay) ↓ O$_2$ stores	Normal or ↓	N1/N2
Medical disorder without CSB	Hypercapnic/Hypoventilation	↓ Chemoresponsiveness	Normal or ↑	REM
Medication or substance	Hypercapnic/Hypoventilation	↓ Chemoresponsiveness	Normal or ↑	Non-REM, including N3
High-altitude periodic breathing	Nonhypercapnic/Hyperventilation	↑ Chemoresponsiveness (for hypoxia) ↑ Ventilatory drive ↓ O$_2$ stores	Normal or ↓	N1/N2
Treatment-emergent	Nonhypercapnic/Hyperventilation	↓ Upper airway resistance ↑ Chemoresponsiveness ↓ Arousal threshold ↓ HAT/PaCO$_2$ difference	Normal or ↓	N1/N2

Note. ↑ =increased; ↓ =decreased; CSB=Cheyne-Stokes breathing; CO$_2$=carbon dioxide; HAT=hypocapnic-apneic threshold; HCO$_3$=serum bicarbonate; PaCO$_2$=arterial partial pressure of carbon dioxide.
*Not a comprehensive list. The most prominent mechanisms are included.

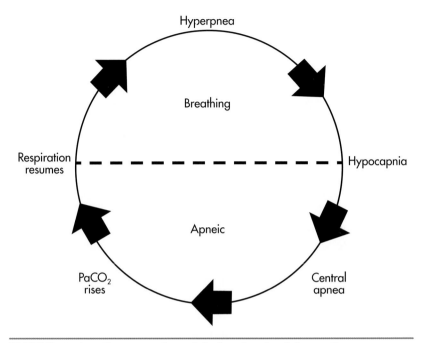

FIGURE 11–1. **Conceptual model of pathophysiology of nonhypercapnic central sleep apnea disorders.**

Circle represents carbon dioxide levels, and *dashed line* represents apneic threshold. Various stimuli can trigger hyperpnea (e.g., arousals, hypoxia, pulmonary congestion, increased sympathetic tone), which may cause ventilatory overshoot and hypocapnia, particularly with increased ventilatory drive. Arterial partial pressure of carbon dioxide ($PaCO_2$) levels drop below apneic threshold, inducing central apnea. This is more likely if sleeping $PaCO_2$ levels are close to the threshold. $PaCO_2$ then rises above the threshold, and respiration resumes. Hyperpnea recurs because of increased chemoresponsiveness.

percapnia and hypoxemia, increased ventilatory drive, unstable sleep with a low arousal threshold, a small difference between the apneic threshold and $PaCO_2$ levels during sleep, and decreased oxygen stores (Figure 11–1). A factor specific to CSA due to CSB contributing to high loop gain is delayed circulatory time, which may result from decreased cardiac output due to heart failure or atrial fibrillation. The other CSA disorders listed in ICSD-3 that are a result of high loop gain include primary CSA, HAPB, and TE-CSA.

Loop gain is higher when the ventilatory control system is unstable, which is more common during sleep-wake transitions as well as during non-REM (NREM) sleep, particularly stages N1 and N2 sleep. This applies to additional CSA subtypes not listed in ICSD-3—sleep-onset and postarousal central apneas—which are not necessarily pathological unless they lead to symptoms, such as sleep disturbance or insomnia. In contrast, CSA is less common during REM sleep due to an increased neurally mediated ventilatory drive but decreased chemoresponsiveness to $PaCO_2$, as well as increased separation between the apneic threshold and eucapnic $PaCO_2$ levels. Collectively, these CSA subtypes caused by high loop gain and hyperventilation are classified as nonhypercapnic CSA disorders, and the relevant pathophysiology is discussed in further detail in subsequent sections. The patient's awake $PaCO_2$ level is normal or may be decreased in such conditions, and the serum bicarbonate level may be low due to metabolic compensation for chronic respiratory alkalosis.

In contrast, CSA disorders due to hypoventilation during sleep are classified as hypercapnic CSA disorders, which are a result of decreased ventilatory response to hypercapnia. $PaCO_2$ is increased during sleep and possibly during wakefulness as well. The relevant subtypes include CSA due to medical disorders without CSB, such as functional or structural abnormalities of ventilatory control centers, and CSA due to a medication or substance (i.e., narcotics). These are further reviewed later in the chapter. Primary alveolar hypoventilation due to decreased chemoreceptor responsiveness may also induce central apnea. Sleep-related hypoventilation disorders are covered in Chapter 10.

Primary CSA

The etiology of primary CSA is unknown (i.e., idiopathic). Alternative classification should be used if a known medical/neurological disorder or medication is thought to be responsible, and no evidence of daytime or nocturnal hypoventilation should be present. Thus, primary CSA is a diagnosis of exclusion. Increased ventilatory drive and responsiveness to hypercapnia are believed to be the main predisposing factors for primary CSA. Other suspected mechanisms include frequent awakenings from sleep (i.e., a low arousal threshold), which lead to ventilatory instability with increased ventilation as well as a small difference between the apneic threshold and sleeping $PaCO_2$ levels. The end result is a decrease in $PaCO_2$ below the apneic threshold, resulting in central apnea. Awake $PaCO_2$ values are also often low (<40 mm Hg; American Academy of Sleep Medicine 2014). Central apneas occur most commonly during stages N1 and N2 sleep, when the respiratory control system is more unstable, as opposed to stage N3 or REM sleep.

CSA With Cheyne-Stokes Breathing

The most common cause of CSA with CSB is congestive heart failure with either systolic or diastolic dysfunction. Other etiologies include stroke (especially in the acute period), other neurological disorders, renal failure, and idiopathic CSA. The major mechanisms responsible for ventilatory instability in CSA with CSB include high ventilatory drive and hypercapnic chemosensitivity, as well as circulatory delay due to low cardiac output (i.e., increased circulation time). The former is thought to be related to pulmonary congestion causing stimulation of vagal irritant receptors, as well as reduced carotid artery blood flow causing increased sympathetic tone. The latter mechanism results in delayed detection of increased $PaCO_2$ in the lungs by the central chemoreceptors in the carotid bodies and brain stem, causing "ventilatory overshoot" and periodic breathing. Lower $PaCO_2$ levels during wakefulness and sleep (<40 mm Hg), with values closer to the apneic threshold, also contribute to CSA with CSB. Low oxygen stores play a role as well. The CSB pattern occurs more commonly during transition from wakefulness to NREM sleep and during stages N1 and N2 sleep.

CSA Due to a Medical Disorder Without Cheyne-Stokes Breathing

The most common disorders causing CSA without CSB are brain stem lesions, which may be due to various conditions. Stroke, Chiari malformation, malignancy, and multiple system atrophy are notable examples of neurological disorders that can produce CSA. Dysfunction of the respiratory control centers in the CNS, resulting in failure of ventilatory effort, is the underlying mechanism of CSA. Although sometimes present while awake, this may only be evident during sleep due to loss of wakefulness stimulus to breathe. Hypoventilation during sleep and at times during wakefulness results in hypercapnia. Blunted ventilatory response to elevated $PaCO_2$ (i.e., pathologically low loop gain) is present. Hypercapnic CSA may be more common in REM sleep due to atonia of accessory respiratory muscles.

CSA Due to a Medication or Substance

The most common medications that induce CSA are opiates, including methadone, long-acting forms of morphine and oxycodone, fentanyl patches, continuous narcotic infusions, buprenorphine, and naloxone. These medications and other respiratory depressants are thought to blunt chemoreflexes due to direct effects on respiratory centers in the brain stem, such as the μ-receptors of the ventral medulla. Depression of hypercapnic and hypoxic respiratory drive, which may be apparent during wakefulness in addition to sleep, is often dose dependent. Central apneas occur mainly during NREM sleep, including during stage N3, unlike other CSA subtypes.

CSA Due to High Altitude Periodic Breathing

Recent ascent to altitude is the main precipitating factor for developing HAPB, and it is universal at higher altitudes (>4,000 m). About one-quarter of people experience periodic breathing at 2,500 m altitude, and some as low as 1,500 m (American Academy of Sleep Medicine 2014). An increased hypoxic ventilatory drive is thought to be responsible in predisposed individuals. Hypoxemia from decreased atmospheric pressure stimulates hyperventilation and thus hypocapnia, with $PaCO_2$ levels dropping below apneic threshold and producing central apneas. Ventilation resumes when $PaCO_2$ rises during central apneas, but periodic breathing recurs. Central apneas occur predominantly during NREM sleep and improve during REM sleep as a result of decreased ventilatory responsiveness to hypoxia and hypercapnia in this stage.

Treatment-Emergent CSA

TE-CSA is characterized by the development of central apneas when PAP without a backup rate is applied in patients with predominantly underlying OSA. It is also described in patients with OSA treated with upper airway surgery, tracheostomy, or an oral appliance. Relief of upper airway resistance by PAP therapy leads to enhanced elimination of carbon dioxide, potentially inducing central apneas if levels fall below apneic threshold. Other putative factors include a high ventilatory response to $PaCO_2$, a small difference between sleeping $PaCO_2$ values and the apneic threshold, and a low arousal threshold. Also, PAP therapy activates stretch receptors in the lung, which inhibits central respiratory output to prevent overinflation of the lung (i.e., Hering-Breuer inflation reflex). Central apneas in this condition are more common in sleep stages N1 and N2 and improve during stage N3 and REM sleep.

Epidemiology (Prevalence and Risk Factors)

CSA is present in about 1% of the general population, with about half of cases related to CSB (Donovan and Kapur 2016). CSA accounts for 5%–10% of all sleep-disordered breathing, most of which is due to OSA (Muza 2015). Overall, central apneas are more common in men (7.8%) than in women (0.3%) and in those older than 65 years of age (1.1%) than in younger adults (0.4%) (Bixler et al. 1998, 2001).

PRIMARY CSA

Primary CSA is believed to be a rare condition more common in males and older individuals who are not typically obese (Muza 2015). Elevated ventilatory chemoresponsiveness is the only identified risk factor.

CSA WITH CHEYNE-STOKES BREATHING

CSA with CSB is common in patients with congestive heart failure, ranging from 27% in those with preserved ejection fraction (Herrscher et al. 2011) to 44% in those with reduced ejection fraction among those with stable, compensated heart failure (Solin et al. 1999). There is a notable male predominance. Other risk factors in this group include age >60 years, presence of atrial fibrillation, and daytime hypocapnia (Pa-CO_2 <38 mm Hg) (Sin et al. 1999).

CSA DUE TO A MEDICAL DISORDER WITHOUT CHEYNE-STOKES BREATHING

Prevalence and affected age groups depend on the etiology of the underlying medical disorder. In addition to the conditions mentioned earlier (see "Pathophysiology"), other conditions associated with this CSA subtype include renal failure, pulmonary hypertension, chronic obstructive pulmonary disease, and interstitial lung disease.

CSA DUE TO A MEDICATION OR SUBSTANCE

Chronic use of long-acting, potent opiates is the main risk factor for CSA due to a medication or substance, affecting about one-quarter of patients. The opioid dose seems to be directly associated with severity of CSA (Correa et al. 2015). No age or sex predilection has been identified.

CSA DUE TO HIGH-ALTITUDE PERIODIC BREATHING

As previously mentioned, HAPB occurs in essentially everyone at higher altitudes, but some individuals are predisposed to developing it at lower elevations. Other possible risk factors include faster speed of ascent, male sex, and older age.

TREATMENT-EMERGENT CSA

The prevalence of TE-CSA is 5%–20% among patients with OSA treated with PAP during either a titration or split-night sleep study (Nigam et al. 2016). Risk factors include male sex, higher baseline OSA severity, presence of central apneas during initial diagnostic study, higher continuous positive airway pressure (CPAP), use of bilevel positive airway pressure (BPAP), supine sleep position, and high altitude.

Clinical Presentation, Course, and Complications

CLINICAL PRESENTATION

Patients with CSA may present with symptoms similar to OSA, with hypersomnia or insomnia phenotypes. Symptoms may include excessive daytime sleepiness, fatigue, sleep fragmentation with poor subjective sleep quality, frequent awakenings (sometimes with shortness of breath), nonrestorative sleep, snoring, witnessed apneas, and morning headaches. Patients may also report symptoms of the underlying disorder associated with development of CSA. Central apneas may be observed in asymptomatic individuals, but symptoms are required to make a diagnosis of a CSA disorder, per ICSD-3 criteria (American Academy of Sleep Medicine 2014).

COURSE

Prospective longitudinal studies evaluating the natural history of CSA are lacking. CSA with or without CSB may develop abruptly after stroke, but this is often self-limited, with transition to OSA. Opioid-induced CSA typically develops with 2 months or more of chronic medication use, and it may improve after 5–8 months of continued use (American Academy of Sleep Medicine 2014). HAPB is usually most prominent the first night at elevation. Symptoms may improve with acclimatization at lower altitudes. Based on observational studies, TE-CSA persists in 14%–46% of patients who demonstrate this finding on initial PAP treatment and develops weeks to months later in 1%–4% of patients who did not initially have it. The overall prevalence of persistent TE-CSA among those treated for OSA is 1%–3% (Nigam et al. 2018).

COMPLICATIONS

Little evidence has shown that CSA, other than when associated with CSB, is associated with significant adverse outcomes, such as increased mortality, development of pulmonary hypertension or cor pulmonale, or other adverse cardiovascular effects. Evidence for adverse outcomes among patients with CSB is conflicting, but some studies demonstrate an increased mortality in the setting of systolic dysfunction and CSA with CSB (Javaheri et al. 2007). Increased mortality is also associated with opioid use, but this has not been demonstrated to be specifically due to CSA.

Diagnostic Procedures and Testing

Polysomnography is mandatory for a diagnosis of CSA, with an overnight, attended sleep study being the gold standard. Home sleep testing has not been validated for diagnosis of CSA.

GENERAL POLYSOMNOGRAPHY FEATURES

Central apnea in adults is defined as a decrease in peak airflow amplitude by ≥90% compared with baseline breathing that lasts ≥10 seconds, with respiratory effort absent throughout , although cardioballistic artifact or oscillations may be observed (Figure 11–2A). Polysomnography demonstrates five or more central apneas or hypopneas per hour of sleep, with the number being >50% of the total number of apneas and hypopneas. Scoring hypopneas as obstructive or central is optional, per the American Academy of Sleep Medicine (AASM) scoring manual (Berry et al. 2018). To score a hypopnea as central, *all* of the following must be *absent*: 1) snoring during event, 2) increased inspiratory flattening of nasal pressure or PAP device flow signal compared with baseline breathing, and 3) thoracoabdominal paradox during event (Berry et al. 2018). Oxygen desaturation in CSA tends to be less severe than in OSA.

SPECIFIC POLYSOMNOGRAPHY FEATURES

In addition to the general polysomnographic features of CSA, CSB requires three or more consecutive central apneas or hypopneas separated by a crescendo-decrescendo airflow pattern, with a cycle length (interval between onsets of consecutive apneas) of ≥40 seconds (Figure 11–2B) (American Academy of Sleep Medicine 2014; Berry et al. 2018). The longer cycle time of CSB (typically 60–90 seconds) distinguishes it from other CSA subtypes, which have cycle times of <40 seconds, with HAPB being close to 20 seconds (apnea duration about 10 seconds). The circulation time (interval from apnea termination to nadir in oxygen saturation) is also prolonged in CSB and directly proportional to the cycle length. Both intervals are inversely related to systolic function. Arousals in CSB typically occur at the peak of the hyperpnea, versus at apnea termination in other CSA disorders. In primary CSA and CSA due to a medical disorder without CSB, five or fewer breaths separate periods of recurrent central apnea (i.e., periodic breathing). Opioid-induced CSA may present with an even shorter ventilatory phase of two to four breaths, bradypnea, or ataxic (Biot) breathing, which is characterized by an irregular respiratory rhythm and variable tidal volume (see Figure 11–2C).

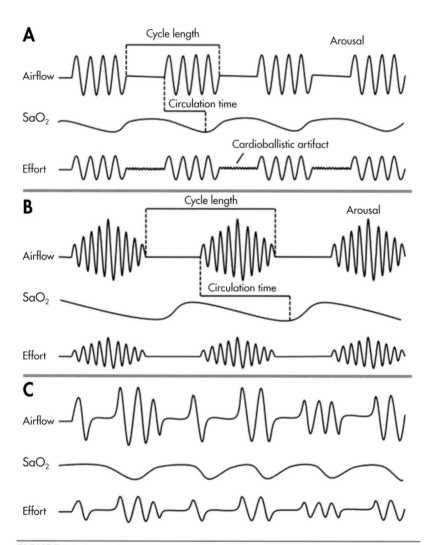

FIGURE 11–2.   Polysomnography findings in *A*, primary central sleep apnea (CSA); *B*, Cheynes-Stokes breathing (CSB); and *C*, ataxic breathing.

CSB has a crescendo-decrescendo airflow pattern, a longer cycle length (>40 seconds) and circulation time, and arousals occurring at the peak of the hyperpnea, as opposed to the shorter intervals and arousals occurring at the termination of the apnea in other CSA disorders. Cardioballistic artifact can be seen in any CSA disorder (only depicted for primary CSA), and it may be seen in the airflow, nasal pressure, esophageal pressure monitoring (if present), and electroencephalogram channels, in addition to the effort belt signals. Note the irregular cycle length and tidal volume of ataxic breathing.

SaO_2=oxygen saturation.

Differential Diagnosis

The main differential diagnoses to consider for CSA disorders are other sleep-related breathing disorders, namely OSA and sleep-related hypoventilation.

OBSTRUCTIVE SLEEP APNEA

Symptoms alone cannot differentiate CSA from OSA; the similarities between these disorders were discussed earlier (see "Clinical Presentation, Course, and Complications"). Although conventional polysomnography distinguishes CSA from OSA by absence of respiratory effort in the former, this distinction is not always unequivocal. That is, the frequency of CSA may be overestimated, cardioballistic artifact may be mistaken for effort, and differentiating obstructive and central hypopneas may be challenging. Chest wall or diaphragmatic electromyography as well as esophageal pressure monitoring may supplement respiratory inductance plethysmography in making this distinction (Berry et al. 2016; Luo et al. 2009). Furthermore, OSA commonly coexists with CSA (i.e., the disorders are not mutually exclusive), but CSA may not be apparent until OSA is treated.

SLEEP-RELATED HYPOVENTILATION

Patients with sleep-related hypoventilation present with $PaCO_2$ levels >45 mm Hg during wakefulness or purely sleep-related hypoventilation, along with a readily apparent neuromuscular or chest wall disorder, parenchymal lung disease, or abnormality in ventilatory control (see Chapter 10).

CSA SUBTYPES

CSA disorders must also be differentiated from one another. Distinctive polysomnographic findings were discussed earlier (see "Diagnostic Procedures and Testing"). An underlying cause of CSA may be apparent, such as heart failure, neurological disorder, renal failure, opioid use, or ascent to altitude. Without such identifiable risk factors, primary CSA may be diagnosed. However, this is a rare condition and a diagnosis of exclusion. An underlying disorder may not be apparent in some cases, so a high index of suspicion should be maintained, with consideration of additional testing (e.g., MRI for Chiari malformation). TE-CSA also seems to be readily apparent, with CSA emerging in patients with underlying OSA treated with PAP therapy. However, CSB and opioid-induced

CSA may present as predominantly OSA during a diagnostic study, and CSA may not be apparent until PAP titration/treatment and resolution of OSA. If these risk factors are present, the diagnosis should be CSB or CSA related to opioid use, rather than TE-CSA that is not better explained by another CSA disorder. *Complex sleep apnea* is a term that encompasses TE-CSA as well as other CSA disorders due to underlying etiologies that present as predominantly obstructive events during a diagnostic study, with CSA not becoming apparent until application of PAP therapy.

Treatment

High-quality evidence demonstrating meaningful clinical benefits of treating CSA disorders is limited. The largest randomized controlled trials have focused on patients with CSB, so extrapolating results to other CSA subtypes is beset with uncertainty. Moreover, cumulative evidence demonstrates not only a lack of benefit of PAP therapy in CSB but also potential for harm (Bradley et al. 2005; Cowie et al. 2015). Despite these caveats, smaller studies suggest treatments for CSA can improve apnea-hypopnea index (AHI), CAHI, oxygenation, cardiac function, exercise capacity, sleep quality, sleepiness, and quality-of-life measures. However, underlying disorders (e.g., heart failure, Chiari malformation) should be sought and appropriately treated, and risk factors (e.g., high altitude, use of potent opioids at high doses) should be addressed, because this may improve or resolve the CSA condition. Asymptomatic patients without significant desaturation (e.g., possibly sleep-onset central apneas and TE-CSA) may not require any treatment and can be reassured.

POSITIVE AIRWAY PRESSURE THERAPY

Various PAP modalities have been used to treat the different CSA disorders. However, the two largest randomized controlled trials focused on patients with heart failure who have CSA (Bradley et al. 2005; Cowie et al. 2015). These studies were not only negative trials but also indicated potential harm from use of PAP therapy in this population. Therefore, use of PAP therapy in CSA disorders should be pursued with caution. In general, performing attended in-laboratory PAP titration is desired to determine optimal PAP modality and pressure settings to minimize AHI, CAHI, and oxygen desaturation.

Continuous Positive Airway Pressure

CPAP is typically the first-line PAP modality tried for nonhypercapnic CSA disorders. Most clinical evidence supporting use of CPAP in such conditions comes from studies evaluating its efficacy in patients with heart failure. Controlled studies of CPAP in this population have demonstrated a reduction in AHI by 21 events per hour and an increase in left ventricular ejection fraction (LVEF) by 6% (Aurora et al. 2012). The Canadian Continuous Positive Airway Pressure for Patients with Central Sleep Apnea and Heart Failure trial is the largest study, and it demonstrated a similar reduction in AHI, along with a mild increase in nocturnal oxygen saturation, LVEF, and 6-minute walk distance (Bradley et al. 2005). However, the primary outcome of transplant-free survival was not met. In addition, no differences were found in hospitalization rates or quality of life. The trial was stopped prematurely due to an early divergence in survival favoring the control group, thereby limiting its power for detecting an effect on the primary outcome. Additional trial limitations included poor adherence to and lack of titration of CPAP. A post hoc analysis suggested that achieving suppression of AHI with CPAP may improve transplant-free survival and result in greater increase in LVEF (Arzt et al. 2007).

CPAP is thought to improve CSA by stabilizing the upper airway (Khayat and Abraham 2016). Hyperpnea, ventilatory overshoot, and hypocapnia are averted by preventing the pharyngeal narrowing and occlusion that may occur with accompanying OSA. The AASM has designated CPAP therapy targeted to normalize AHI as the standard initial treatment for CSA associated with heart failure, whereas PAP therapy is considered optional treatment for primary CSA, due to the lack of direct evidence for the condition (Aurora et al. 2012). Expectant management of TE-CSA with CPAP is also reasonable, because most patients experience resolution after a few months.

Bilevel Positive Airway Pressure

When treating CSA, BPAP is typically employed in the spontaneous timed (ST) mode (i.e., with a backup rate). Use of spontaneous mode may worsen CSA with or without CSB, although CSB may still persist despite use of BPAP-ST (Johnson and Johnson 2005). BPAP-ST can be considered for treating CSA if CPAP is not effective or tolerated. Small, nonrandomized, and mostly uncontrolled studies suggest that BPAP-ST may improve AHI and LVEF in CSA related to heart failure (Aurora et al. 2012). A small randomized crossover trial showed that CPAP and BPAP-ST were equally effective in lowering AHI, improving sleep quality, reducing daytime fatigue, and lowering New York Heart Association class in CSA with CSB and low LVEF (Köhnlein et al. 2002). However, caution should be employed when considering BPAP-ST in this population given the findings of the Treatment of Sleep-Disordered Breathing with Predominant Central Sleep Apnea by Adaptive Servo Ventilation in Patients with Heart Failure (SERVE-HF) trial (Cowie et al. 2015), which is discussed later.

The mechanism of BPAP-ST in treating CSA is presumably similar to that of CPAP regarding stabilization of the upper airway (Khayat and Abraham 2016) while also providing inspiratory support and backup respirations. The AASM has designated BPAP-ST therapy targeted to normalize AHI as an optional treatment for CSA associated with heart failure if CPAP and supplemental oxygen are ineffective (Aurora et al. 2012). BPAP-ST can also be considered in primary CSA, CSA related to use of narcotics, and TE-CSA, although evidence for these subtypes is sparse.

Adaptive Servo Ventilation

Although an update to the 2012 AASM guidelines on treatment of CSA reports that adaptive servo ventilation (ASV) reduces AHI by 30 events per hour and increases LVEF by about 5% in CSA and heart failure, it also indicates that ASV is contraindicated in individuals with an LVEF ≤45% (Aurora et al. 2016). This standard level recommendation against use of ASV in this group of patients is based on the results of the SERVE-HF trial, which compared ASV with medical therapy in patients with CSA and heart failure and an LVEF below 45% (Cowie et al. 2015). No difference was found in the primary end point of death from any cause, need for lifesaving cardiovascular intervention, or unplanned hospitalization for worsening heart failure. However, all-cause and cardiovascular mortality were both higher in patients treated with ASV. The main risk was of sudden cardiac death (possibly related to coexisting arrhythmias), and a significant association was found between risk of mortality and lower ejection fraction. Although ASV was effective at lowering AHI and decreasing sleepiness compared with baseline, no difference was seen in quality of life measures or exercise capacity compared with control subjects.

ASV uses expiratory PAP to maintain airway patency, similar to CPAP, as well as variable inspiratory pressure support to counterbalance ventilatory instability (i.e., low-pressure support during hyperpnea and high-pressure support during central apneas and hypopneas). The objective is to stabilize ventilation and prevent ventilatory overshoot and hypocapnia. The AASM designates ASV therapy targeted to normalize

AHI as an optional treatment for CSA associated with heart failure in adults with an ejection fraction >45% (Aurora et al. 2016). ASV also resolves opioid-associated CSA that persists despite continued use of CPAP (Javaheri et al. 2014). It is more effective in reducing AHI and CAHI as well as improving sleep quality and daytime sleepiness compared with BPAP-ST in patients with opioid-related CSA (Cao et al. 2014). Likewise, ASV is more effective in relieving TE-CSA compared with persistent use of CPAP (Morgenthaler et al. 2014) or BPAP-ST (Dellweg et al. 2013). Given the findings of SERVE-HF, caution should be exercised when using ASV for any indication.

NOCTURNAL SUPPLEMENTAL OXYGEN

Nocturnal supplemental oxygen is an alternative treatment option in patients with nonhypercapnic CSA, particularly in those who do not tolerate or benefit from PAP therapy or for whom harm from PAP therapy is a concern. Supplemental oxygen can also be used in conjunction with PAP therapy in patients with sustained hypoxemia. It should not be used alone in patients with hypercapnic CSA due to the possibility of carbon dioxide retention. Controlled trials in CSA due to heart failure demonstrate an increase in LVEF by about 5% and reduction in AHI by about 15 events per hour (Aurora et al. 2012). Small sample sizes limit the quality of evidence. Proposed mechanisms by which supplemental oxygen improves CSA include reduction in chemoresponsiveness to carbon dioxide and increased cerebral carbon dioxide levels. The AASM designates nocturnal supplemental oxygen as a standard treatment for CSA associated with heart failure (Aurora et al. 2012).

PHARMACOLOGICAL THERAPY

After optimization of underlying medical conditions and elimination of risk factors to the extent possible, medications may be considered when patients with CSA are unable to tolerate PAP therapy, if benefit from either PAP therapy or nocturnal supplemental oxygen is lacking, or if harm from use of PAP therapy is a concern. The main categories of medications that have demonstrated benefit in CSA are respiratory stimulants and hypnotic agents, both of which address the underlying pathophysiology of hypercapnic CSA due to carbon dioxide dysregulation by stabilizing ventilation.

Respiratory Stimulants

Acetazolamide is a carbonic anhydrase inhibitor and weak diuretic that stimulates ventilation by inducing a mild metabolic acidosis. This medication has been used to treat periodic breathing at high altitude, and it can normalize AHI as well as improve oxygenation during sleep in this situation (Fischer et al. 2004). It has also been demonstrated to reduce overall AHI due to a decrease in CAHI by >20 events per hour, as well as improve nocturnal oxygenation, subjective sleep quality, daytime sleepiness, and fatigue in CSA with CSB (Javaheri 2006). The AASM designates acetazolamide as an optional treatment for CSA associated with heart failure as well as primary CSA (Aurora et al. 2012). Side effects include electrolyte imbalance, parasthesias, altered taste perception, polyuria, gastrointestinal symptoms, and tinnitus.

Theophylline is another respiratory stimulant that has been used to treat CSA. Similar to acetazolamide, it has been used to treat HAPB, with normalization of AHI and improvement in oxygenation during sleep (Fischer et al. 2004). It has also been demonstrated to reduce overall AHI by nearly 30 events per hour and CAHI by 20 events per hour, as well as improve nocturnal oxygenation in CSA with CSB (Javaheri et al. 1996). The AASM has designated theophylline as an optional treatment for CSA associated with heart failure (Aurora et al. 2012). Theophylline has a narrow therapeutic window, with side effects including cardiac arrhythmias, CNS excitation, and gastrointestinal symptoms.

Hypnotics

Zolpidem has been demonstrated to reduce AHI by 30 events per hour and CAHI by 26 events per hour, as well as to improve sleep efficiency and daytime sleepiness among patients with primary CSA (Quadri et al. 2009). Triazolam has also been demonstrated to reduce central apneas by about 50%, as well as to reduce arousals, increase total sleep time, and improve daytime psychomotor performance and alertness (Bonnet et al. 1990). The proposed mechanism by which sedative-hypnotics treat CSA is reduction in arousals, resulting in more stable sleep and decreased ventilatory overshoot and hypocapnia. The AASM designates zolpidem and triazolam as optional treatments for primary CSA in the absence of underlying risk factors for respiratory depression (Aurora et al. 2012).

PHRENIC NERVE STIMULATION

Unilateral transvenous phrenic nerve stimulation for selected patients with CSA is a promising novel therapy that can reduce overall AHI and CAHI by about 25 events per hour and also reduce oxygen desaturation events and sleepiness, as well as improve quality of life (Costanzo et al. 2016). An implantable device approved by the FDA causes diaphragmatic contraction and restoration of normal breathing during central apneas through negative intrathoracic pressure, thus mimicking normal breathing. Transvenous neurostimulation appears to be well tolerated, with an acceptable safety profile. However, studies comparing it with PAP therapy and other CSA therapies, as well as evaluating long-term safety data, are needed.

Conclusion

Although CSA is relatively uncommon, especially in comparison with OSA, concerns remain about adverse outcomes, such as increased cardiovascular complications and mortality, particularly with CSB. Whether central apneas in such patients are a risk factor or a marker of poor prognosis remains to be elucidated. Prior to considering specific therapies for CSA, it is prudent to evaluate for and treat underlying conditions, as well as eliminate to the extent possible any risk factors that may be predisposing the patient to central apneas, because this may improve or resolve the CSA condition. Although uncertainty persists concerning the harms of CSA and benefits of treatment, emerging evidence has demonstrated harm with particular PAP modalities in specific populations, namely ASV and possibly CPAP in patients with CSA related to heart failure and low LVEF. Extrapolating available evidence to other PAP modalities and CSA disorders is questionable. Studies of CSA are generally sparse and often quite small. Better evidence is clearly needed to help guide management decisions. Until more data are available, a reasonable approach may be to address underlying etiologies and pursue treatment in the setting of persistent, prominent symptoms, including disrupted sleep or excessive daytime sleepiness, as well as concerning physiological consequences of CSA, such as significant oxygen desaturation during sleep.

KEY CLINICAL POINTS

- Central sleep apnea (CSA) is characterized by recurring periods of absent airflow during sleep due to a reduction or loss of respiratory effort. Polysomnography is required to identify these features.

- Symptoms cannot be used to differentiate CSA from obstructive sleep apnea (OSA), because they are essentially identical for both disorders, including snoring, witnessed apneas, frequent nocturnal awakenings with or without shortness of breath, insomnia, nonrestorative sleep, morning headaches, daytime sleepiness, and fatigue.

- CSA is a relatively uncommon disorder, especially primary CSA, but its prevalence is higher in men, older adults, and those with certain medical disorders or risk factors, such as heart failure, stroke, use of long-acting opiates, ascent to high altitude, and use of positive airway pressure (PAP) therapy for underlying OSA.

- A common classification system of CSA disorders is based on carbon dioxide levels and degree of ventilation, with nonhypercapnic subtypes resulting from hyperventilation and high loop gain and hypercapnic subtypes resulting from hypoventilation.

- Nonhypercapnic CSA disorders include primary CSA, Cheyne-Stokes breathing (CSB), high-altitude periodic breathing, and treatment-emergent CSA; hypercapnic CSA disorders include medical disorders without CSB and use of a medication or substance.

- Identifying and addressing underlying conditions and risk factors for central apneas is essential, because this may resolve or improve the CSA disorder, and evidence that specifically treating CSA improves relevant clinical outcomes is limited.

- Adaptive servo ventilation (ASV) is contraindicated in CSA with CSB in the setting of systolic dysfunction (i.e., left ventricle ejection fraction <45%), and continuous PAP (CPAP) targeted to normalized apnea-hypopnea index is the preferred PAP modality in this population, whereas bilevel PAP (BPAP) in either the spontaneous or timed mode should be used with caution.

- Although data regarding treatment of other CSA disorders are limited, CPAP targeted to normalize apnea-hypopnea index is also the preferred PAP modality for other nonhypercapnic CSA subtypes, including those with treatment-emergent CSA, because this usually resolves after a few months; a trial of ASV or spontaneous timed BPAP after laboratory titration can be considered for those who fail or do not tolerate CPAP, including in those with heart failure with preserved ejection fraction.

- Spontaneous timed BPAP is typically the preferred PAP modality for hypercapnic CSA disorders, although BPAP in the spontaneous mode or even CPAP can be considered.

- Alternative treatments to PAP therapy for patients who fail or do not tolerate it include nocturnal oxygen therapy, medications (i.e., respiratory stimulants and hypnotics), and phrenic nerve stimulation, although data regarding these treatments are limited.

References

American Academy of Sleep Medicine: International Classification of Sleep Disorders, 3rd Edition. Darien, IL, American Academy of Sleep Medicine, 2014

Arzt M, Floras JS, Logan AG, et al: Suppression of central sleep apnea by continuous positive airway pressure and transplant-free survival in heart failure: a post hoc analysis of the Canadian Continuous Positive Airway Pressure for Patients with Central Sleep Apnea and Heart Failure trial (CANPAP). Circulation 115(25):3173–3180, 2007 17562959

Aurora RN, Chowdhuri S, Ramar K, et al: The treatment of central sleep apnea syndromes in adults: practice parameters with an evidence-based literature review and meta-analyses. Sleep (Basel) 35(1):17–40, 2012 22215916

Aurora RN, Bista SR, Casey KR, et al: Updated adaptive servo-ventilation recommendations for the 2012 AASM guideline: "The treatment of central sleep apnea syndromes in adults: practice parameters with an evidence-based literature review and meta-analyses." J Clin Sleep Med 12(5):757–761, 2016 27092695

Berry RB, Ryals S, Girdhar A, et al: Use of chest wall electromyography to detect respiratory effort during polysomnography. J Clin Sleep Med 12(9):1239–1244, 2016 27306391

Berry RB, Albertario CL, Hardin SM, et al: The AASM Manual for Scoring of Sleep and Associated Events: Rules, Terminology and Technical Specifications, Version 2.5. Darien, IL, American Academy of Sleep Medicine, 2018

Bixler EO, Vgontzas AN, Ten Have T, et al: Effects of age on sleep apnea in men: I. Prevalence and severity. Am J Respir Crit Care Med 157(1):144–148, 1998 9445292

Bixler EO, Vgontzas AN, Lin HM, et al: Prevalence of sleep-disordered breathing in women: effects of gender. Am J Respir Crit Care Med 163(3 Pt 1):608–613, 2001 11254512

Bonnet MH, Dexter JR, Arand DL: The effect of triazolam on arousal and respiration in central sleep apnea patients. Sleep 13(1):31–41, 1990 2406849

Bradley TD, Logan AG, Kimoff RJ, et al: Continuous positive airway pressure for central sleep apnea and heart failure. N Engl J Med 353(19):2025–2033, 2005 16282177

Cao M, Cardell CY, Willes L, et al: A novel adaptive servoventilation (ASVAuto) for the treatment of central sleep apnea associated with chronic use of opioids. J Clin Sleep Med 10(8):855–861, 2014 25126031

Correa D, Farney RJ, Chung F, et al: Chronic opioid use and central sleep apnea: a review of the prevalence, mechanisms, and perioperative considerations. Anesth Analg 120(6):1273–1285, 2015 25988636

Costanzo MR, Ponikowski P, Javaheri S, et al: Transvenous neurostimulation for central sleep apnoea: a randomised controlled trial. Lancet 388(10048):974–982, 2016 27598679

Cowie MR, Woehrle H, Wegscheider K, et al: Adaptive servo-ventilation for central sleep apnea in systolic heart failure. N Engl J Med 373(12):1095–1105, 2015 26323938

Dellweg D, Kerl J, Hoehn E, et al: Randomized controlled trial of noninvasive positive pressure ventilation (NPPV) versus servoventilation in patients with CPAP-induced central sleep apnea (complex sleep apnea). Sleep (Basel) 36(8):1163–1171, 2013 23904676

Donovan LM, Kapur VK: Prevalence and characteristics of central compared to obstructive sleep apnea: analyses from the Sleep Heart Health study cohort. Sleep (Basel) 39(7):1353–1359, 2016 27166235

Fischer R, Lang SM, Leitl M, et al: Theophylline and acetazolamide reduce sleep-disordered breathing at high altitude. Eur Respir J 23(1):47–52, 2004 14738230

Herrscher TE, Akre H, Øverland B, et al: High prevalence of sleep apnea in heart failure outpatients: even in patients with preserved systolic function. J Card Fail 17(5):420–425, 2011 21549300

Javaheri S: Acetazolamide improves central sleep apnea in heart failure: a double-blind, prospective study. Am J Respir Crit Care Med 173(2):234–237, 2006 16239622

Javaheri S, Parker TJ, Wexler L, et al: Effect of theophylline on sleep-disordered breathing in heart failure. N Engl J Med 335(8):562–567, 1996 8678934

Javaheri S, Shukla R, Zeigler H, et al: Central sleep apnea, right ventricular dysfunction, and low diastolic blood pressure are predictors of mortality in systolic heart failure. J Am Coll Cardiol 49(20):2028–2034, 2007 17512359

Javaheri S, Harris N, Howard J, et al: Adaptive servoventilation for treatment of opioid-associated central sleep apnea. J Clin Sleep Med 10(6):637–643, 2014 24932143

Johnson KG, Johnson DC: Bilevel positive airway pressure worsens central apneas during sleep. Chest 128(4):2141–2150, 2005 16236867

Khayat RN, Abraham WT: Current treatment approaches and trials in central sleep apnea. Int J Cardiol 206(suppl):S22–S27, 2016 26961738

Köhnlein T, Welte T, Tan LB, et al: Assisted ventilation for heart failure patients with Cheyne-Stokes respiration. Eur Respir J 20(4):934–941, 2002 12412686

Luo YM, Tang J, Jolley C, et al: Distinguishing obstructive from central sleep apnea events: diaphragm electromyogram and esophageal pressure compared. Chest 135(5):1133–1141, 2009 19118271

Morgenthaler TI, Kuzniar TJ, Wolfe LF, et al: The complex sleep apnea resolution study: a prospective randomized controlled trial of continuous positive airway pressure versus adaptive servoventilation therapy. Sleep (Basel) 37(5):927–934, 2014 24790271

Muza RT: Central sleep apnoea: a clinical review. J Thorac Dis 7(5):930–937, 2015 26101651

Nigam G, Pathak C, Riaz M: A systematic review on prevalence and risk factors associated with treatment-emergent central sleep apnea. Sleep Breath 20(3):957–964, 2016 26815045

Nigam G, Riaz M, Chang ET, et al: Natural history of treatment-emergent central sleep apnea on positive airway pressure: a systematic review. Ann Thorac Med 13(2):86–91, 2018 29675059

Quadri S, Drake C, Hudgel DW: Improvement of idiopathic central sleep apnea with zolpidem. J Clin Sleep Med 5(2):122–129, 2009 19968044

Sin DD, Fitzgerald F, Parker JD, et al: Risk factors for central and obstructive sleep apnea in 450 men and women with congestive heart failure. Am J Respir Crit Care Med 160(4):1101–1106, 1999 10508793

Solin P, Bergin P, Richardson M, et al: Influence of pulmonary capillary wedge pressure on central apnea in heart failure. Circulation 99(12):1574–1579, 1999 10096933

CHAPTER 12

Delayed and Advanced Sleep-Wake Phase Disorders

Daniella Palermo, M.D.

Katherine M. Sharkey, M.D., Ph.D., FAASM

Delayed Sleep-Wake Phase Disorder

Delayed sleep-wake phase disorder (DSWPD) is a circadian rhythm sleep-wake disorder characterized by sleep onset and wake times that occur much later than socially conventional times. When patients with DSWPD are allowed to sleep at their internally driven preferred times, sleep duration and quality are similar to those of healthy sleepers. To adhere to conventional schedules, however, these patients frequently are forced to awaken earlier than their body clocks' endogenously driven wake times, and because they cannot fall asleep at typical bedtimes, they do not accumulate sufficient sleep. Thus, these patients accrue significant sleep debt. This chronic insufficient sleep, combined with circadian misalignment, can result in profound daytime sleepiness and impairment.

DIAGNOSTIC CRITERIA

The *International Classification of Sleep Disorders*, 3rd Edition (ICSD-3; American Academy of Sleep Medicine 2014), requires that the following five conditions be present to diagnose this disorder:

1. The phase of the major sleep episode shows a significant delay in relation to desired or required sleep and wakeup times, as evidenced by a chronic or recurrent complaint by patient or a caregiver of inability to fall asleep and difficulty awakening at desired or required clock times.

2. When allowed to choose their *ad libitum* schedule, patients exhibit improved sleep quality and duration for age and maintain delayed phase of the 24-hour sleep-wake pattern.
3. Symptoms must be present for at least 3 months.
4. Sleep diary or actigraphy monitoring for at least 7–14 days that includes both work/school days and free days demonstrates delay in timing of habitual sleep period.
5. Sleep disturbance is not better explained by another sleep disorder, medical or neurological disorder, mental disorder, medication use, or substance use disorder.

PATHOPHYSIOLOGY

The etiology of DSWPD is multifactorial and heterogeneous, and the various aspects of DSWPD discussed here may impact some patients more than others. Nevertheless, evidence supports a pathophysiological role of each of these features in DSWPD (Micic et al. 2016).

Circadian Phase Delay

Circadian rhythms strongly influence a person's experience of sleepiness, as well as the timing of habitual sleep onset and awakening. Given their association with endogenous circadian drive, two circadian markers are used frequently to assess internal biological time: 1) pattern of melatonin secretion, and 2) circadian rhythm of core body temperature. Melatonin-based circadian measures include the time of melatonin onset (most common), melatonin offset, and melatonin synthesis offset (also called the SynOff). In those with normally timed circadian rhythms, the beginning of the biological night is associated with a significant evening rise in melatonin secretion from the pineal gland. Blood or saliva samples used to measure this rapid rise must be collected in dim light because melatonin secretion is suppressed acutely by bright light exposure. Hence, the time of the beginning of nightly melatonin secretion is termed the *dim light melatonin onset* (DLMO). In the circadian rhythm of core body temperature, the time of minimum core body temperature, also referred to as Tmin, usually occurs about 2 hours before habitual wake time in normally entrained adults and is associated with the maximum circadian drive for sleep.

These phase markers have been used to examine individual differences in sleep timing, and both Tmin and DLMO demonstrate significant delays in patients with DSWPD. For example, one study found that subjects with DSWPD reached Tmin at 7:17 A.M. ± 47 minutes, whereas control subjects reached Tmin at 4:56 A.M. ± 19 minutes. Melatonin onset also occurred approximately 4 hours later in patients with DSWPD compared with control subjects (Ozaki et al. 1996). Given the strong and positive correlation of phase markers with sleep onset and wake time, DSWPD is hypothesized to arise from a circadian phase delay.

Longer Circadian Period

Due to Earth's solar rotation, virtually all organisms exposed to natural light and dark have adapted to living in a cycling 24-hour environment. However, in most people, the internal day length is not exactly 24 hours. Indeed, wide individual differences have been observed in circadian period length, also known as "tau." Tau has been shown to be as short as 23.3 hours and as long as 24.64 hours in different people. When an individual's tau is not exactly 24 hours, the endogenous circadian rhythms must make small daily adjustments to stay synchronized or "entrained" to 24-hour clock time. A longer tau requires a larger adjustment and increases the likelihood of circadian rhythm delay. If the daily resetting does not occur or is incomplete, this can result in delayed wake and sleep times. The delay in sleep onset, in particular, leads to later evening light exposure as well as delayed morning light exposure, further perpetuating phase delay (Micic et al. 2016). This is particularly relevant for adolescents, who experience both developmental lengthening in tau (slightly >24 hours) and delays that are partly attributable to puberty-related changes in the adolescent circadian system (Richardson et al. 2017).

Differences in Homeostatic Sleep Drive

The homeostatic sleep-wake drive and the circadian system work together to influence sleep timing. First described by Borbély et al. (2016), the interaction of these elements is referred to as the "two-process model of sleep regulation." Consistent with our understanding of biological homeostatic regulation, the drive for sleep increases with time spent awake and decreases during sleep. As shown in Figure 12–1, synchrony between homeostatic drive and circadian rhythms leads to optimal sleep in healthy sleepers.

Dysfunction of homeostatic sleep-wake mechanisms can contribute to DSWPD. It has been hypothesized that homeostatic drive accumulates more slowly during wakefulness among individuals with DSWPD when compared with control subjects (Duffy et al. 2001). The reduced rate of sleep drive accumulation is also evident around puberty and may explain why DSWPD is commonly diagnosed in adolescence (Campbell et al. 2011; Carskadon 2011). Additional data indicate that patients with DSWPD experience not only a slower accumulation of sleep drive but also a slower dissipation during sleep (Uchiyama et al. 1999). The resul-

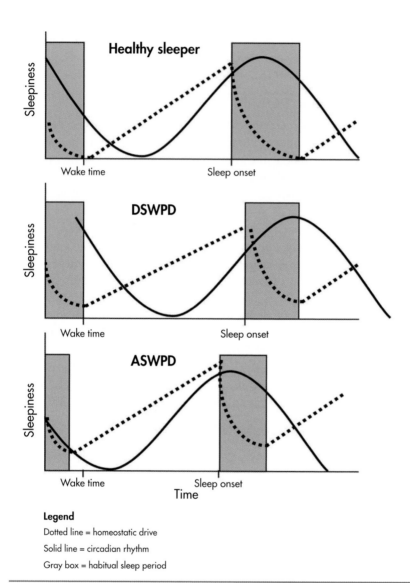

Legend

Dotted line = homeostatic drive

Solid line = circadian rhythm

Gray box = habitual sleep period

FIGURE 12–1.   Two-process model of sleep regulation.

The interaction of homeostatic and circadian processes drives sleep timing and duration. The *top panel* depicts a healthy sleeper whose homeostatic drive and circadian rhythms are synchronized, producing optimal sleep timing and duration. The *middle panel* shows the interaction of the two sleep regulatory processes in a patient with delayed sleep-wake phase disorder (DSWPD). Homeostatic drive builds up more slowly, and circadian phase is delayed with respect to clock time. As a result, sleep onset is delayed, but it also occurs *earlier* with respect to the internal biological clock. Sleep duration is curtailed by adherence to the socially required wake time. Advanced sleep-wake phase disorder (ASWPD) is illustrated in the *bottom panel*, which shows earlier sleep onset that occurs later with respect to the internal circadian clock and an early wake time that results in insufficient sleep duration.

tant decrease or later timing of morning light exposure likely also contributes to delayed sleep timing.

Sensitivity to Light

DSWPD may occur as a result of abnormalities in the phase response curve to light, in which individuals with DSWPD are hypersensitive to light in the late evening (potentiating phase delay) or less sensitive to light upon awakening (diminishing phase advance). Research comparing patients with DSWPD and control subjects with regard to sensitivity of melatonin suppression in response to light exposure found greater melatonin suppression in DSWPD (Aoki et al. 2001), consistent with a hypersensitivity mechanism.

Additionally, reduced exposure to sunlight and the widespread use of electrical lighting, particularly after sunset, alters human circadian physiology, diminishing the environmental zeitgeber's ("time giver's") strong influence and, in turn, increasing the likelihood of phase delays. For example, in a study of healthy young adults with *ad libitum* access to artificial light, the circadian low point in brain arousal, as defined by cognitive performance level or physiological markers of sleepiness, occurred approximately 2 hours after habitual wake time and was accompanied by a delay in melatonin offset compared with measurements made in the same individuals after living for a week in natural lighting conditions (Wright et al. 2013).

Behavioral and Physiological Interactions

Patients with DSWPD appear to experience heightened alertness in the evening in comparison with healthy control subjects, with 75% reporting subjective alertness after dinner (Gradisar et al. 2011). This, along with depressed alertness in the first hours after awakening, may predispose patients with DSWPD to behaviorally avoid mornings by sleeping in late and extend their positive experiences in the evening by delaying bedtime (Lack and Wright 2012). This tendency to avoid morning light has also been reported in 85% of adolescents diagnosed with DSWPD (Gradisar et al. 2011).

Role of Psychoactive Medications

Based on animal models designed to investigate the interaction of circadian rhythms and psychoactive substances, including medications, alcohol, and recreational substances, bidirectional influences between these domains are likely, but this area has little research in humans. More work has been done on the effects of psychiatric medications on sleep stages than on circadian rhythms. In the absence of strong data, a reasonable clinical strategy for treating DSWPD in patients who take psychoactive medications is to consider the medications carefully in light of their timing with respect to the patient's sleep-wake cycle.

EPIDEMIOLOGY

Prevalence

DSWPD is the most common circadian rhythm sleep-wake phase disorder. The true prevalence of DSWPD is difficult to estimate, ranging from 0.2% to 10% depending on the diagnostic sample (Micic et al. 2016). Although prevalence varies by country, studies have consistently shown a higher prevalence among adolescents, with no suggestion of sex difference.

Personality and Psychosocial Aspects

Personality traits underwrite attitudes and influence behaviors, which suggests that they can also cause or contribute to circadian misalignment. In a recent study, Micic et al. (2017) used the Revised NEO Personality Inventory to explore the personality factors most associated with DSWPD. Individuals with DSWPD reported higher neuroticism and significantly lower extraversion, conscientiousness, and agreeableness, suggesting that personality factors may also drive sleep timing. From a clinical perspective, these findings highlight the role of motivational interviewing as a therapeutic intervention for those who are low on conscientiousness and lack motivation for change, placing them at increased risk of circadian delays. Additionally, optimizing a patient's competency for social inclusion and building interpersonal trust could aid in addressing the low extraversion and agreeableness factors that further perpetuate sleep phase disturbances.

Genetic Predisposition

Interest has been intense, but evidence limited, for the role of genetic differences related to circadian phase, most predominantly polymorphisms in the human Period 3 (*hPER3*) genes (Jones et al. 2013). Polymorphisms in *hPER1* (Carpen et al. 2006), *hPER2* (Carpen et al. 2005), and *CLOCK* genes (Katzenberg et al. 1998) have also been associated with DSWPD, whereas mutations in S408N in *hCK1ε* have been deemed protective (Takano et al. 2004).

CLINICAL PRESENTATION

DSWPD is characterized by delayed sleep onset and wake times that result in sleep insufficiency and functional impairment due to a circadian rhythm that is incompatible with social norms. Individuals with DSWPD display preference for "eveningness," delaying sleep time by ≥2 hours. They experience later awakenings, likely associated with sleep inertia and delayed endogenous circadian phase. When attempting to comply with societal obligations, these individuals fail to obtain adequate sleep. This is particularly apparent among adolescents, with 70% reporting insufficient sleep on school nights, according to data from the Centers for Disease Control and Prevention (Eaton et al. 2010). School start times that fail to account for the developmental changes in sleep and circadian rhythms that occur during adolescence contribute to insufficient sleep in teens even in the absence of DSWPD and in those with DSWPD can also contribute to truancy and school avoidance.

Negative Effects on Executive Functioning

DSWPD is associated with negative cognitive outcomes, including reduced daytime performance and difficulties with treatment adherence, both of which are mediated by impairments in working memory and attention (Wilhelmsen-Langeland et al. 2019).

Mental Health and Delayed Sleep Phase

DSWPD is associated with poorer mental health outcomes. For instance, a population-based Norwegian study compared mental health and resilience in adolescents with and without DSWPD and found that delays in sleep onset were associated with symptoms of depression, anxiety, and ADHD as well as lower levels of resilience (Sivertsen et al. 2015).

DIAGNOSTIC PROCEDURES, TESTS, AND QUESTIONNAIRES

DSWPD is a clinical diagnosis that should be considered in individuals who report difficulty with sleeping at desired or socially accepted times to fulfill daytime obligations while also obtaining sufficient night sleep. Patients' most common concerns are difficulty falling asleep or waking at the time required for social obligations. In most patients, thorough history taking, supplemented by data acquired from sleep diaries and actigraphy when available, is sufficient to confirm the DSWPD diagnosis.

Sleep History

Sleep and wake time data are of particular importance and should be inclusive of both school/work and off days. According to a poll conducted by the National Sleep Foundation (2006), sleep onset at or after 11 P.M. in children younger than 14 years of age or after midnight in individuals older than 14 years of age should be considered as a deviation from the norm. Of note, both sleep and wake times are likely to be delayed during off days in individuals with DSWPD, reflective of their endogenous circadian clock. Clinical history should also include inquiry into sleep quality and other possible sleep disturbances that could be suggestive of other sleep disorders, because individuals with DSWPD are unlikely to report these when sleep is reflective of their circadian preference. Close attention should also be paid to behavioral as well as environmental factors that may impact sleep quality, with particular attention to the period between sunset and sleep onset. Practitioners should inquire about evening exercise, exposure to light-emitting electronics, and medication and caffeine intake, all of which can delay sleep time.

Sleep Diary and Actigraphy

As noted in ICSD-3, 1–2 weeks of quantitative data regarding sleep-wake times are required to make a diagnosis of DSWPD. When available, an actigraph device can provide objective data for patients who may otherwise have difficulty completing a sleep log. An example of actigraphy in a patient with DSWPD is shown in Figure 12–2.

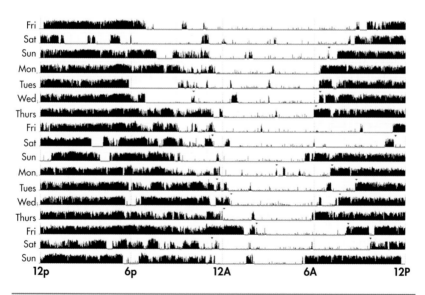

FIGURE 12–2.   Actigraph recording in a patient with delayed sleep-wake phase disorder (DSWPD).

This wrist actigraphy plot shows sleep patterns over 17 days in an adult woman with DSWPD. Her work schedule requires her to start her day at 6 A.M., but on free days, she routinely sleeps until 10–11 A.M. She attempts to fall asleep at around 10 P.M. on the nights before she has to work but is restless and reports that she often just lays quietly without falling asleep until 2–3 A.M.

Questionnaires

Self-administered chronotype questionnaires help differentiate DSWPD from other sleep disorders that also impact sleep onset. For example, the Horne-Östberg Morningness-Eveningness Questionnaire is a 19-item scale that assesses preference for timing of sleep and other activities and has been shown to correlate with circadian phase (Baehr et al. 2000). The Munich ChronoType Questionnaire assesses timing of behavior rather than preference (Roenneberg et al. 2004). Finally, the Children's Chronotype Questionnaire is a 27-item parental-report instrument that has been validated with actigraphy and can be used to discern chronotype in prepubertal children ages 4–11 (Werner et al. 2009).

Phase Markers

Although DLMO and Tmin are frequently measured in research, they currently serve a limited role in the clinical diagnosis of DSWPD because clinical testing is not available at most centers.

DIFFERENTIAL DIAGNOSIS

Insomnia

Patients with DSWPD and patients with insomnia (see Chapter 3) both describe difficulties with sleep initiation. However, individuals with DSWPD can readily initiate and maintain sufficient sleep when their sleep timing is not influenced by societal obligations. The etiology of sleep-onset insomnia is likely multifactorial, including both chronobiological and cognitive/behavioral components. As such, it is important to consider delayed sleep onset itself as something that could further perpetuate the disturbance. Anxiety associated with delayed sleep onset can result in chronic psychophysiological insomnia by perpetuating a delay in sleep onset (Lack and Wright 2007). Furthermore, light exposure at night in patients with sleep-onset insomnia can delay circadian rhythms and increase arousal before sleep. In these cases, cognitive-behavioral therapy for insomnia (CBT-I) should be used to address the sleep disturbance (see Chapter 5).

Depression and Anxiety

As evidenced by the DSM-5 (American Psychiatric Association 2013) criteria for both depression and anxiety disorders, sleep disturbances are a common symptom and can include delayed onset, impaired maintenance insomnia, or hypersomnia. Additionally, both depression and anxiety are common comorbidities encountered in DSWPD. As such, careful screening for psychiatric illness can aid in accurate diagnosis and management, because neither the circadian disorder nor the mood disturbance will fully improve unless both comorbid issues are treated.

In a meta-analysis of 49 randomized controlled trials that included nearly 6,000 patients, nonpharmacological sleep interventions such as stimulus control therapy, relaxation training, sleep restriction therapy, biofeedback, paradoxical intention, and multicomponent CBT-I were effective in reducing the severity of depression, particularly in clinical populations (Gee et al. 2019). Addressing sleep disturbances offers a relatively low-stigma means of reducing depressive symptoms in individuals who have both sleep and mental health difficulties.

Attention-Deficit/Hyperactivity Disorder

The behavioral and cognitive consequences that arise in DSWPD as a result of excessive daytime sleepiness could emerge as behaviors characteristic of ADHD. The risk of misdiagnosing DSWPD as ADHD and vice versa is, therefore, presumably high and may potentially lead to erroneous treatment (Wilhelmsen-Langeland et al. 2019). Therefore, it is important to assess sleep patterns before diagnosing or testing cognitive function in patients who are concerned about deficits in attention and concentration or are experiencing hyperactivity.

TREATMENT

Behavioral Modifications

Providers should encourage patients to adhere to a fixed sleep-wake schedule and to avoid daytime naps. One study found that significant advances in salivary DLMO can be achieved with strict adherence to a fixed earlier sleep-wake schedule in those with subclinical DSWPD resulting in misalignment between their usual sleep schedule and school/work obligations (Sharkey et al. 2011). Additionally, patients should be encouraged to moderate or eliminate caffeine, alcohol, and nicotine use. Finally, driving safety should be addressed with these patients because circadian misalignment and chronic insufficient sleep can contribute to increased risk of automobile accidents (Kosmadopoulos et al. 2017).

Bright Light Therapy

Light is the most potent zeitgeber, and appropriately timed bright light exposure can be used to correct circadian rhythm disturbances. Bright light exposure after the Tmin results in a phase advance, whereas light before Tmin results in a phase delay. The degree of the phase change is impacted by the proximity of light exposure to Tmin, light intensity, and duration (Lack and Wright 2007).

To phase-advance circadian rhythms, patients with DSWPD should use a bright light with ultraviolet filtering and an intensity of 2,500–10,000 lux for 30–120 minutes upon awakening (Auger et al. 2015). Patients should be told to place the bright light source 12–24 inches from their face directed toward their visual gaze. The length of therapy necessary to correct circadian delay and sustain the response has not been studied, so patients should be monitored clinically to gauge response. Although bright light therapy is usually well tolerated and risks are low, patients should be cautioned about the following side effects: headaches, eye strain, nausea, agitation, and hypomania. Caution should be used in patients with ophthalmological or dermatological conditions.

Chronotherapy

Chronotherapy aims to reset a patient's circadian clock by slowly delaying bedtime by 1–3 hours on successive days. This strategy is used less frequently than bright light therapy. The disadvantage is that it disrupts the individual's normal schedule of activity during the shift, when day and night are reversed.

Exogenous Melatonin

In people with typical sleep timing, melatonin secretion from the pineal gland begins around 9:00 P.M. on average, preceding habitual sleep onset by about 2 hours and wakeup time by about 10 hours. Secretion peaks between 2:00 and 4:00 A.M. Exogenous melatonin administered 4–8 hours prior to onset of endogenous melatonin will phase-advance circadian rhythms, with optimal phase advances occurring when exogenous melatonin overlaps endogenous onset (Lack and Wright 2007). Doses ranging from 0.3 mg to 5.0 mg have been used in most studies of melatonin treatment for DSWPD, and although doses up to 10 mg have a reassuring safety profile, optimal dosing parameters are not well established and controversy remains about chronic melatonin use in children and adolescents (Auger et al. 2015). Treatment with exogenous melatonin is more straightforward in patients who are shift workers or are experiencing jet lag than in patients with DSWPD because it is difficult to determine the proper time to administer melatonin in the latter without accurate information about the timing of their endogenous melatonin production.

Exercise

Nocturnal exercise can impact circadian timing by delaying or possibly reducing melatonin secretion. Additionally, nocturnal exercise may delay sleep propensity by increasing core body temperature and arousal (Richardson et al. 2017). However, not enough data are available yet to support the use of morning exercise for phase advances. Practitioners should inquire about the types of activities patients are engaging in before to bedtime while encouraging them to limit their physical activity in the evening in order to reduce the risk of increasing their circadian phase delay.

Pharmacological Treatment

Limited data support the use of hypnotics in the treatment of DSWPD. Therefore, their use is discouraged.

CONCLUSION

DSWPD is the most common circadian rhythm disorder, with its highest prevalence in the adolescent and young adult populations. It is characterized by delayed sleep onset and wake times resulting in sleep insufficiency and functional impairment due to a circadian rhythm that is not compatible with social norms. Both physiological and environmental factors lead to the emergence of DSWPD. In most patients, a thorough history, supplemented by data acquired from sleep diaries and actigraphy, is sufficient to confirm the DSWPD diagnosis. Although DSWPD is often confused with sleep-onset insomnia, when patients with DWSPD are released from their schedule constraints, their only sleep disturbance is delayed sleep onset and offset, with normal sleep quality and duration. The goal of treatment is to "reset" the individual's internal clock to a schedule that is more compatible with the demands of school or work. This can be achieved through improved sleep hygiene practices, chronotherapy, bright light therapy, or exogenous melatonin use.

Advanced Sleep-Wake Phase Disorder

Advanced sleep-wake phase disorder (ASWPD) is a circadian rhythm sleep-wake disorder that presents with symptoms that are the opposite of those experienced by patients with DSWPD. Characterized by biologically driven sleep timing that occurs earlier than either desired or conventional sleep-wake times, patients with ASWPD naturally awaken at early clock times but often force themselves to stay awake past when they feel sleepy at night in order to meet social or occupational obligations, resulting in insufficient sleep duration and subsequent daytime sleepiness.

DIAGNOSTIC CRITERIA

ICSD-3 requires the following five criteria be met to diagnose ASWPD:

1. An advance (early timing) in the phase of major sleep episode in relation to desired/required sleep and wakeup times, as evidenced by chronic or recurrent complaints of difficulty staying awake until the required or desired conventional bedtime and an inability to remain asleep until the required or desired time for awakening.
2. Symptoms must be present for at least 3 months.
3. When allowed to sleep in accordance with their internal biological clock, patients' sleep quality and duration are improved, with consistent but advanced timing of the major sleep episode.
4. Sleep log and, whenever possible, actigraphy monitoring for at least 7 days (and preferably 14 days) demonstrate a stable advance in timing of the habitual sleep period. Both work/school days and free days must be included within this monitoring.
5. Sleep disturbance is not better explained by another current sleep disorder, medical or neurological disorder, mental disorder, medication use, or substance use disorder.

PATHOPHYSIOLOGY

As in DSWPD, multiple endogenous and exogenous factors may contribute to the syndrome of ASWPD, and all elements may not be relevant in an individual patient. Nevertheless, various lines of research indicate that the processes described in the following discussion contribute to ASWPD.

Clock Gene Polymorphisms

Circadian clock gene polymorphisms have been implicated in the pathophysiology of ASWPD in families with multiple affected relatives. Pedigrees indicate that familial inheritance of ASWPD occurs in a highly penetrant, autosomal dominant manner. Mutations in the human Period 2 (*hPER2*) clock gene (Toh et al. 2001), casein kinase 1 delta (*CK1δ*; Brennan et al. 2013; Xu et al. 2005), and cryptochrome 2 (Hirano et al. 2016) all have been shown to play a role in familial ASWPD.

Circadian Phase Advance

As in DSWPD, abnormal internal circadian timing has been observed in patients with ASWPD (see Figure 12–1). One study that measured sleep timing and endogenous circadian phase showed that compared with control subjects, patients with ASWPD had earlier mean sleep onset times (7:25 P.M. vs. 11:10 P.M.) and wake times (4:18 A.M. vs. 7:44 A.M.) as well as earlier DLMOs (5:31 P.M. vs. 9:21 P.M.) and Tmin (11:22 P.M. vs. 3:35 A.M.) (Jones et al. 1999).

Shorter Circadian Period

Genetic and behavioral evidence support a shorter tau (period length) as an etiology of ASWPD. At least two gene mutations in familial ASWPD are thought to shorten tau. A serine-to-glycine mutation in the CK1ε binding region of the *hPER2* clock gene was found in one family, and the homologous gene in *Drosophila* shortens the circadian period in the fruit fly (Toh et al. 2001). Similarly, a cryptochrome 2 missense mutation identified in another family with inherited ASWPD has been shown to shorten tau and to decrease evening light sensitivity in mice (Hirano et al. 2016).

Behavioral data from a patient with ASWPD showed a period length of 23.3 hours (Jones et al. 1999). Just as a longer tau predisposes individuals to have delayed circadian phase, a shorter tau increases the likelihood of circadian phase advance because it is difficult for the internal circadian clock to entrain to 24-hour clock time, resulting in an "internal day" that ends before 24 hours have elapsed and manifests as earlier timing of biological night and sleep patterns.

Premature Birth

In rodents, patterns of light-dark exposure early in development can affect circadian behavior in mature animals. The underlying mechanisms of this phenomenon are not known. However, adults who were born prematurely and with low birth weights have been observed to have earlier sleep timing than control subjects born full term (Björkqvist et al. 2014). It is speculated that light exposure during neonatal intensive care may alter circadian responsiveness in adults.

Sensitivity to Light

As in DSWPD, the advanced sleep-wake patterns and circadian rhythms in ASWPD may be due to altered sensitivity to the entraining effects of light-dark exposure, specifically decreased sensitivity to phase-delaying effects of evening light or increased sensitivity to phase-advancing effects of morning light. In older adults, cataracts have been identified as a possible contributing factor in ASWPD because the yellowing of the lens diminishes light exposure and filters the wavelengths of light with the greatest circadian effects (Yan and Wang 2016).

EPIDEMIOLOGY

ASWPD is believed to be relatively uncommon, although precise prevalence estimates are not known. In a study of approximately 4,000 New Zealand adults between the ages of 20 and 59 years, self-reported symptoms yielded prevalence estimates ranging from <1% up to 7%, depending on the symptoms used to define the diagnosis (Paine et al. 2014). ASWPD is more common among older adults (e.g., Ando et al. 2002), but no clear sex or gender differences have been established.

CLINICAL PRESENTATION

Excessive evening sleepiness with an inability to stay awake until a conventional bedtime and chronic early morning awakenings are the hallmarks of ASWPD. Patients report that they become so sleepy that they cannot participate in evening activities or do so with great difficulty. Furthermore, they state that they cannot sleep past their earlier-than-desired wake time regardless of the time they fell asleep the night before. Delaying bedtime past the time that they desire to sleep contributes to chronic insufficient sleep in patients with ASWPD, which can impact daytime functioning.

DIAGNOSTIC PROCEDURES, TESTS, AND QUESTIONNAIRES

ASWPD is a clinical diagnosis, because no biomarkers or genetic tests are available at this time. As with DSWPD, a diagnosis of ASWPD can be confirmed with a thorough history and documentation of sleep patterns with sleep diaries or actigraphy. The ICSD-3 recommends that sleep and wake times be recorded for at least 7 days, and ideally at least 14 days, including work/school days and free days. Further details of diagnostic procedures are described earlier in the DSWPD section on diagnostic tools.

DIFFERENTIAL DIAGNOSIS

Insomnia

ASWPD must be distinguished from chronic sleep maintenance insomnia (see Chapter 3). One factor is that patients with ASWPD are more likely to report a preference for beginning their nighttime sleep episode in the early evening than are individuals with insomnia. Patients with insomnia are more likely to report multiple awakenings at night rather than a single terminal awakening and may also experience more hyperarousal and perpetuating behaviors than those with ASWPD. Psycho-physiological insomnia can overlap with ASWPD. For instance, patients whose sleep difficulties start with an advanced circadian phase may develop a psychophysiological component due to the recurrent experience of waking earlier than expected. Similarly, repetitive exposure to light in the morning hours may advance circadian rhythms among patients whose sleep difficulties begin with psychophysiological insomnia.

Other Sleep and Circadian Disorders

When approaching a patient with evening sleepiness and early morning awakenings, it is critical that other common sleep disorders are considered and excluded. For instance, sleep-disordered breathing results in sleep fragmentation and physiological changes that can lead to sleepiness in the daytime or evening and nighttime awakenings. Testing for sleep apnea and other sleep disorders is warranted when suggested by history and physical examination findings (see Chapter 8). ASWPD is distinguished from irregular sleep-wake rhythm disorder (ISWRD; see Chapter 13) by the mostly consolidated sleep periods in ASWPD compared with ISWRD and from non-24-hour sleep-wake phase disorder (see Chapter 13) by lack of free-running circadian rhythms and sleep-wake patterns.

Psychiatric Disorders

Early morning awakenings are a marker of one clinical phenotype of major depressive disorder (Benca et al. 1992), and most patients with anxiety disorders experience sleep maintenance insomnia (Monti and Monti 2000). PTSD is also associated with various sleep disturbances that can include early morning awakenings (Ohayon and Shapiro 2000). Indeed, circadian dysfunction likely plays an important role in many psychiatric disorders. As described earlier, a meta-analysis performed by Gee et al. (2019) indicated that addressing sleep disturbances in psychiatric disorders significantly reduces depressive symptoms. Nevertheless, although abnormal sleep timing can occur in patients with mental health difficulties and may exacerbate those syndromes, ASWPD can and should be distinguished from a primary psychiatric illness so that targeted therapies can be offered.

TREATMENT

Bright Light Therapy

Evening bright light therapy is the main treatment for ASWPD, and its use is supported by two clinical trials. One trial showed a circadian phase delay of Tmin and an increase in sleep duration after 12 days of exposure to 4,000 lux light for 2 hours between 8 P.M. and 11 P.M. (Campbell et al. 1993). The other showed an improvement in patient-reported sleepiness after exposure to 250 lux for 2–3 hours per night but no shift in circadian phase or sleep improvements (Palmer et al. 2003). Bright light exposure should be timed to begin at the onset of evening sleepiness for approximately 1–3 hours. Other than the timing, parameters for treating ASWPD with bright light are the same as in DSWPD.

Behavioral Modifications

Chronotherapy could also be employed to treat ASWPD. This strategy has been described in one case study (Moldofsky et al. 1986) wherein a man in his 60s progressively moved his bedtime earlier by 3 hours every 2 days, and ultimately advanced his bedtime 19.5 hours from 6:30 P.M. to 11:00 P.M.

Exogenous Melatonin

Based on published melatonin phase response curves (e.g., Lewy et al. 1998), melatonin administration late in the biological night or early in the morning would be expected to produce phase delays. Evidence that exogenous melatonin can produce reliable phase delays is weaker than data supporting phase advances, and no studies show efficacy or safety of melatonin to treat ASWPD. Thus, exogenous melatonin administration is not recommended.

Pharmacological Treatment

Although short-acting hypnotics might help some patients with ASWPD fall back to sleep after awakening too early in the morning, these medications do not work through the circadian system and would not be expected to correct the underlying circadian dysregulation in this disorder. In addition, hypnotics can be associated with adverse effects and are not recommended to treat ASWPD.

CONCLUSION

ASWPD is a rare circadian rhythm sleep disorder that affects mostly older individuals and manifests as excessive sleepiness and a desire to begin the nightly sleep period in the late afternoon/early evening. Patients with ASWPD struggle to stay awake to attend to end-of-the-day personal responsibilities and social obligations. Several clock gene mutations have been identified in families with inherited forms of ASPWD and provide clues to the underlying pathophysiology, including the contributions of a relatively advanced circadian phase, a circadian period less than 24 hours, and decreased responsiveness to evening light exposure. Diagnosis is made clinically after documenting at least 3 months of sleep patterns that are earlier than desired/conventional sleep times. First-line treatment for ASWPD is evening bright light exposure to delay circadian rhythms.

Summary

DSWPD and ASWPD are disorders of circadian timing that yield sleep-wake patterns that do not conform to desired or socially acceptable times. Genetics, circadian physiology, and individual behaviors and routines contribute to the development of DSWPD and ASWPD. Persons with DSWPD and ASWPD often obtain insufficient sleep resulting in daytime impairment and further exacerbation of their circadian misalignment. The most promising treatment at this time is the use of light-dark exposure to realign endogenous circadian rhythms to yield a more conventional sleep-wake schedule.

KEY CLINICAL POINTS

- Thorough assessment is critical to differentiating features of delayed sleep-wake phase disorder (DSWPD) from other common sleep problems. Individuals who report difficulties with sleep onset are commonly misdiagnosed with primary insomnia and are prescribed hypnotic drugs. However, the data supporting this as an effective intervention in DSWPD are limited.

- Nonpharmacological sleep interventions are effective in reducing the severity of depression in the context of circadian dysfunction. Treating sleep may offer a relatively low-stigma means of reducing depressive symptoms in individuals who have both DSWPD and mental health difficulties.

- The lack of public awareness of DSWPD contributes to the difficulties experienced by affected individuals. Parents may be chastised for not imposing acceptable sleep patterns on their children, and schools and workplaces rarely tolerate chronic lateness or absenteeism, failing to appreciate the etiology of DSWPD.

- Early morning obligations play a significant role in the onset of DSWPD in adolescents in particular, making it that much more important to advocate for later school start times that can translate to improvements in nocturnal sleep while reducing the risk of functional impairments that often result from sleep insufficiency.

- Many individuals with DSWPD attempt to address their sleep disorder by forcing themselves to keep a normal schedule, which results in a chronic sleep deficit. These symptoms can mimic depression, anxiety, or ADHD.

- A diagnosis of advanced sleep-wake phase disorder (ASWPD) should be considered in older adults who report falling asleep and waking too early. Documentation of advanced sleep timing with sleep diaries or actigraphy for 7–14 days is needed to confirm the diagnosis.

- Sleep quality and duration are normal in ASWPD when patients are allowed to sleep at their preferred, biologically driven times, but many patients force themselves to stay awake in the evening to fulfill work, family, or social obligations and accumulate sleep debt because they cannot stay asleep late enough in the morning to obtain adequate sleep.

- Studies of familial ASWPD have identified mutations in several clock genes, and the homologous genes in animal models have been shown to shorten the circadian period or reduce sensitivity to light, revealing important clues to the underlying pathophysiology of circadian rhythm sleep-wake disorders.

- Bright light therapy in the evening is the first-line treatment to phase-delay endogenous circadian rhythms, promote alertness in the evening, and facilitate later wake times in patients with ASWPD. Neither melatonin nor hypnotics have been shown to be effective in treating this disorder, and their use is discouraged.

References

American Academy of Sleep Medicine: International Classification of Sleep Disorders, 3rd Edition. Darien, IL, American Academy of Sleep Medicine, 2014

American Psychiatric Association: Diagnostic and Statistical Manual of Mental Disorders, 5th Edition. Arlington, VA, American Psychiatric Association, 2013

Ando K, Kripke DF, Ancoli-Israel S: Delayed and advanced sleep phase symptoms. Isr J Psychiatry Relat Sci 39(1):11–18, 2002 12013705

Aoki H, Ozeki Y, Yamada N: Hypersensitivity of melatonin suppression in response to light in patients with delayed sleep phase syndrome. Chronobiol Int 18(2):263–271, 2001 11379666

Auger RR, Burgess HJ, Emens JS, et al: Clinical practice guideline for the treatment of intrinsic circadian rhythm sleep-wake disorders: advanced sleep-wake phase disorder (ASWPD), delayed sleep-wake phase disorder (DSWPD), non-24-hour sleep-wake rhythm disorder (N24SWD), and irregular sleep-wake rhythm disorder (ISWRD). An update for 2015. J Clin Sleep Med 11(10):1199–1236, 2015 26414986

Baehr EK, Revelle W, Eastman CI: Individual differences in the phase and amplitude of the human circadian temperature rhythm: with an emphasis on morningness–eveningness. J Sleep Res 9(2):117–127 2000 10849238

Benca RM, Obermeyer WH, Thisted RA, et al: Sleep and psychiatric disorders. A meta-analysis. Arch Gen Psychiatry 49(8):651–670, 1992 1386215

Björkqvist J, Paavonen J, Andersson S, et al: Advanced sleep-wake rhythm in adults born prematurely: confirmation by actigraphy-based assessment in the Helsinki Study of Very Low Birth Weight Adults. Sleep Med 15(9):1101–1106, 2014 24980065

Borbély AA, Daan S, Wirz-Justice A, et al: The two-process model of sleep regulation: a reappraisal. J Sleep Res 25(2):131–143, 2016 26762182

Brennan KC, Bates EA, Shapiro RE, et al: Casein kinase 1δ mutations in familial migraine and advanced sleep phase. Sci Transl Med 5(183):1–11, 2013 23636092

Campbell IG, Darchia N, Higgins LM, et al: Adolescent changes in homeostatic regulation of EEG activity in the delta and theta frequency bands during NREM sleep. Sleep (Basel) 34(1):83–91, 2011 21203377

Campbell SS, Dawson D, Anderson MW: Alleviation of sleep maintenance insomnia with timed exposure to bright light. J Am Geriatr Soc 41(8):829–836, 1993 8340561

Carpen JD, Archer SN, Skene DJ, et al: A single-nucleotide polymorphism in the 5′-untranslated region of the hPER2 gene is associated with diurnal preference. J Sleep Res 14(3):293–297, 2005 16120104

Carpen JD, von Schantz M, Smits M, et al: A silent polymorphism in the PER1 gene associates with extreme diurnal preference in humans. J Hum Genet 51(12):1122–1125, 2006 17051316

Carskadon MA: Sleep in adolescents: the perfect storm. Pediatr Clin North Am 58(3):637–647, 2011 21600346

Duffy JF, Rimmer DW, Czeisler CA: Association of intrinsic circadian period with morningness-eveningness, usual wake time, and circadian phase. Behav Neurosci 115(4):895–899, 2001 11508728

Eaton DK, McKnight-Eily LR, Lowry R, et al: Prevalence of insufficient, borderline, and optimal hours of sleep among high school students—United States, 2007. J Adolesc Health 46(4):399–401, 2010 20307832

Gee B, Orchard F, Clarke E, et al: The effect of non-pharmacological sleep interventions on depression symptoms: a meta-analysis of randomised controlled trials. Sleep Med Rev 43:118–128, 2019 30579141

Gradisar M, Dohnt H, Gardner G, et al: A randomized controlled trial of cognitive-behavior therapy plus bright light therapy for adolescent delayed sleep phase disorder. Sleep (Basel) 34(12):1671–1680, 2011 22131604

Hirano A, Shi G, Jones CR, et al: A cryptochrome 2 mutation yields advanced sleep phase in humans. eLife 5:e16695, 2016 27529127

Jones CR, Campbell SS, Zone SE, et al: Familial advanced sleep-phase syndrome: a short-period circadian rhythm variant in humans. Nat Med 5(9):1062–1065, 1999 10470086

Jones CR, Huang AL, Ptácek LJ, et al: Genetic basis of human circadian rhythm disorders. Exp Neurol 243:28–33, 2013 22849821

Katzenberg D, Young T, Finn L, et al: A CLOCK polymorphism associated with human diurnal preference. Sleep 21(6):569–576, 1998 9779516

Kosmadopoulos A, Sargent C, Zhou X, et al: The efficacy of objective and subjective predictors of driving performance during sleep restriction and circadian misalignment. Accid Anal Prev 99(Pt B):445–451, 2017

Lack LC, Wright HR: Treating chronobiological components of chronic insomnia. Sleep Med 8(6):637–644, 2007 17383935

Lack L, Wright H: Circadian rhythm disorders 1: phase-advanced and phase-delayed disorders, in Oxford Handbook on Sleep and Sleep Disorders. Edited by Espie C, Morin C. New York, Oxford University Press, 2012, pp 597–625

Lewy AJ, Bauer VK, Ahmed S, et al: The human phase response curve (PRC) to melatonin is about 12 hours out of phase with the PRC to light. Chronobiol Int 15(1):71–83, 1998

Micic G, Lovato N, Gradisar M, et al: The etiology of delayed sleep phase disorder. Sleep Med Rev 27:29–38, 2016 26434674

Micic G, Lovato N, Gradisar M, et al: Personality differences in patients with delayed sleep-wake phase disorder and non-24-h sleep-wake rhythm disorder relative to healthy sleepers. Sleep Med 30:128–135, 2017 28215235

Moldofsky H, Musisi S, Phillipson EA: Treatment of a case of advanced sleep phase syndrome by phase advance chronotherapy. Sleep 9(1):61–65, 1986 3961368

Monti JM, Monti D: Sleep disturbance in generalized anxiety disorder and its treatment. Sleep Med Rev 4(3):263–276, 2000 12531169

National Sleep Foundation: Sleep in America Poll: 2006 Teens and Sleep. Washington, DC, 2006. Available at: https://www.sleepfoundation.org/professionals/sleep-americar-polls/2006-teens-and-sleep. Accessed April 22, 2020.

Ohayon MM, Shapiro CM: Sleep disturbances and psychiatric disorders associated with posttraumatic stress disorder in the general population. Compr Psychiatry 41(6):469–478, 2000 11086154

Ozaki S, Uchiyama M, Shirakawa S, et al: Prolonged interval from body temperature nadir to sleep offset in patients with delayed sleep phase syndrome. Sleep 19(1):36–40, 1996 8650460

Paine SJ, Fink J, Gander PH, et al: Identifying advanced and delayed sleep phase disorders in the general population: a national survey of New Zealand adults. Chronobiol Int 31(5):627–636, 2014 24548144

Palmer CR, Kripke DF, Savage HC Jr, et al: Efficacy of enhanced evening light for advanced sleep phase syndrome. Behav Sleep Med 1(4):213–226, 2003 15602801

Richardson CE, Gradisar M, Short MA, et al: Can exercise regulate the circadian system of adolescents? Novel implications for the treatment of delayed sleep-wake phase disorder. Sleep Med Rev 34:122–129, 2017 27546185

Roenneberg T, Kuehnle T, Pramstaller PP, et al: A marker for the end of adolescence. Curr Biol 14(24):R1038–R1039, 2004 15620633

Sharkey KM, Carskadon MA, Figueiro MG, et al: Effects of an advanced sleep schedule and morning short wavelength light exposure on circadian phase in young adults with late sleep schedules. Sleep Med 12(7):685–692, 2011 21704557

Sivertsen B, Harvey AG, Pallesen S, et al: Mental health problems in adolescents with delayed sleep phase: results from a large population-based study in Norway. J Sleep Res 24(1):11–18, 2015 25358244

Takano A, Uchiyama M, Kajimura N, et al: A missense variation in human casein kinase I epsilon gene that induces functional alteration and shows an inverse association with circadian rhythm sleep disorders. Neuropsychopharmacology 29(10):1901–1909, 2004 15187983

Toh KL, Jones CR, He Y, et al: An *hPer2* phosphorylation site mutation in familial advanced sleep phase syndrome. Science 291(5506):1040–1043, 2001 11232563

Uchiyama M, Okawa M, Shibui K, et al: Poor recovery sleep after sleep deprivation in delayed sleep phase syndrome. Psychiatry Clin Neurosci 53(2):195–197, 1999 10459687

Werner H, Lebourgeois MK, Geiger A, et al: Assessment of chronotype in four- to eleven-year-old children: reliability and validity of the Children's Chronotype Questionnaire (CCTQ). Chronobiol Int 26(5):992–1014, 2009 19637055

Wilhelmsen-Langeland A, Saxvig IW, Johnsen EH, et al: Patients with delayed sleep-wake phase disorder show poorer executive functions compared to good sleepers. Sleep Med 54:244–249, 2019

Wright KP Jr, McHill AW, Birks BR, et al: Entrainment of the human circadian clock to the natural light-dark cycle. Curr Biol 23(16):1554–1558, 2013 23910656

Xu Y, Padiath QS, Shapiro RE, et al: Functional consequences of a CKIdelta mutation causing familial advanced sleep phase syndrome. Nature 434(7033):640–644, 2005 15800623

Yan SS, Wang W: The effect of lens aging and cataract surgery on circadian rhythm. Int J Ophthalmol 9(7):1066–1074, 2016 27500118

Irregular Sleep-Wake, Non-24-Hour Sleep-Wake, Jet Lag, and Shift Work Sleep Disorders

Daniel Jin Blum, Ph.D.

Jamie M. Zeitzer, Ph.D.

This chapter rounds out the remaining four circadian rhythm sleep-wake disorders. We begin with the rare irregular sleep-wake rhythm disorder (ISWRD) and non-24-hour sleep-wake disorder (N24SWD), and follow with the increasingly more common jet lag and shift work sleep disorder (SWSD). Whereas both advanced sleep-wake phase disorder (ASWPD) and delayed sleep-wake phase disorder (DSWPD; see Chapter 12) are generally considered to be stable, naturally occurring circadian rhythms that occur significantly earlier or later than the social clock, respectively, the four conditions discussed in this chapter are characterized by their instability in sleep-wake patterns. Biological factors drive underlying circadian disruptions in ISWRD and N24SWD, whereas behavioral patterns largely dictate jet lag and SWSD. However, both biological and behavioral dimensions contribute to the development and maintenance of these circadian rhythm disorders.

Irregular Sleep-Wake Rhythm Disorder

DIAGNOSTIC CRITERIA

ISWRD is characterized by the absence of a well-defined circadian pattern to the sleep-wake cycle. Although the patient's total amount of sleep could be comparable with a healthy same-age peer, no major sleep period occurs across the 24-hour day. Instead, at least three sleep episodes occur, varying between 1 and 4 hours in length, with the longest period typi-

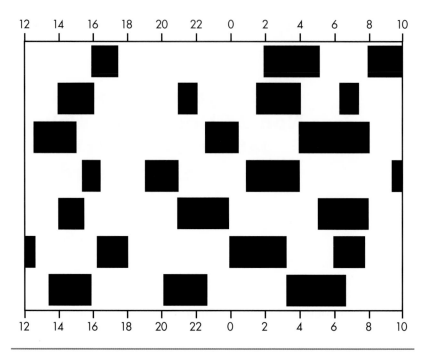

FIGURE 13–1.   Irregular sleep-wake rhythm disorder sample sleep log (7 days depicted vertically).

Sleep-wake pattern characterized by at least three sleep episodes (*black bars*) that vary between 1 and 4 hours in length across a 24-hour period (represented horizontally).

cally occurring between 2 A.M. and 6 A.M. (Figure 13–1) (Wagner 1996; Zee and Vitiello 2009). Symptoms must be present for at least 3 months and not be better explained by medication use or by another sleep, medical, neurological, mental, or substance use disorder (American Academy of Sleep Medicine 2014).

PATHOPHYSIOLOGY

The typical pattern of sleep in adult humans is a single consolidated, approximately 8-hour nighttime sleep period each day. In individuals with ISWRD, however, sleep bouts can be highly fragmented, occurring seemingly sporadically throughout the day. It has been speculated that ISWRD is secondary to a deficit in the circadian component of sleep and wake regulation. The timing and consolidation of sleep are regulated by an interplay between two systems: the sleep homeostat (Process S) and the circadian timing system (Process C) (Borbély 1982). The sleep homeostat—the physiological equivalent of which is unknown, although it is hypothesized to be excess adenosine release in the basal forebrain (Porkka-Heiskanen et al. 1997)—is an appetitive process such that the longer you are awake, the more tired you become, and the longer you are asleep, the less sleep you need.

The circadian timing system provides two separable signals. The first is a wake-promoting signal that rises throughout the normal waking day and peaks in the hours just before expected bedtime (Dijk and Czeisler 1994). The second is a sleep-promoting signal that rises throughout the normal sleep period and peaks in the hours just before expected wake time (Dijk and Czeisler 1994). In this manner, the sleep homeostat is *responsive* to sleep behavior, whereas the circadian system is *predictive* of sleep behavior. The interaction of these two signals leads to the consolidation of sleep and wake into single daily periods. With a decrease in the amplitude of the circadian component, the timing of sleep would primarily be driven by the sleep homeostat. Thus, as homeostatic pressure for sleep increased with time awake, no circadian wake-promoting signal would be sent to offset the drive for sleep, and sleep would be initiated after only a few hours of wakefulness. Sleep and wake would thereby cycle more frequently over the course of a single day. Non-circadian-related causes of ISWRD are also possible, including the use of medication that can alter normal sleep processes, specific types of brain injuries, and both internal (e.g., pain) and external (e.g., ambient sound or light) stimuli that can fragment nocturnal sleep.

EPIDEMIOLOGY

The prevalence of ISWRD is unknown, but it is thought to be relatively rare. No accurate statistics are available on sex, cultural, or racial correlations. Patients with associated risk factors include institutionalized older adults as well as individuals with neurodegenerative disorders such as Alzheimer's disease; neurodevelopmental disorders such as intellectual disability; psychiatric disorders such as schizophrenia; or traumatic brain injury. ISWRD is most common in Alzheimer's disease, but it can also be observed in other neurodegenerative diseases as well as in normal aging. ISWRD may also be found in some hospital environments, notably intensive care and rehabilitation units. In the latter situation, the diminished circadian drive may be secondary to acute neural damage (e.g., traumatic brain injury) (Baumann et al. 2007) or due to the continuous lighting and loud or disruptive environment found in many intensive care units (Jewett et al. 1994). Continuous lighting or the lack of outdoor light exposure may be partially responsible for the irregular sleep-wake pattern often observed among elderly patients in institutional settings. No other genetic patterns to ISWRD have been documented, other than those associated with neurodegenerative and neurodevelopmental disorders.

CLINICAL PRESENTATION, COURSE, AND COMPLICATIONS

ISWRD is more frequently seen in older individuals and can occur at any age. People who present with ISWRD often describe symptoms of maintenance insomnia due to fragmented nocturnal sleep and excessive daytime sleepiness (EDS) related to frequent napping during the day. Even patients with minimal or mild cognitive impairment may appear unmotivated or resistant to treatment—clearly understanding the interventions and rationale in sessions but failing to track their sleep or implement the strategies consistently. Due to the frequently associated cognitive component, treatment success can often be contingent upon caregiver support and engagement. Caregiver burden and burnout can be high for those caring for this population, so it is important to address this issue early in treatment.

DIAGNOSTIC PROCEDURES, TESTS, AND QUESTIONNAIRES

Diagnosis of ISWRD is based on a thorough clinical interview accompanied by at least 1 week (preferably 2 weeks) of sleep logs or continuous actigraphic monitoring. Analysis of sleep data should indicate at least one 24-hour period that has three or more bouts of sleep between 1 and 4 hours in duration. When selecting an appropriate method for sleep tracking, consider the degree of cognitive impairment of the presenting individual. Given that ISWRD is frequently associated with disorders involving significant cognitive impairment (e.g., dementia, intellectual disability), actigraphy may provide a more accurate assessment of a patient's baseline sleep-wake behaviors from diagnosis through treatment.

DIFFERENTIAL DIAGNOSIS

ISWRD can be differentiated from other factors that contribute to irregular sleep schedules, such as poor sleep hygiene, shift work, and other sleep disorders, based on the number of distinct sleep bouts (three or more) that regularly recur over a 24-hour period. The relatively low prevalence rates in the general public combined with the association with significant cognitive impairment can also help alert a clinician to include ISWRD as a possible differential diagnosis when working with individuals with neurodegenerative disorders.

TREATMENT

Clinical management of ISWRD seeks to consolidate sleep during a patient's circadian night by increasing the amplitude and regularity of his or her circadian rhythms.

Light Therapy

Most treatments of ISWRD have focused on regularizing the timing of light during the day and minimizing nocturnal light exposure. These treatments have been variable in their success. No consensus has been found on the specific amounts or pattern of light, or whether just morning light is necessary or if light throughout the day is more beneficial. It is important to recognize that treatments for ISWRD should be specific to the etiology of the disorder. If nocturnal sleep fragmentation is caused by a noncircadian cause (e.g., pain), circadian-based treatments such as phototherapy will be unlikely to have a successful outcome.

Melatonin

Evening melatonin can enhance treatment by reducing sleep latency and increasing total sleep time for pediatric and adolescent populations. Although research examining doses is inconclusive (ranging from 2 mg to 20 mg), it is likely that lower doses (0.1–3 mg) could be more effective in stabilizing the patient's circadian phase. However, more research is needed to determine the effective doses and timing. Additionally, when melatonin is used as a monotherapy for ISWRD, these benefits are offset by the negative impact it may have on mood (Riemersma-van der Lek et al. 2008).

Multimodal Approaches

Multimodal approaches have the strongest evidence base (Morgenthaler et al. 2007) and include improving sleep hygiene (e.g., regular bedtimes and rise times, maintaining a consistent bedtime routine, decreasing evening light and noise), using light therapy in the morning, increasing light during the day (duration and intensity), and increasing structured social and physical activity. Clinicians can consider melatonin as an adjunctive therapy on a case-by-case basis while being cognizant of possible adverse effects.

Hypnotics

Hypnotic medications are not recommended in the treatment of ISWRD in elderly or cognitively impaired patients due to increased risk for falls, headaches, cognitive impairment, and medication interactions (Morgenthaler et al. 2007).

CONCLUSION

Rigorous studies examining ISWRD are scarce, likely due in part to the predominant focus on the comorbid disorders (i.e., severe developmental delay, dementia) when individuals with ISWRD are seen in clinics. As such, diagnosis and subsequent treatment of ISWRD can often be overlooked, given that sleep is often thought of as secondary to these other health issues. As with many circadian rhythm disorders, a multimodal approach that focuses on increasing circadian amplitude (i.e., creating greater contrasts between light and dark, sleep and wake, activity and rest, feeding and fasting) has the largest evidence base. For ISWRD, this typically includes increasing daytime light (duration and intensity) and social and physical activities along with decreasing evening light and activities. Melatonin has also been used successfully in conjunction with daytime light and social rhythm therapy but is not recommended as a solo intervention for any age. Additionally, it is not recommended for older adults with ISWRD even in multicomponent treatment.

Due to the associated level of cognitive impairment, ISWRD can be a challenging disorder for a patient to manage alone. Thus, an ecological approach to identifying social, familial, and institutional structures and constraints can be vital for implementing interventions successfully. Future directions could examine melatonin doses and timing, light intensity, caregiver training for implementing interventions, reducing associated caregiver burnout, and interventions targeting the food entrained oscillator to stabilize peripheral clocks.

Non-24-Hour Sleep-Wake Disorder

DIAGNOSTIC CRITERIA

N24SWD, also referred to as "free-running disorder," "nonentrained disorder," or "hypernychthemeral syndrome," describes a chronic desynchrony between the sleep-wake cycle and 24-hour light-dark cycle (Zhu and Zee 2012). This pattern of circadian misalignment typically presents as a relatively steady, continual delay in sleep-wake timing and should be apparent on daily sleep logs or actigraphy for at least 14 days (Figure 13–2). Symptoms must be present for at least 3 months and not be better explained by medication or another sleep, medical, neurological, psychological, or substance use disorder (American Academy of Sleep Medicine 2014).

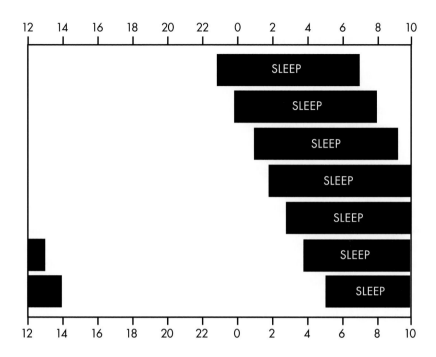

FIGURE 13–2. **Non-24-hour sleep-wake disorder sample sleep log (7 days depicted vertically).**

Sleep-wake pattern characterized by a relatively steady, continual delay in the sleep-wake timing. Sleep episodes depicted as *black bars*, with 24-hour time represented horizontally.

PATHOPHYSIOLOGY

Central Circadian Clock and Light Signal

N24SWD is characterized by a lack of synchronization between the internal circadian clock and 24-hour solar day. In the parlance of the field, the circadian clock is "free running." The human circadian clock has a near, but not exactly, 24-hour rhythm, reported to average 24 hours and 12 minutes (Czeisler et al. 1999). Thus, on a daily or near-daily basis, in most individuals the clock is synchronized or entrained to an external stimulus to keep this non-24-hour rhythm aligned with the 24-hour solar day. The most robust entraining signal is light. In mammals, light signals to the central circadian clock, located in the suprachiasmatic nucleus (SCN) of the anterior hypothalamus, are mediated by a pathway originating at the retina (Moore 1995). A specialized set of retinal ganglion cells express light-sensitive melanopsin, which creates a retinohypothalamic tract connecting the retina with the SCN (Gooley et al. 2001). These cells integrate information from both rod and cone pathways as well as from intrinsic signals arising from light-induced melanopsin activation (Ruby et al. 2002). When the light signal is absent or inadequate, the internal circadian clock is not aligned to the solar day and free runs. In the complete absence of a light signal, such as occurs in many blind individuals, the circadian clock would run at its intrinsic period and signal approximately 12 minutes later each day. Thus, every 5 days, the internal clock becomes misaligned by about 1 hour—in essence, the brain shifts one time zone every 5 days.

Non-24-Hour Sleep-Wake Disorder in the Blind

N24SWD is most commonly observed in blind individuals, although not all blind individuals have this disorder. This can best be explained by the varied biological causes of blindness as well as a difference between the biological and legal definitions of blindness. If individuals who are blind have any residual perception of images, even if it is insufficient to read or recognize objects, they typically have no significant impediment to normal circadian entrainment through light. Although the formation of images depends upon a dense network of retinal neurons, the conveyance of light information from the retina to the SCN can be accomplished with a sparse network that is missing many photoreceptive elements, such as occurs in many forms of blindness. Cortical causes of blindness would also allow for relatively normal circadian entrainment by light (Flynn-Evans et al. 2014).

EPIDEMIOLOGY

N24SWD is most commonly found in individuals who are blind, with prevalence rates ranging from 13% to 50%. N24SWD has also been reported in sighted individuals, but this is considered extremely rare and has no reported prevalence statistics (Abbott et al. 2017). It is controversial as to whether N24SWD in sighted individuals is etiologically similar to that found in those who are blind. N24SWD in sighted individuals is often found comorbid with psychiatric disorders such as schizophrenia and unipolar and bipolar depression, likely due to the general circadian desynchrony (e.g., irregular light exposure) associated with these disorders (Uchiyama and Lockley 2015).

N24SWD may also be found in sighted individuals with DSWPD (see Chapter 12) who have a very long intrinsic circadian period, reduced responsivity to light, or a combination, such that the synchronizing signal that light provides is insufficient to overcome the >24-hour period. For example, an individual with a 25-hour circadian period who is exposed to a daily light schedule that can provide at most a 45-minute change in circadian timing would still experience a 15-minute delay each day. In sighted individuals fitting this phenotype, patients present with highly delayed sleep times that can be maintained for weeks or even months at a time and suddenly devolve into N24SWD. It is likely that the light that they are receiving is the exact amount necessary to synchronize their circadian clock with the solar day, and any deviation from this pattern will cause the clock to become desynchronized until it free runs back into the proper alignment with light exposure. Aside from compromised photoreception, other risk factors that may contribute to the development or maintenance of N24SWD include insufficient daytime light (duration or intensity), poor sleep hygiene, and irregularly timed nonphotic zeitgebers (e.g., exercise, social rhythms, meal timing).

Case reports have been made of patients with DSWPD and long intrinsic circadian periods developing N24SWD after receiving chronotherapy (Oren and Wehr 1992). Given this, clinicians should discuss this potential side effect with patients who have DSWPD and are considering chronotherapy. No sex, racial, or ethnic differences of N24SWD are known.

CLINICAL PRESENTATION, COURSE, AND COMPLICATIONS

Due to the progressive circadian drift, N24SWD can present as periods of insomnia, as EDS, or be asymptomatic depending upon when the individual is trying to sleep relative to his or her circadian period (Uchiyama and Lockley 2015). Individuals will have 1) no difficulties with sleep when their internal clock is aligned with the desired social or waking rhythm, 2) sleep initiation difficulties as their clock starts to drift later into the evening, and 3) EDS (often accompanied by napping) as their clock pushes the circadian night into the social daytime. Each period (i.e., insomnia, EDS, asymptomatic) can last several days to weeks depending upon the length of the circadian period, taking as little as 3 weeks to cycle through the 24-hour day with a particularly long circadian period (i.e., >25 hours) to as long as 6 months for an average circadian period (i.e., approximately 24.2 hours).

Although this constantly shifting pattern of sleep and wake can be highly disruptive to occupational, social, and academic functioning, diagnosis and treatment of N24SWD is typically delayed several years after initial symptoms appear. The onset of N24SWD can occur at any age in blind individuals and is often temporally linked to the loss of photoreception (Lockley et al. 1997).

In sighted patients with N24SWD, this pattern follows a relatively consistent "free-running" cadence when the start of the endogenous circadian night overlaps with the evening to early morning. These individuals typically have a long circadian period leading to 1-hour delays every day. As sleep initiation approaches 8–10 A.M., their sleep pattern becomes more disrupted, accelerating their endogenous clock quickly through the daylight hours within a few days before resuming the "free-running" rhythm. These phase-delay "jumps" occur in approximately one-half of sighted individuals with N24SWD.

Blind individuals with N24SWD fall across the spectrum of short to lengthy daily delays, with a small minority experiencing continual phase advances instead of delays. Sleep rhythms in blind individuals also show a steady "free-running" pattern, while sleep initiation occurs during the circadian evening and early morning. Sleep becomes fragmented into longer naps as the circadian night enters the morning and daytime (e.g., when endogenous melatonin peaks during daylight hours) until the endogenous clock realigns with the light-dark cycle. Phase "jumps" starting in the morning have also been observed in some blind individuals, although not as commonly as in sighted individuals with N24SWD.

DIAGNOSIS

Diagnosis of N24SWD is conducted primarily with a thorough clinical interview, a detailed sleep history, and sleep logs or actigraphy for at least 14 days. Estimating circadian phase using serial measurements of 6-sulfatoxymelatonin, the primary urine metabolite of melatonin, or time of core body temperature minimum (Tmin) can be helpful to confirm the continual circadian desynchrony, although these are not routinely available. Polysomnography is also not routinely used in the treatment or diagnosis of N24SWD (Sack et al. 2007).

DIFFERENTIAL DIAGNOSIS

Differentiating N24SWD from other sleep and circadian rhythm disorders can be nuanced but is important. A patient with N24SWD could appear to have insomnia (see Chapter 3), DSWPD, ASWPD (see Chapter 12), or EDS or be asymptomatic depending upon the time he or she is assessed by a clinician (i.e., phase alignment of the endogenous clock relative to light-dark cycle). As such, inquiring about the nature of the sleep disturbances (e.g., precipitating factors for sleep difficulties, cyclical vs. persistent symptoms) can help elucidate whether someone has a cyclical history of these symptoms. For example, unlike DSWPD or ASWPD, an individual with N24SWD cannot maintain a stable delayed or advanced sleep-wake pattern (Zee et al. 2013).

It is unclear whether sighted individuals with N24SWD (who typically have a long circadian period) are different from individuals with

DSWPD (see Chapter 12), who also have a long intrinsic circadian period (i.e., >25 hours). Because the treatments for both are similar, distinguishing between these two phenotypes is currently less important than adequate treatment.

TREATMENT

For Sighted Individuals

In sighted individuals with N24SWD, the most effective treatments are the same as for DSWPD (see Chapter 12), although they are likely to be less effective in N24SWD than would be expected in DSWPD. In some, a very regular schedule can help keep the circadian clock aligned with the solar day (Klerman et al. 1998). This will only likely be effective in individuals who are able to maintain a highly rigorous schedule and are fortunate enough to have an endogenous circadian period very close to 24 hours. Nonphotic signals can generate relatively little change in circadian timing, at best around 30 minutes per day (Lewy et al. 1998). It may be possible the impact of nonphotic cues on circadian timing is greater in individuals who are blind because the loss of input from light pathways may upregulate the strength of nonphotic inputs to the SCN (e.g., serotonin from the dorsal raphe, neuropeptide Y from the intergeniculate leaflet nucleus of the thalamus).

For Blind Individuals

In blind individuals with N24SWD, light is not likely to be an effective treatment because these individuals are unlikely to have the photoreception necessary to transmit light information to the circadian clock. The most robust treatment for blind individuals with N24SWD is low-dose melatonin or melatonin agonists. Properly timed, this treatment can generate changes in the acute timing of the circadian clock. Under normal, entrained conditions in sighted individuals, melatonin administered before bedtime can cause phase advances of the circadian clock, whereas melatonin administered during the early morning can cause phase delays (Lewy et al. 1998). Thus, evening administration can be helpful to synchronize the SCN (to offset the natural delay caused by the >24-hour endogenous period).

In individuals with N24SWD, however, the position of the circadian clock, which is likely free running, is unknown. Thus, administering melatonin or a melatonin agonist (e.g., ramelteon, tasimelteon) in the evening is not likely to work immediately because it may take weeks or months for the circadian clock to achieve the proper alignment with the solar day to make this timing effective. Nevertheless, because we have no current mechanism to determine circadian phase in real time, this remains the best solution. If melatonin and not an agonist is used, a low dose of melatonin (<300 µg) should be administered (Lewy et al. 2002). Higher doses will remain in the circulation for longer periods of time and cause both phase advances and delays (sum phase change of zero), thereby negating the therapeutic value of the melatonin. Treatment using a melatonin receptor agonist or melatonin begins by administering it 1–2 hours before the desired bedtime. Once entrainment is established over the course of a month, it is appropriate to switch to a low dose of melatonin (≤0.5 mg) 2–6 hours before bedtime to maintain entrainment. Evidence supporting the regular use of other sleep medications, such as benzodiazepines or benzodiazepine receptor agonists, for the treatment of N24SWD is insufficient.

CONCLUSION

N24SWD is characterized by an inability to sleep during a consistent time in the 24-hour period. Although N24SWD is very common among totally blind individuals and caused by the inability of light stimulation to reach the SCN, it is rare in sighted individuals, likely due to a combination of circadian (period length, photosensitivity to light) and irregular behavioral factors. Treatment for N24SWD centers around regularly timed entrainment of the internal pacemaker using either a melatonin receptor agonist or pharmaceutical-grade melatonin 1–2 hours before the desired bedtime. Engaging individuals in regular structured social and physical activities (and bright light at rise time for sighted individuals with N24SWD) can be very important for treatment beyond simply acting as peripheral zeitgebers (external cues that entrain an organism's biological clocks to the 24-hour day). N24SWD can be incredibly debilitating, so understanding and experiencing the power and limitations of different strategies can help individuals feel a greater sense of agency in managing this condition. Future investigations could explore the additive benefit of food oscillator entrainment (e.g., time-restricted feeding) and maximizing the phase-advance portion of the phase response curve (e.g., timed light pulses in the early morning).

Jet Lag Disorder

DIAGNOSTIC CRITERIA

Jet lag disorder is defined as complaints of insomnia or EDS along with reduced total sleep time associated with jet travel across at least two time zones. Onset of associated daytime impairment (e.g., fatigue, general malaise, compromised decision making, delayed reaction times, reduced athletic performance) or somatic complaints (e.g., gastrointestinal disruptions) occurs within 1–2 days after travel and is not better explained by another sleep, medical, neurological, psychological, medication, or substance use disorder (American Academy of Sleep Medicine 2014).

PATHOPHYSIOLOGY

Jet lag occurs when the timing of the internal circadian clock and timing of behavior, notably sleep and wake, are misaligned. During travel across multiple time zones, individuals often attempt to sleep at the same clock time as in their home time zone; however, their internal clock may be many hours out of sync with the new time zone. For example, a person who normally sleeps from 11 P.M. to 7 A.M. in California flies to New York and attempts to sleep the same hours. Without any adjustment to his circadian clock, sleeping from 11 P.M. to 7 A.M. in New York would be like attempting to sleep from 8 P.M. to 4 A.M. vis-à-vis circadian time. With regard to sleep, a strong circadian drive for wake occurs in the hours before normal bedtime and a strong circadian drive for sleep occurs near the end of normal sleep time (Dijk and Czeisler 1994). Thus, this hypothetical traveler would be attempting to go to sleep in New York just when his circadian system has a strong wake-promoting drive (making it difficult to initiate sleep) and would be waking up just when the circadian system has a strong sleep-promoting drive (making it difficult to wake up alert). In addition to driving the timing of sleep and wake, the central circadian clock acts as a kind of conductor for clocks found in tissues throughout the body (Welsh et al. 2010). These clocks are synchronized to each other and to the outside world through signals from the central circadian clock. During jet travel across time zones, these clocks can become desynchronized from one another due to competing misaligned signaling from the clock and behavior. For example, the liver may receive time cues from the central circadian clock and misaligned time cues from food intake patterns, which are often adjusted immediately. This desynchrony may contribute to some of the other symptoms commonly associated with jet lag (e.g., digestive problems, weakened immune response).

EPIDEMIOLOGY

More than 11 million airline passengers are estimated to travel each day (International Air Transport Association 2018), and although many fly within their home time zones, a substantial number of passengers cross time zones. In addition to jet travel, many individuals willingly put themselves into a pattern in which their sleep timing is adjusted by several hours each week, changing between off days and workdays. This has been described as "social jet lag" and may be even more problematic because frequent shifting of sleep timing could lead to a diminished amplitude of circadian rhythms (Jewett et al. 1994). Such a reduced amplitude has been posited to be linked to increased metabolic, immune, and memory difficulties, similar to those found in SWSD (Abbott et al. 2020).

Demographic factors, including sex, culture, and race, do not appear to affect susceptibility to jet lag. Limited data suggest the reported severity of symptoms increases for middle-age and older adults (>50 years) compared with younger adults (<30 years) despite similarities in the rate of physiological adjustment (e.g., Tmin, circadian amplitude). These differences are likely due to the effects of age, slowing down global physiological recovery and reducing the compensatory response to sleep deprivation (Moline et al. 1992). Other notable risk factors include alcohol use during flights, due to its effects on sleep fragmentation, and frequency of transmeridian travel (e.g., pilots), as well as a prior history of a mood disorder. Limited data suggest that jet lag could precipitate a relapse of a depressive episode (for westward travel) or a hypomanic episode (for eastward travel) (Inder et al. 2016).

CLINICAL PRESENTATION, COURSE, AND COMPLICATIONS

Jet lag is typically a temporary condition that often resolves within a few days in the absence of intervention. The severity and duration of symptoms worsen in relation to the number of time zones crossed, the direction of travel (i.e., westward travel is easier than eastward), the amount of sleep obtained during travel, and the timing, intensity, and duration of various zeitgebers in the arrival time zone (Drake and Wright 2017). Symptoms of jet lag for eastward travel mimic those of DSWPD (i.e., difficulties with sleep initiation, increased sleep inertia upon awakening) and generally persist longer and are more severe. Gastrointestinal disturbance (e.g., diarrhea, constipation), caused by trying to eat during the biological night, and cognitive impairments (e.g., slowed reaction times, decreased attention, irritability, increased errors), caused by trying to drive or work during the Tmin when these functions are at their weakest, can be more pronounced for eastward travel. Westward travel is often easier due to the natural propensity to stay awake longer each day. However, when traveling westward across numerous time zones, associated impairment mimics symptoms of ASWPD (i.e., increased sleepiness in the early evening, difficulties with early morning awakening). Similar to ASWPD, the associated impairment is often less disruptive to daytime functioning because social rhythms are based on a neutral phase (see Chapter 12). Frequency of travel has also been cited as a contributing factor to the severity and duration of jet lag symptoms as well as disruptions in menstrual functioning (Cho et al. 2000).

It takes approximately 24 hours for the average person to adjust for each time zone difference (i.e., 48 hours to adjust after traveling across two time zones, 72 hours to adjust after three time zones). Flying east is generally more challenging than flying west due to the length of the average circadian period being slightly longer than the 24-hour day (approximately 24.2 hours). That extra fraction makes it easier to delay (as happens during westward travel) but harder to advance sleep (as happens during eastward travel). However, for those with circadian periods <24 hours (e.g., ASWPD), flying east will likely be easier.

Getting insufficient sleep during jet travel, or exposure to circadian cues at inopportune times (e.g., bright light, food, caffeine, exercise), can exacerbate the circadian desynchrony and increase the severity and duration of jet lag symptoms. The subsequent sleep initiation or maintenance difficulties that can arise from jet travel can eventually lead to the development of chronic insomnia.

DIAGNOSIS

Diagnosis of jet lag is performed by clinical interview. If social jet lag is suspected, the addition of sleep logs or actigraphy can help confirm this variant.

DIFFERENTIAL DIAGNOSIS

The key feature of jet lag is its temporal association with transmeridian jet travel across two or more time zones. A thorough clinical interview and physical examination can help distinguish whether the associated symptoms are temporally related to jet travel, were present prior to jet travel, or are persistent beyond the expected time frame.

TREATMENT

Light Therapy

The most robust treatment for jet lag is the use of properly timed light exposure, with the timing specific to the direction and history of travel. For westward travel, the treatment description is similar to that for delaying sleep (e.g., seek evening light exposure that approaches the Tmin to provide the greatest delaying effects, avoid bright light in the morning for the first few days in the new time zone). For eastward travel, countermeasures are similar to those for advancing sleep (e.g., avoid bright light in the evening, seek bright light in the morning). When eastward travel exceeds nine time zones, it becomes more advantageous to make any adjustments as though the trip were a 14-hour westward journey.

As a general rule for infrequent travelers, light exposure (especially sunlight) should be maximized during the daytime of the new time zone, especially when it overlaps with the nighttime of the previous time zone. Problematically for many who are frequent travelers, the precise position of the circadian clock cannot readily be determined in the field; thus, the timing of light to maximize readjustment can only be estimated, with mathematical approximations available in some mobile applications.

Melatonin

Low-dose melatonin may also be used to treat jet lag, although its potency is nearly 10-fold less than light. As with treatment for delayed or advanced sleep, the timing of melatonin is opposite to that of light (e.g., evening melatonin and morning light generate advances in the timing of the circadian system). Low doses (<300 µg) are advised because higher doses can lead to both phase advances and delays, canceling out the impact of the drug.

Hypnotics

Although no drugs have been approved by the FDA for jet lag, hypnotics are often prescribed to facilitate sleep during jet travel or upon arrival. Research evaluating benzodiazepine receptor agonists suggests some positive effects on sleep duration during jet travel but no significant effects on wakefulness or daytime functioning. Along with associated side effects (e.g., cognitive impairment, sleep-related automatic complex behaviors, tolerance, withdrawal), risks and benefits should be carefully considered before recommending any over-the-counter or prescription sleep aids.

Wake-Promoting Drugs

Wake-promoting medications modafinil and armodafinil have also been studied in the treatment of jet lag. Although both have shown to provide modest benefits in terms of subjective ratings of jet lag severity, side effects include increased wakefulness after sleep onset, insomnia, headaches, nausea, and palpitations.

Time-Restricted Eating

An emerging therapy for jet lag uses a time-restricted feeding protocol to leverage entrainment by the food-entrained oscillator. Based on work by Fuller et al. (2008), strategic timing of a 16-hour fast may facilitate the adjustment of peripheral clocks and reduce symptoms of jet lag. In this experimental strategy, an individual who is traveling across multiple time zones should eat a large breakfast in the morning in the destination time zone and fast for 16 hours before that meal. For flight itineraries that land in the morning, this means eating the large meal upon arrival; for afternoon arrivals, eating a few hours before landing; and for evening arrivals, sleeping upon arrival and eating the following morning. This one-time extended period of fasting appears to help quickly reset peripheral clocks to the morning of the new time zone and to reduce jet lag, especially when combined with appropriate light exposure.

CONCLUSION

Jet lag is a ubiquitous response to transmeridian jet travel that can have serious consequences for individuals who cannot afford travel-related performance decrements (e.g., pilots, professional athletes, business travelers). Because the circadian disruptions are mechanistically similar to those in shift work, habitual jet lag may contribute to the development of long-term health consequences (e.g., metabolic disorders, cardiovascular disease, obesity) (Arble et al. 2010). Fortunately, jet lag can be quickly and effectively managed, predominantly via behavioral strategies. Although strategic exposure to bright and dim light is the most effective strategy, leveraging peripheral oscillators for jet lag and circadian rhythm disorders more broadly (e.g., time-restricted feeding) may provide additional benefits for resynchronizing endogenous rhythms. Optimal timing of bright and dim light can easily be calculated using one of the numerous smartphone applications available and is often most effective when done in session with an individual prior to travel.

Shift Work Sleep Disorder

DIAGNOSTIC CRITERIA

SWSD is characterized by complaints of insomnia or EDS along with insufficient total sleep time caused by a work schedule that routinely occurs during habitual sleep time. The diagnosis should be confirmed by at least 14 days of sleep logs or actigraphy (Figure 13–3). Symptoms must be present for at least 3 months and are not better explained by another sleep, medical, neurological, psychological, medication or substance use disorder (American Academy of Sleep Medicine 2014).

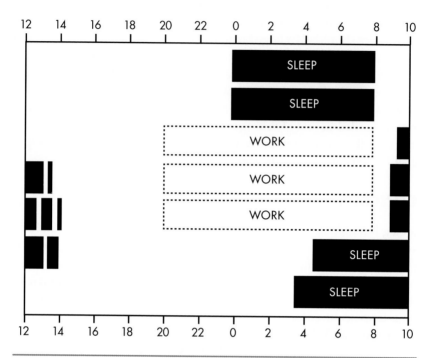

FIGURE 13–3.   Shift work sleep disorder sample sleep log (7 days depicted vertically).

Difficulties with sleep (*black bars*) are caused by a work schedule (*dotted bars*) that routinely occurs during habitual sleep time; 24-hour time depicted horizontally.

PATHOPHYSIOLOGY

Shift work is often broadly defined as work that takes place outside of the traditional 9 A.M.–5 P.M. working hours. This can constitute fixed nonstandard work hours, rotating shift schedules, or erratic schedules. It is common for individuals doing shift work to have difficulty sleeping during the daytime between shifts and during the nighttime on their off days (many shift workers switch to nighttime sleep during off days to coincide with the social schedules of family and friends). This difficulty is in part due to the misalignment of the timing of sleep and the timing of the internal circadian clock. Depending on the regularity of the shift work and the specific pattern of light to which a person is exposed, the circadian clock will have a fairly robust wake-promoting signal during the time many shift workers attempt to sleep (Dijk and Czeisler 1994). This wake-promoting signal will often get stronger as the sleep episode continues, making it difficult to obtain sufficiently prolonged sleep.

This difficulty may be further compounded by development of a new insomnia "mindset" (e.g., excessive worry about difficulties sleeping) spurred by this inability to remain asleep, causing a positive loop and self-sustaining insomnia.

EPIDEMIOLOGY

According to the U.S. Bureau of Labor Statistics (2005), 13.5% of the U.S. work force in 2004 was engaged in shift work. Among these individuals, 35% worked regular afternoon/evening shifts (starting between 2 P.M. and 6 P.M.), 24% worked regular overnight shifts (starting between 6 P.M. and 4 A.M.), 23% worked employer-scheduled irregular shifts, and 18% worked rotating shift schedules. With current labor force estimates, this indicates approximately 22 million shift workers in the United States alone (U.S. Bureau of Labor Statistics 2018). Prevalence rates of SWSD among shift workers range from 8% to 54% (American Academy of Sleep Medicine 2014; Di Milia et al. 2013; Flo et al. 2012).

Several scheduling factors influence the risk for developing SWSD, including the type of shift (from most harmful to least: night shift, rotating, early morning, afternoon/evening, daytime); duration of shift work, both in terms of hours per shift (>12 hours per shift) and number of years engaged in regular shift work (in a dose-dependent response); direction of rotation (counterclockwise is worse than clockwise); and speed of shift rotation (faster rotation—i.e., multiple rotations within 1 week—may have a more negative impact than slower rotation) (Bambra et al. 2008; Drake and Wright 2017). Circadian tendency may affect the ease with which an individual can adapt to shift work (e.g., evening types may be more able to adapt to night shifts or shift work that rotates in the clockwise direction), whereas medical and psychological conditions that are vulnerable to irregular sleep schedules (e.g., bipolar disorder, sleep apnea) may constitute increased risks for developing SWSD.

Age may impact the propensity to develop SWSD, with older shift workers indicating more difficulties with daytime sleepiness, fatigue, and disrupted sleep. Contributing factors related to age may include reduced capacity to accumulate sleep pressure, blunted circadian rhythms, shift toward morningness, and reduced sensitivity to the phase-shifting effects of light.

Sex has also been studied as a possible factor in tolerance to shift work. Although research has generally suggested that males show fewer negative effects of shift work, confounding factors for females such as additional social and familial responsibilities outside of work may account for these differences (Saksvik et al. 2011; Wickwire et al. 2017).

CLINICAL PRESENTATION, COURSE, AND COMPLICATIONS

In addition to symptoms of insomnia or EDS, the negative impact of SWSD can present as poor cognitive performance, increased rates of errors and accidents during shift work, sleep-related motor vehicle accidents post shift, absenteeism, social isolation, fatigue, irritability, mood swings, or increased substance use. Overnight and early morning shift workers (starting between 4 A.M. and 7 A.M.) have the highest risk for accidents and errors due to the overlap of Tmin/performance nadir with their work shift and work commute, respectively. Symptoms may ebb and flow as an individual moves between shift work and off-day schedules, with general trends toward remission the longer the individual is able to maintain a consistent sleep-wake-work schedule.

Complications associated with habitual shift work include increased risk for metabolic, cardiovascular, reproductive, gastrointestinal, mood, substance use, and other sleep disorders, along with all-cause mortality. Long-term shift work is also associated with an increased risk of several types of cancer, with breast cancer presenting the highest risk, and was declared to be a "known probable carcinogen" in 2007 by the International Agency for Research on Cancer, a part of the World Health Organization.

DIAGNOSTIC PROCEDURES, TESTS, AND QUESTIONNAIRES

Diagnosis of SWSD is typically conducted via a thorough clinical interview, a detailed sleep history, and sleep and work logs or actigraphy for at least 14 days. Similar to other circadian rhythm sleep disorders, polysomnography is not indicated to diagnose SWSD.

In clinical practice, general measures of sleep quality and daytime functioning (e.g., Insomnia Severity Index, Epworth Sleepiness Scale, Pittsburgh Sleep Quality Index, Fatigue Severity Scale) can help confirm the presence of daytime sleepiness and difficulties with sleep initiation or maintenance seen in SWSD. In terms of SWSD-specific measures, Barger et al. (2012) validated the Shiftwork Disorder Screening Questionnaire. This four-item screener demonstrated acceptable positive and negative predictive values to justify use in primary care clinics to help clinicians identify at-risk individuals who may be appropriate for additional evaluation by a sleep specialist. However, it is insufficient to diagnose SWSD on its own.

DIFFERENTIAL DIAGNOSIS

Sleep initiation and maintenance difficulties should be differentiated from insomnia or another circadian rhythm disorder, whereas daytime sleepiness should be distinguished from sleep-disordered breathing or hypersomnia. Careful assessment via clinical interview can illuminate a temporal relationship between shift work and associated impairments in sleep and performance. If a comorbid sleep disorder is suspected, polysomnography is recommended when diagnostically appropriate (e.g., sleep-disordered breathing).

TREATMENT

The most effective treatment for SWSD is cessation of shift work. Most individuals experience symptom remission as they return to a daytime work schedule. For those unable or unwilling to change work schedules, SWSD countermeasures can include differential lighting, napping, the FDA-approved wake-promoting agent modafinil, fasting overnight, or modified sleep-wake schedules.

Although lighting could be used to synchronize the circadian clock of a night shift worker, this is often an insufficient solution because those who are working night shifts often elect to stay awake during the day on their off days. Current lighting interventions are unable to shift the circadian system the necessary 8–12 hours in a single day to keep the circadian system aligned with rapid changes in schedule. As such, current treatments focused solely on lighting mainly consist of making the sleeping environment as dark and quiet as possible.

Modified Off-Day Schedule

Shifting the circadian phase in a manner that preserves Tmin within the sleep window across shift work and off-day schedules has been proposed as a method for managing the negative impacts of shift work. For a night shift worker, this protocol has an individual oscillate between the shift schedule and a modified off-day schedule that is delayed a few hours into the evening (e.g., bedtime of 3 A.M. instead of 11 P.M. on off days; bedtime upon arrival at home on shift work days). Adding a prophylactic nap (duration of 60–120 minutes) that ends 60 minutes prior to the start of the shift can help reduce sleep pressure while minimizing sleep inertia during transit to work; caffeine or stimulants within the first 2 hours of the shift can improve alertness during work; bright light during the first half of the shift enhances alertness; and dim light (e.g., wearing sunglasses) during the commute home facilitates sleep (Burgess 2011). Experimental evidence suggests that fasting rather than eating during a night shift may help preserve metabolic functioning while enhancing cognitive functioning and reaction times during and after the shift (Grant et al. 2017).

Regular Off-Day Schedule

For shift workers who prefer to resume regular daytime hours during off days, the use of mild hypnotics, such as melatonin or antihistamines, may provide small improvements in daytime sleep during shift schedules and nighttime sleep during off schedules. However, improvements in daytime sleep duration or continuity have no effect on performance decrements during nighttime shift work. As such, pharmacologically enhanced sleep is not advisable as a long-term solution when coupled with the associated health consequences of common sleep aids.

CONCLUSION

Shift work and SWSD are becoming increasingly common in the modern workforce. The subsequent disease risk associated with habitually and dramatically shifting circadian phases from work days to off days necessitates continued research to alleviate the burden on performance, health, and the health care system.

Although permanently switching to a normal work schedule is ideal, it is not realistic for many industries, including health care. Currently available countermeasures can be effective in minimizing the circadian disruptions but require commitment from both the clinician and the patient. Designing a realistic and executable treatment plan for SWSD in clinical settings requires adequate time to establish rapport, understand the available support structures, and incorporate the individual's expectations of successful treatment (e.g., desire to return to a normal schedule on off days). Accountability to the clinician or social supports is essential to adherence, especially when attempting to manage the regular shifts in circadian phases on a chronic basis.

As with other circadian rhythm disorders, future treatments could benefit from exploring the potency of leveraging peripheral clocks via food-entrained oscillators, not just the central SCN clock. If circadian desynchrony (internal or external) is a primary cause of many of the associated illnesses (e.g., metabolic, cardiovascular, cancer), interventions designed to quickly resynchronize these two major clocks could be an important aspect of symptom and disease management.

Summary

Despite their etiological differences, the irregularity of circadian rhythmicity apparent in ISWSD, N24SWD, jet lag, and SWSD offers a glimpse into the shared treatment philosophy: strengthening the consistency and amplitude of a patient's circadian rhythms. Whether through strategic timing of light-dark (or melatonin in the case of blind individuals with N24SWD), activity-rest, or social rhythms, enhancing the predictability of daily activities will be an important aspect of maintaining consistent periods of sleep and wake. Continuing this theme, leveraging the other master oscillator, the food-entrained oscillator, is a promising direction for enhancing circadian entrainment that warrants future research. As a final note, it is important to remember that sedatives are not indicated for the treatment of any of these disorders.

KEY CLINICAL POINTS

Irregular Sleep-Wake Rhythm Disorder

- When treating irregular sleep-wake rhythm disorder (ISWRD), providers should design treatment that maximizes circadian amplitude and leverages social and institutional support structures.

- Multicomponent treatments should include sleep hygiene, light therapy (bright upon awakening and during the day), dim light at night, and social rhythm therapy.

- Melatonin may help with entrainment but should be used with caution because it may exacerbate mood symptoms and should not be used with older adults.

- Benzodiazepines or nonbenzodiazepine receptor agonists are contraindicated in the treatment of ISWRD.

Non-24-Hour Sleep-Wake Phase Disorder

- Regularly timed melatonin or melatonin agonists 1–2 hours prior to bedtime is the standard treatment for non-24-hour sleep-wake phase disorder (N24SWD).

- Once sleep-wake rhythms have been stabilized for a month, entrainment can be maintained by switching to a low dose of melatonin (≤ 0.5 mg) 2–6 hours before bedtime.

- Consistent adherence to daily rhythms (e.g., exercise, nutrition, occupation, social/familial, sleep hygiene) can provide additional support for entrainment to a 24-hour cycle.

- Sleep logs or actigraphy can illuminate the approximate length of an individual's circadian period, which can help with prognosis (e.g., a very long period of 24.8 hours will be more challenging to entrain than a "normal" period of 24.2 hours).

- Evidence supporting the use of benzodiazepines or nonbenzodiazepine receptor agonists in the treatment of N24SWD is insufficient at this time.

Jet Lag Disorder

- Standard treatment for jet lag centers around switching sleep-wake rhythm to the destination time zone upon arrival.

- Westward travel is generally easier, particularly for individuals with a neutral or delayed phase. Eastward travel is generally more difficult, except for individuals with an advanced phase.

- Eastward travel across ≥10 time zones should be treated like westward travel of ≥14 hours to enhance entrainment.

- Wake-promoting agents (e.g., modafinil, armodafinil) may provide modest benefits in terms of subjective ratings of jet lag but not objective performance.

- Hypnotic drugs (e.g., zolpidem, eszopiclone) may produce small increases in sleep duration without improving objective performance.

- Consider a strategic 16-hour fast for rapid entrainment in individuals healthy enough for sustained fasting.

Shift Work Sleep Disorder

- Developing a modified sleep schedule can be effective in preserving sleep ability without the use of medications but requires significant commitment from both patient and provider to apply consistently.

- A light-centric approach should focus on maintaining a very dark and quiet sleep environment.

- Napping (duration of at least 1 hour, ending at least 1 hour before the start of the shift) prior to a night shift can reduce fatigue and improve cognition during the shift.

- Although the use of FDA-approved alerting medication may be helpful, the use of hypnotics is not recommended to treat shift work sleep disorder.

- Strategic use of time-restricted feeding schedules (e.g., fasting over a night shift) may preserve metabolic and cognitive functioning during and after the shift.

- Permanently switching to a non–shift work schedule for several years can reverse the adverse health effects of shift work.

References

Abbott SM, Reid KJ, Zee PC: Circadian disorders of the sleep-wake cycle, in Principles and Practice of Sleep Medicine, 6th Edition. Edited by Kryger M, Roth T, Dement WC. Philadelphia, PA, Elsevier, 2017, pp 414–424

Abbott SM, Malkani RG, Zee PC: Circadian disruption and human health: a bidirectional relationship. Eur J Neurosci 51(1):567–583, 2020 30549337

American Academy of Sleep Medicine: International Classification of Sleep Disorders, 3rd Edition. Darien, IL, American Academy of Sleep Medicine, 2014

Arble DM, Ramsey KM, Bass J, et al: Circadian disruption and metabolic disease: findings from animal models. Best Pract Res Clin Endocrinol Metab 24(5):785–800, 2010 21112026

Bambra CL, Whitehead MM, Sowden AJ, et al: Shifting schedules: the health effects of reorganizing shift work. Am J Prev Med 34(5):427–434, 2008 18407011

Barger LK, Ogeil RP, Drake CL, et al: Validation of a questionnaire to screen for shift work disorder. Sleep (Basel) 35(12):1693–1703, 2012 23204612

Baumann CR, Werth E, Stocker R, et al: Sleep-wake disturbances 6 months after traumatic brain injury: a prospective study. Brain 130(pt 7):1873–1883, 2007

Borbély AA: A two process model of sleep regulation. Hum Neurobiol 1(3):195–204, 1982

Burgess HJ: Using bright light and melatonin to adjust to night work, in Behavioral Treatments for Sleep Disorders: Practical Resources for the Mental Health Professional. Edited by Perlis M, Aloia M, Kuhn B. Cambridge, UK, Academic Press, 2011, pp 159–165

Cho K, Ennaceur A, Cole JC: Chronic jet lag produces cognitive deficits. J Neurosci 20(6):RC66, 2000

Czeisler CA, Duffy JF, Shanahan TL, et al: Stability, precision, and near-24-hour period of the human circadian pacemaker. Science 284(5423):2177–2181, 1999

Di Milia L, Waage S, Pallesen S, et al: Shift work disorder in a random population sample—prevalence and comorbidities. PLoS One 8(1):e55306, 2013 23372847

Dijk DJ, Czeisler CA: Paradoxical timing of the circadian rhythm of sleep propensity serves to consolidate sleep and wakefulness in humans. Neurosci Lett 166(1):63–68, 1994

Drake CL, Wright KP: Shift work, shift-work disorder, and jet lag, in Principles and Practice of Sleep Medicine, 6th Edition. Edited by Kryger M, Roth T, Dement WC. Philadelphia, PA, Elsevier, 2017, pp 714–725

Flo E, Pallesen S, Magerøy N, et al: Shift work disorder in nurses—assessment, prevalence and related health problems. PLoS One 7(4):e33981, 2012 22485153

Flynn-Evans EE, Tabandeh H, Skene DJ, et al: Circadian rhythm disorders and melatonin production in 127 blind women with and without light perception. J Biol Rhythms 29(3):215–224, 2014 24916394

Fuller PM, Lu J, Saper CB: Differential rescue of light- and food-entrainable circadian rhythms. Science 320(5879):1074–1077, 2008 18497298

Gooley JJ, Lu J, Chou TC, et al: Melanopsin in cells of origin of the retinohypothalamic tract. Nat Neurosci 4(12):1165, 2001 11713469

Grant CL, Coates AM, Dorrian J, et al: Timing of food intake during simulated night shift impacts glucose metabolism: a controlled study. Chronobiol Int 34(8):1003–1013, 2017 28635334

Inder ML, Crowe MT, Porter R: Effect of transmeridian travel and jetlag on mood disorders: evidence and implications. Aust NZ J Psychiatry 50(3):220–227, 2016 26268923

International Air Transport Association: World Air Transport Statistics. Montréal, Canada, International Air Transport Association, 2018

Jewett ME, Kronauer RE, Czeisler CA: Phase-amplitude resetting of the human circadian pacemaker via bright light: a further analysis. J Biol Rhythms 9(3–4):295–314, 1994

Klerman EB, Rimmer DW, Dijk DJ, et al: Nonphotic entrainment of the human circadian pacemaker. Am J Physiol 274(4 pt 2):R991–R996, 1998 9575961

Lewy AJ, Bauer VK, Ahmed S, et al: The human phase response curve (PRC) to melatonin is about 12 hours out of phase with the PRC to light. Chronobiol Int 15(1):71–83, 1998 9493716

Lewy AJ, Emens JS, Sack RL, et al: Low, but not high, doses of melatonin entrained a free-running blind person with a long circadian period. Chronobiol Int 19(3):649–658, 2002 12069043

Lockley SW, Skene DJ, Arendt J, et al: Relationship between melatonin rhythms and visual loss in the blind. J Clin Endocrinol Metab 82(11):3763–3770, 1997 9360538

Moline ML, Pollak CP, Monk TH, et al: Age-related differences in recovery from simulated jet lag. Sleep 15(1):28–40, 1992 1557592

Moore RY: Organization of the mammalian circadian system, in Circadian Clocks and Their Adjustment. Edited by Chadwick DJ, Ackrill K. Chichester, UK, Wiley, 1995, pp 88–106

Morgenthaler TI, Lee-Chiong T, Alessi C, et al: Practice parameters for the clinical evaluation and treatment of circadian rhythm sleep disorders. An American Academy of Sleep Medicine report. Sleep 30(11):1445–1459, 2007 18041479

Oren DA, Wehr TA: Hypernyctohemeral syndrome after chronotherapy for delayed sleep phase syndrome. N Engl J Med 327(24):1762, 1992 1435929

Porkka-Heiskanen T, Strecker RE, Thakkar M, et al: Adenosine: a mediator of the sleep-inducing effects of prolonged wakefulness. Science 276(5316):1265–1268, 1997 9157887

Riemersma-van der Lek RF, Swaab DF, Twisk J, et al: Effect of bright light and melatonin on cognitive and noncognitive function in elderly residents of group care facilities: a randomized controlled trial. JAMA 299(22):2642–2655, 2008 18544724

Ruby NF, Brennan TJ, Xie X, et al: Role of melanopsin in circadian responses to light. Science 298(5601):2211–2213, 2002 12481140

Sack RL, Auckley D, Auger RR, et al: Circadian rhythm sleep disorders: part II, advanced sleep phase disorder, delayed sleep phase disorder, free-running disorder, and irregular sleep-wake rhythm. An American Academy of Sleep Medicine review. Sleep 30(11):1484–1501, 2007 18041481

Saksvik IB, Bjorvatn B, Hetland H, et al: Individual differences in tolerance to shift work—a systematic review. Sleep Med Rev 15(4):221–235, 2011 20851006

Uchiyama M, Lockley SW: Non-24-hour sleep-wake rhythm disorder in sighted and blind patients. Sleep Med Clin 10(4):495–516, 2015 26568125

U.S. Bureau of Labor Statistics: Workers on Flexible and Shift Schedules in May 2004. Report #USDL 05-1198. Washington, DC, U.S. Bureau of Labor Statistics, 2005

U.S. Bureau of Labor Statistics: Civilian Labor Force Level. Report #LNS11000000. Washington, DC, U.S. Bureau of Labor Statistics, 2018

Wagner DR: Disorders of the circadian sleep-wake cycle. Neurol Clin 14(3):651–670, 1996 8871981

Welsh DK, Takahashi JS, Kay SA: Suprachiasmatic nucleus: cell autonomy and network properties. Annu Rev Physiol 72:551–577, 2010 20148688

Wickwire EM, Geiger-Brown J, Scharf SM, et al: Shift work and shift work disorder: clinical and organizational perspectives. Chest 151(5):1156–1172, 2017 28012806

Zee PC, Vitiello MV: Circadian rhythm sleep disorder: irregular sleep wake rhythm type. Sleep Med Clin 4(2):213–218, 2009 20160950

Zee PC, Attarian H, Videnovic A: Circadian rhythm abnormalities. Continuum 19(1):132–147, 2013

Zhu L, Zee PC: Circadian rhythm sleep disorders. Neurol Clin 30(4):1167–1191, 2012 23099133

CHAPTER 14

Non-REM Parasomnias

Muna Irfan, M.D.

Carlos H. Schenck, M.D.

Michael J. Howell, M.D.

Parasomnias are characterized by undesirable motor, experiential, and autonomic nervous system activities that occur during any stage of sleep. Such abnormal events arising out of non-REM (NREM) sleep are called *non-REM parasomnias*. Termed "disorders of arousal" (DOAs), NREM parasomnias occur as partial awakenings from sleep with a spectrum of clinical behaviors, such as ambulation, feeding, sexual activity, and talking, as well as autonomic symptoms. These nocturnal episodes can lead to sleep disruption and can have physical, psychological, social, and forensic implications. The general diagnostic criteria for NREM parasomnias according to the *International Classification of Sleep Disorders*, 3rd Edition (ICSD-3; American Academy of Sleep Medicine 2014), are listed in Table 14–1.

Of note, sleep-related eating disorder (SRED) is not considered a DOA in the ICSD-3 but rather a separate NREM parasomnia. Recent discoveries since publication of the ICSD-3 in 2014, however, suggest that SRED is, in effect, sleepwalking with eating and is thus a DOA, with a frequent atypical feature being that eating episodes often emerge from stage N2 sleep rather than the usual N3 sleep for DOA. Because of this, we consider SRED a DOA for the rest of this chapter.

Pathophysiology

The DOAs or NREM parasomnias include confusional arousals, sleepwalking, sleep terrors, SRED, and, less commonly, sleep-related sexual behaviors. These parasomnias share the same underlying pathophysiology of sleep-wake boundary dysregulation. NREM parasomnias offer a unique neurobiological substrate for focal sleep and wake activity occur-

TABLE 14–1.   Diagnostic criteria for disorders of arousal

1. Recurrent episodes of partial awakenings from sleep
2. Lack of/Inappropriate response to intervention during episodes
3. Limited/No cognition or dream content
4. Partial/Complete amnesia for the event
5. Nocturnal disturbance not explained by other disorders or medication/ substance use

ring simultaneously in the brain, evidenced by electroencephalographic activity commensurate with these states. Physiologically, this represents a dissociation between behavior and state of consciousness, manifested as release of primeval behaviors of locomotion, feeding, aggression, and sex emanating from sleep (Castelnovo et al. 2018). The transition from NREM sleep to wake state is incomplete, resulting in emergence of phenotypic nocturnal behaviors without recollection. They generally emanate from the N3 stage of sleep (slow-wave sleep [SWS]), although they can also occur in N2 (Joncas et al. 2002).

Pressman (2007) conceptualized the model for NREM parasomnias, theorizing that an individual with an intrinsic predisposition can be primed by factors, such as a sedating medication, to impair normal cortical arousals. Subsequently, precipitating factors such as obstructive sleep apnea (OSA) events and periodic limb movements (PLMs), or other disruptions such as external stimuli, can lead to disordered, incomplete arousals. The higher prevalence of DOAs in the pediatric population points to neurodevelopmental immaturity of sleep-wake state boundary regulation as an additional susceptibility factor. Studies have also demonstrated SWS instability, reflected by a dysregulation of the cyclic alternating pattern and propensity for greater arousal oscillations (Guilleminault 2006). Genetic elements have been incriminated in addition to environment factors. Studies have established a high prevalence of human leukocyte antigens *HLA-DQB1*05:01* and *HLA-DQB1*04* in various NREM parasomnias (Heidbreder et al. 2016). An autosomal dominant trait for sleepwalking has also been identified on chromosome 20 (Licis et al. 2011). Factors and conditions associated with DOAs are listed in Table 14–2.

Clinical Manifestation

The clinical presentation of various DOA phenotypes comprises recurrent episodes of partial arousal from sleep with diminished or absent re-

TABLE 14–2.   Pathophysiology of disorders of arousal

Predisposing factors	Priming/precipitating factors
Genetic factors	Enhancement of slow-wave sleep
HLA-DQB1*05 and *HLA DQB1*04* alleles	Sleep deprivation
	Circadian misalignment
Chromosome 20q12–q13.12 locus	Impairment of cortical arousal
Maturational factors	CNS suppressant drugs
Pediatric age	Sleep fragmentation
Ambulating disorders	Extrinsic stimuli
Restless legs (for sleepwalking)	Periodic limb movements
	Obstructive sleep apnea
	Medical disorders such as gastroesophageal reflux disease
	Psychiatric disorders

sponsiveness, restricted cognition, and partial or complete amnesia for the event. DOAs tend to occur during the first third of nocturnal sleep (typically the first 60–90 minutes) as the higher density of SWS in earlier ultradian sleep cycles raises the threshold for arousal. The individual fails to emerge to full consciousness and may exhibit amnestic automatic complex behaviors such as ambulation, feeding, vocalization, and sexual behaviors with autonomic activation. They typically occur around the time of transition from one sleep state to another or during rapid oscillation between sleep stages. Attempts at redirection are usually futile.

DOAs are on a spectrum of clinical complexity, with frequent occurrence of more than one type of DOA in an individual's life span. Various clinical DOA phenotypes are described in the following sections.

CONFUSIONAL AROUSALS

Confusional arousals, also known as sleep drunkenness or Elpenor syndrome, are episodes of partial awakenings from sleep in which the patient is usually disoriented and confused. They are characterized by incomplete arousal from sleep, during which time the individual may sit up, appear startled or disoriented, or exhibit automatic behavior with mumbling or minor motoric behaviors without ambulation but associated with sympathetic hyperactivity. The individual usually has partial or no recollection of the episode. Episodes can be minutes long in duration but are occasionally more prolonged, especially in cases in which drugs are implicated.

TABLE 14–3.   Diagnostic criteria for confusional arousal

1. Condition fulfills the general criteria for non-REM disorders of arousal

2. Episodes consist of patient exhibiting confused behavior after arousal in bed

3. Absence of terror or ambulation out of bed

The prevalence of confusional arousals is higher in the pediatric population at 17% and decreases in adults to about 3%–4% (Wills and Garcia 2002). The diagnostic criteria for confusional arousals are listed in Table 14–3.

SLEEPWALKING

Sleepwalking is a DOA associated with recurrent ambulatory behavior. The clinical manifestation may vary from the simple motoric behavior of aimless wandering to complex learned behavior with ambulation such as driving a vehicle or bizarre situations such as peeing in the closet or exiting the house disrobed in extreme weather conditions (Arnulf 2018). Thus, the risk of potential injury to the patient and others during these episodes is significant. Redirecting endeavors can be counterproductive and may lead to aggressive behaviors exhibited by the sleeper.

A large prospective study revealed the overall pediatric prevalence (ages 2.5–13 years) of sleepwalking to be 29.1%, with the peak observed at age 10 (Petit et al. 2015). The prevalence is higher at 47.4% for children who have one parent with a history of sleepwalking and up to 61.5% for children for whom both parents have a history of sleepwalking, signifying a strong genetic influence (Frauscher et al. 2014). The prevalence of sleepwalking is much lower in adults, seen in 1%–4% (Petit et al. 2015), although a study posited that noninjurious sleepwalking may be more prevalent, at 12%, than originally recognized (Frauscher et al. 2014).

Occasionally, a seemingly benign act of sleepwalking can lead to life-threatening circumstances, such as walking out of a top-floor window or driving an automobile in a disoriented state of incomplete arousal, and at times major injuries and extreme violence can also occur (Broughton et al. 1994; Schenck et al. 1989).

Sleepwalking can be aggravated by OSA (see Chapters 8 and 9) and restless legs syndrome (RLS; Chapter 17), as well as by sedative-hypnotic medications such as benzodiazepine receptor agonists (zolpidem). In addition to this class of medication, drugs from other categories incriminated in sleepwalking include antidepressants (amitriptyline, bupropion, paroxetine, mirtazapine), antipsychotics (quetiapine, olanzapine), antihypertensives (propranolol, metoprolol), antiepileptics (topiramate), antiasthmatics (montelukast), and antibiotics (fluoroquinolones) (Howell 2012). Some medical conditions have also been implicated in the occurrence of sleepwalking, such as vitiligo, hyperthyroidism, migraines, febrile illness, head injury, encephalitis, stroke, and chronic pain syndrome (Lopez et al. 2015).

Another clinical scenario worthy of mention is zolpidem-induced sleepwalking and other amnestic sleep-related behaviors. Zolpidem can aggravate motor restlessness in patients with a predisposition to RLS (see Chapters 4 and 17), which leads to the emergence of various DOAs as a complication of sedative-hypnotic therapy. Thus, one should be very cautious and investigate subclinical RLS in patients with insomnia to avoid inadvertent hypnotic-induced sleep ambulatory behaviors (Howell et al. 2010). The FDA recently required a black box warning be added on the prescribing information and the patient medication guides for all "Z" drugs (zolpidem, zaleplon, eszopiclone). The ICSD-3 diagnostic criteria for sleepwalking are listed in Table 14–4.

TABLE 14-4.   Diagnostic criteria for sleepwalking

1. Condition fulfills the general criteria for non-REM disorders of arousal

2. Episodes are marked by ambulation and other complex behaviors

SLEEP TERRORS

Sleep terrors are also known as night terrors, or *pavor nocturnus*. They comprise nocturnal episodes marked by intense fear, with abrupt onset associated with inconsolable crying and sympathetic hyperactivity. The prevalence of sleep terrors in children varies widely, from 14.7% to 56% (American Academy of Sleep Medicine 2014; Petit et al. 2015). In adults, the prevalence decreases substantially to 2.2% (Dolder and Nelson 2008), with a relatively constant rate of 2.3%–2.6% in those 15–64 years of age, decreasing to 1% in those older than 65 years (American Academy of Sleep Medicine 2014).

The occurrence of sleep terrors is marked by partial arousal with physical behaviors reflective of intense fright, demonstrated by screaming and crying that is not amenable to calming efforts. Redirecting attempts only add to the aggression and intensity of patient's behaviors. Sleep terrors are associated with increased autonomic activity in the form of tachypnea, tachycardia, mydriasis, diaphoresis, and increased muscle tone (American Academy of Sleep Medicine 2014). Typically, patients do not have any recollection of the event but occasionally may have vague, fragmented reminiscence of dream mentation of a terrifying situation, such as a tree or ceiling falling. Although the behaviors are noninjurious, they can lead to significant emotional distress in parents and cause disruption of their sleep. The ICSD-3 criteria for these parasomnias are enumerated in Table 14–5.

TABLE 14–5.   Diagnostic criteria for sleep terrors

1. Condition fulfills the general criteria for non-REM disorders of arousal

2. Arousal characterized by fright, manifested as sudden screaming and vocalizations upon awakening

3. Episode consists of signs of intense fear and autonomic arousal, such as mydriasis, tachycardia, tachypnea, and diaphoresis

SLEEP-RELATED EATING DISORDER

SRED is characterized by recurrent episodes arising from NREM sleep during which the individual consumes high-calorie, carbohydrate-rich food items and sometimes ingests strange, pica-like items without any (or only partial) awareness or recollection. The prevalence of SRED is not very well characterized. In a sleep clinic referral population, the prevalence was noted to be 0.5% (Schenck et al. 1991). In a college population, 4.6% of subjects (Brion et al. 2012) were found to have sleep-related eating, whereas 3.4% of the patients in a depression clinic were afflicted by it (Winkelman et al. 1999). This disorder has a 60%–83% female preponderance, which is congruent with other eating disorders but discordant with other DOA phenotypes (Inoue 2015).

The episodes of eating in SRED are not driven by hunger but seem to be resulting from involuntary compulsive eating. The selection of food items also seems to be haphazard, peculiar combinations typically high in carbohydrate content but may also include inedible or noxious items such as raw frozen meat, pet food, buttered cigarettes, or soap. Frequency of these episodes can range from several times a night to a few times a week. Involuntary sleep-related eating can lead to several adverse consequences, such as hyperglycemia in a diabetic, hypercholesterolemia, dental caries, weight gain, and potential injuries sustained from careless handling, cutting, and heating food with impaired consciousness during partial arousal.

TABLE 14–6.   Diagnostic criteria for sleep-related eating disorder

1. Recurrent episodes of amnestic eating occurring after arousal from sleep

   Presence of at least one of the following with automatic eating:
   - Consumption of peculiar forms or combinations of food, inedible, or noxious substances
   - Potentially injurious behavior noted during food preparation/pursuit
   - Adverse consequences from recurrent sleep-related eating

2. Partial or complete loss of awareness during episode with subsequent impaired/absent recall

3. Disturbance not explained by another sleep, mental, or medical disorder or medication/substance use

Heterogeneous factors play a role in causation of sleep-related eating. It is considered by many experts to be a variant of sleepwalking, because it involves partial arousal and ambulatory behaviors culminating with feeding and is affected by the same predisposing and precipitating factors as other DOAs. These patients have a high frequency of prior or concurrent sleepwalking occurrence (60%; Schenck et al. 1991). Misclassification of RLS as insomnia and treatment with sedative-hypnotics, especially zolpidem, can lead to the appearance of amnestic sleep-related eating behaviors. Other psychotropic agents, including benzodiazepines, mirtazapine, quetiapine, lithium carbonate, and anticholinergic drugs, have also been implicated (American Academy of Sleep Medicine 2014). Other associated factors include alcohol and other substance use, smoking cessation, acute stress, onset of narcolepsy, autoimmune hepatitis, and encephalitis. The ICSD-3 criteria for SRED are described in Table 14–6.

SEXSOMNIA

According to ICSD-3, sexsomnia is classified as a subtype of NREM parasomnia ("sleep-related abnormal sexual behaviors"), with sexual behaviors emerging during partial arousals from SWS consistent with other DOAs. The first classification of sexsomnia was published in 2007 (Schenck et al. 2007) and updated in 2015 (Schenck 2015). Sexsomnia and SRED are considered "appetitive" parasomnias, which can occur concurrently.

A series of 49 patients from a world literature review revealed a male preponderance of 75%, with mean age at onset of 28 years and mean age at presentation of 35 years (Schenck 2015). A wide range of sexual behaviors, including intercourse/attempted intercourse, fondling, agitated/assaultive acts, masturbation, vocalizations, and spontaneous sleep orgasms were noted. The same predisposing and precipitating factors as in other DOAs affect the occurrence of these behaviors as well, and hence a common pathophysiology is implicated. Understandably, these behaviors can have grave legal and forensic implications.

Male predominance of sexsomnia was found in two series of sleep clinic patients from the United Kingdom (90% of 41 patients; Muza et al. 2016) and France (71% of 17 patients; Dubessy et al. 2017), with mean ages of 32 years and 37 years, respectively. A range of sexual behaviors (from masturbation to intercourse with orgasm) was reported, along with aggressive or violent sexual behavior toward the bed partner in 27% and 35% of patients, respectively, with legal consequences. A history of comorbid NREM parasomnia was present in 73% and 53% of patients, respectively. Amnesia for the sexsomnia was present in 100% of patients in the first series and most patients in the second series. The findings from these two series reinforce the typical clinical profile of sexsomnia reported in the world literature (Dubessy et al. 2017; Muza et al. 2016).

Diagnosis

CLINICAL EVALUATION

Obtaining a careful collateral historical account from the parents of pediatric patients and from the bed partners of adult patients is pivotal for diagnosis. Inquiry should be focused on the nature of the nocturnal behaviors, their timing in the sleep period night, and whether the behaviors were preceded by any changes in sleep habits, particularly sleep deprivation (Irfan et al. 2017). The Munich Parasomnia Screening Questionnaire is a 21-item self-rating screening tool for various nocturnal behaviors and parasomnias, including NREM. For individual items, the sensitivity and specificity is ≥90% for 19 items (Fulda et al. 2008). The clinician should also ask about predisposing factors, such as family history of parasomnias, and the presence of any symptoms (snoring, witnessed apneas) and signs (crowded oropharynx) suggestive of sleep-disordered breathing. In the setting of sleepwalking- and SRED-specific questions, history should explore whether the patient has underlying RLS, and clinicians should have a low threshold for ordering a serum ferritin level. A ferritin level <50 ng/mL warrants targeted intervention with iron replacement strategies. If the descriptive details are unclear, then video polysomnography (vPSG) with extended electroencephalography can help characterize the nocturnal episodes and identify any aggravating underlying sleep conditions.

POLYSOMNOGRAPHIC CHARACTERISTICS OF PARASOMNIAS

According to the American Academy of Sleep Medicine, comprehensive vPSG is indicated if parasomnias are (Kushida et al. 2005):

- Atypical or unusual in terms of age, onset, duration, or specific behaviors
- Frequent in occurrence (more than two or three times a week)
- Potentially injurious
- Potentially originating from epileptogenic activity, if prior evaluation has been inconclusive

Practice parameters recommend the use of expanded electroencephalographic and electromyographic channels with high-resolution video.

In pediatric patients, comprehensive vPSG with electroencephalographic and electromyographic leads is recommended in cases where OSA is suspected or violent sleep-related arousals are noted. The focus is on diagnosing and treating reversible conditions such as OSA or epilepsy to prevent the nocturnal behaviors from causing injury. Although a single night's study may not record parasomnia episodes, other suggestive features such as sleep state instability, epileptiform activity, and muscle tone changes in REM sleep (as seen in REM sleep behavior disorder [RBD]) can help with diagnosis. Other interventions, such as sleep deprivation before and auditory stimulation during the polysomnogram, can significantly increase the diagnostic yield in capturing events during the polysomnogram. This approach should be applied with proper oversight, such as caution for driving before and after the polysomnogram, and consideration of lowering seizure threshold and thus exercising seizure/injury precautions in the sleep laboratory.

In DOAs, although specific diagnostic criteria on polysomnography are not established, several characteristics have been noted, such as SWS fragmentation and hypersynchronous delta activity. A gradual buildup of synchronous slow delta wave frequency associated with or preceding the arousal-related events can be recorded. Post arousal, persistent slow cortical activity may evolve into awake alpha rhythm or revert to an NREM stage of sleep (Drakatos et al. 2018). A polysomnographic clip of such electrocerebral activity is demonstrated in Figure 14–1.

A recent study analyzing polysomnogram findings revealed that, in comparison with control subjects, patients with DOAs showed significant SWS alterations, with higher fragmentation and a higher proportion of slow/mixed arousal electroencephalographic patterns in SWS.

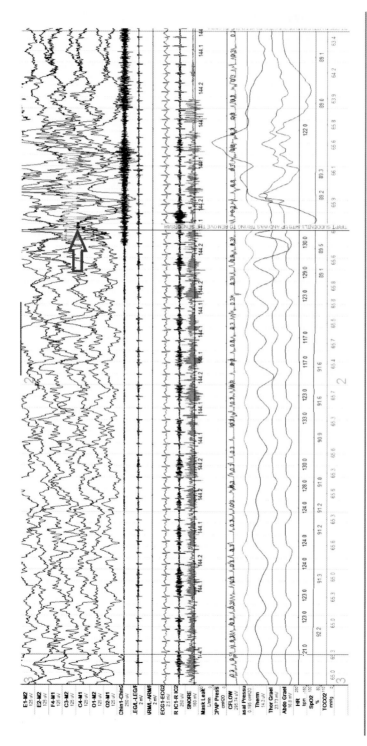

FIGURE 14–1. Polysomnography at the onset of a confusional arousal.

A polysomnographic recording demonstrating hypersynchronous slow-wave activity during a confusional arousal, denoted by the *arrow*. Immediately preceding the arousal, an increase in heart rate is also notable.

TABLE 14–7. Polysomnographic features of various parasomnias

Parasomnia	Sleep stage	NREM sleep instability*	REM sleep atonia	Other features
Confusional arousals	NREM	Present	Present	Hypersynchronous slow-wave EEG activity
Sleepwalking	NREM	Present	Present	Hypersynchronous slow wave, RLS
Sleep terrors	NREM	Present	Present	Increased heart rate, hypersynchronous slow wave
Sleep-related eating	NREM	Present	Present	RLS, PLMs, rhythmic masticatory muscle activity
Sexsomnia	NREM	Present	Present	
REM sleep behavior disorder	REM	Absent	Absent	PLMs, penile erection, irregular heart and respiratory rate

Note. EEG=electroencephalographic; NREM=non-REM; PLM=periodic limb movement; RLS=restless legs syndrome.
*Cyclic alternating pattern.

The designated cutoffs for the SWS fragmentation index (≥6.8 hours) and slow/mixed arousal index (≥2.5 hours) can lead to correct classification rates of DOA between 73.3% and 85.3%. Additionally, inclusion of parasomnia episodes recorded by vPSG improved the classification rate up to 91.3% (Lopez et al. 2018). These results are in accordance with prior studies showing SWS instability in patients with DOAs, based on a visual cyclic alternating pattern or spectral analysis assessment (Terzano et al. 2002). The polysomnographic features of various parasomnias are listed in Table 14–7.

Differential Diagnosis

The NREM DOAs should be distinguished from other sleep-related conditions with similar clinical presentations, such as RBD, sleep-related hypermotor seizures, sleep-related dissociative disorders/psychogenic spells, alcohol- and drug-related behaviors, OSA, and malingering (with identified secondary gain from reported parasomnia symptoms). Some differentiating clinical features of various parasomnias are enumerated in Table 14–8.

REM SLEEP BEHAVIOR DISORDER

RBD (see Chapter 15) can be differentiated from NREM parasomnias by several characteristic features, such as dream enactment behaviors emanating from vivid REM dreams themed at hostile connotations of being chased, attacked, and defending oneself. These behaviors occur in the second half of the night, when REM sleep periods are longer. Polysomnography also can reveal increases in electromyographic tone in REM sleep.

SLEEP-RELATED HYPERMOTOR EPILEPSY

Sleep-related hypermotor seizures are characterized by repetitive, highly stereotypical, bizarre movements such as bicycling, kicking, rocking, and running leg movements. Extended seizure montage with vPSG can not only can capture the stereotypical event but also reveal epileptogenic activity characteristic of seizures. Epilepsy is typically amenable to treatment with antiepileptic agents. Diagnosis and treatment of concurrent OSA and RLS not only improve sleep quality but also can diminish the occurrence of DOAs. Rarely, sexual behaviors can arise from nocturnal seizures, which should be carefully delineated from DOAs by obtaining a meticulous history of the stereotypical nature of the sexual behaviors and semiology and applying a full seizure montage on polysomnography. In such cases, an antiepileptic regimen can control the events with reasonable success.

SLEEP-RELATED DISSOCIATIVE DISORDER

History of significant psychosocial burden, including sexual, physical, and emotional abuse, should raise concern for a possible diagnosis of dissociative disorder.

NIGHTMARE DISORDER

Nightmare disorder occurs primarily as disruptive REM-related nightmares that can lead to arousals from REM sleep and do not have the other characteristic features of DOAs. REM atonia is preserved. DOAs should also be distinguished from parasomnia overlap disorder, which is a condition characterized by the presence of both NREM parasomnia and RBD (see Chapter 15). Historical account usually suggests the occurrence of

TABLE 14–8. Differential diagnosis of various parasomnias

	Confusional arousals	Sleepwalking	Sleep terrors	SRED	Sexsomnia	RBD
Behavior	Disoriented, movements in bed	Ambulation, wandering or leaving bed	Distress, agitated, crying; inconsolable	Carbohydrate-rich or bizarre food intake	Typical or atypical sexual behavior during partial arousal	Dream enacting movements or vocalizations
Timing	First part of night	First part of night	First part of night	Usually first part of night, but can be anytime	Anytime	2 hours after sleep onset or second half of night
Duration	Several minutes; rarely prolonged	Several minutes to prolonged	Several minutes	Several minutes	Seconds to several minutes	Seconds to minutes
Sex	No preference, injurious in males	No preference, injurious in males	No preference, injurious in males	Females>males	Males>females	Males>females
Autonomic symptoms	Absent	Absent	Present	Absent	Absent	Absent
Amnesia	Present	Present	Present	Present, with variable recall	Present	Variable recall
Provoking factors	Sleep deprivation, forced arousals	Sleep deprivation, forced arousals, RLS	Sleep deprivation, forced arousals	Sleep deprivation, RLS	Sleep deprivation	Antidepressants*

Note. RBD=REM sleep behavior disorder; RLS=restless legs syndrome; SRED=sleep-related eating disorder.
*Except bupropion.

both types of parasomnia, and polysomnography also reveals features of sleep-state instability in NREM sleep and increased electromyographic tone in REM sleep, with or without associated behaviors. Parasomnia overlap disorder can also be seen secondary to various disorders such as narcolepsy, multiple sclerosis, brain tumors, rhombencephalitis, brain trauma, spinocerebellar ataxia type 3, psychiatric disorders, substance abuse, and alcohol withdrawal (Mahowald and Schenck 1991).

EATING DISORDERS

SRED should be differentiated from other disorders, such as night eating syndrome, and nocturnal occurrence of other eating disorders, such as bulimia nervosa or intentional binge-eating behavior at night before sleep or after awakening from sleep with full awareness. Daytime eating disorders may be associated with compensatory behaviors, such as purging and induced vomiting, which are not noted in SRED. Kleine-Levin syndrome is a rare disorder of recurrent periodic hypersomnia, cognitive impairment, hypersexuality, and hyperphagia during wakefulness with return to baseline normal cognitive and physical status between episodes and thus can be easily differentiated from SRED.

Treatment

NONPHARMACOLOGICAL THERAPY

The chief goal of treatment is to ensure the safety of the patient and bed partner. Any potential predisposing, priming, and precipitating factors, such as those discussed earlier in the "Pathophysiology" section, should be carefully addressed to reduce the occurrence. Environmental safety should be ensured by removing any sharp objects, furniture items, and weapons from proximity to the patient. Windows and exits to outside should be properly secured with the assistance of alarms, to avoid any injurious consequences. For benign parasomnias, such as confusional arousals and sleep terrors in the pediatric population, parents should be reassured about their generally inconsequential nature, if no physical risk is anticipated. Also, parents should be counseled about children's tendency to outgrow the condition with time.

Other behavioral strategies, such as psychotherapy, have also been attempted, with variable benefit (Galbiati et al. 2015). In pediatric cases of distressing sleep terror episodes, anticipatory awakenings 15–20 minutes before the usual time of episodes can greatly alleviate the frequency of these disordered arousals (Galbiati et al. 2015).

Clinical hypnosis has also been employed in NREM parasomnias with variable success ranging from 27% to 87% according to different case series (Hauri et al. 2007).

TREATMENT OF COMORBIDITIES

Any concurrent sleep disorder such as OSA (Chapters 8, 9, and 10) and RLS/PLM (see Chapter 17) should be adequately treated to minimize disordered arousals. Likewise, any incriminating agent such as sedative-hypnotic medication should be eliminated to reduce the occurrence. As noted earlier, screening for iron deficiency with a serum ferritin should be recommended in the settings of sleepwalking and SRED, especially with patients at risk for iron deficiency, such as vegetarians and premeno-pausal females.

PHARMACOTHERAPY

If, after a trial of the strategies just described, parasomnia behaviors persist and have a negative impact on safety or quality of life, medical intervention is warranted. Evidence in the medical literature is sparse, with the most commonly tried agents being benzodiazepines and antidepressants, depending on the DOA (Manni et al. 2018; Proserpio et al. 2018).

Benzodiazepines

Clonazepam is extensively used as a first-line agent for NREM parasomnias, although short-acting (e.g., triazolam) and intermediate-acting (e.g., temazepam) agents may be considered. A series of 69 patients with somnambulism and sleep terrors showed sustained benefit in 86% of patients with clonazepam and other benzodiazepine use after an average follow-up of 3.5 years, without significant dosage escalation (Schenck and Mahowald 1996).

Serotonergic Antidepressants

Various serotonergic antidepressants have shown benefit in DOAs, especially sleep terrors, presumably attributed to their action on mesencephalic periaqueductal gray matter. A case report showed success in two patients with sleepwalking and sleep terrors treated with imipramine (Cooper 1987), whereas others have demonstrated benefit in sleep terrors with trazodone (Balon 1994) and paroxetine (Wilson et al. 1997).

Other Pharmacotherapy

For SRED, dopamine agonists and topiramate have shown success. Dopamine agonists showed improvement in about 52% (14/27) of patients according to an original case series (Schenck et al. 1993). A randomized controlled trial of pramipexole 0.18–0.36 mg/day showed improvement in nocturnal activity based on actigraphy and subjective improvement in sleep (Provini et al. 2005). Topiramate has been proposed to have anorexinergic effects. According to one study, 68% of patients responded to a mean bedtime dose of 135 mg, but side effects led to high discontinuation rates (Winkelman 2006). Another study demonstrated good response to topiramate, with fewer side effects, over a period of 1.8 years (Schenck and Mahowald 2006). A recently published randomized controlled trial supports the use of topiramate (median dose, 125 mg). In this trial, the group receiving topiramate showed a reduced frequency of episodes by 55% versus 25% in the placebo group (Winkelman et al. 2020).

Conclusion

The NREM parasomnias, also known as DOAs, comprise sleepwalking, confusional arousals, sleep terrors, sleep-related eating, and sexsomnia. They arise from partial arousal from the N3 and N2 stages of NREM sleep, which are associated with lack of orientation and restricted cognition. Although generally benign in pediatric cases, in adults these behaviors not only have negative consequences on quality of life but also can lead to potential injuries. Management is mainly aimed at addressing the priming and precipitating factors, treating comorbid sleep disorders, counseling patients, and ensuring environmental safety, although pharmacological agents can be tried if the nocturnal behaviors continue to be injurious/potentially injurious or distressing.

KEY CLINICAL POINTS

- Disorders of arousal (DOAs) are characterized by partial awakening from non-REM (NREM) stages of sleep and are associated with amnestic automatic ambulation, feeding, or sexual behaviors, with decreased responsiveness to external stimuli, lack of recall, and enhanced autonomic activity.

- DOAs include confusional arousals, sleepwalking, sleep terrors, sleep-related eating, and sexsomnia.

- Nocturnal behaviors emanate predominantly from N3 sleep but can also occur in N2 sleep.

- Predisposing factors that increase homeostatic drive and precipitating factors that fragment sleep can lead to emergence of these behaviors.

- Meticulous history taking, examination, and polysomnography with extended electroencephalographic and extra electromyographic leads can facilitate diagnosis.

- Polysomnography can reveal slow-wave sleep instability in the form of an abnormal cyclic alternating pattern, hypersynchronous delta, and slow/mixed arousal pattern.

- The involuntary sleep-related behaviors with impaired consciousness can lead to potential injuries and forensic implications.

- Treatment of underlying aggravating factors such as restless legs syndrome, periodic limb movements, and obstructive sleep apnea can decrease the occurrence of NREM parasomnias.

- Elimination of inciting agents, such as sedative-hypnotics, and other priming factors, such as insufficient sleep, can help diminish the frequency of NREM parasomnias.

- Reassurance, counseling, behavioral modification, and pharmacological agents such as clonazepam or serotonergic antidepressants are used to successfully manage these disorders.

References

American Academy of Sleep Medicine: International Classification of Sleep Disorders, 3rd Edition. Darien, IL, American Academy of Sleep Medicine, 2014

Arnulf I: Sleepwalking. Curr Biol 28(22):R1288–R1289, 2018 30458142

Balon R: Sleep terror disorder and insomnia treated with trazodone: a case report. Ann Clin Psychiatry 6(3):161–163, 1994 7881496

Brion A, Flamand M, Oudiette D, et al: Sleep-related eating disorder versus sleepwalking: a controlled study. Sleep Med 13(8):1094–1101, 2012 22841035

Broughton R, Billings R, Cartwright R, et al: Homicidal somnambulism: a case report. Sleep 17(3):253–264, 1994 7939126

Castelnovo A, Lopez R, Proserpio P, et al: NREM sleep parasomnias as disorders of sleep-state dissociation. Natl Rev 14(8):470–481, 2018

Cooper AJ: Treatment of coexistent night-terrors and somnambulism in adults with imipramine and diazepam. J Clin Psychiatry 48(5):209–210, 1987

Dolder CR, Nelson MH: Hypnosedative-induced complex behaviours: incidence, mechanisms, and management. CNS Drugs 22(12):1021–1036, 2008 18998740

Drakatos P, Marples L, Muza R, et al: Video polysomnographic findings in non-rapid eye movement parasomnia. J Sleep Res 28(2):E12772, 2018 30295353

Dubessy AL, Leu-Semenescu S, Attali V, et al: Sexsomnia: a specialized non-REM parasomnia? Sleep (Basel) 40(2):2017 28364495

Frauscher B, Mitterling T, Bode A, et al: A prospective questionnaire study of 100 healthy sleepers: non-bothersome forms of recognizable sleep disorders are still present. J Clin Sleep Med 10(6):623–629, 2014

Fulda S, Hornyak M, Müller K, et al: Development and validation of the Munich Parasomnia Screening (MUPS). Somnologie (Berl) 12:56–65, 2008

Galbiati A, Rinaldi F, Giora E, et al: Behavioural and cognitive-behavioural treatments of parasomnias. Behav Neurol 2015:786928, 2015 26101458

Guilleminault C: Hypersynchronous slow delta, cyclic alternating pattern and sleepwalking. Sleep 29(1):14–15, 2006 16453974

Hauri PJ, Silber MH, Boeve BF: The treatment of parasomnias with hypnosis: a 5-year follow-up study. J Clin Sleep Med 3(4):369–373, 2007

Heidbreder A, Frauscher B, Mitterling T, et al: Not only sleepwalking but NREM parasomnia irrespective of the type is associated with *HLA DQB1*05:01*. J Clin Sleep Med 12(4):565–570, 2016

Howell MJ: Parasomnias: an updated review. Neurotherapeutics 9(4):753–775, 2012

Howell MJ, Schenck CH, Larson S, et al: Nocturnal eating and sleep-related eating disorder (SRED) are common among patients with restless legs syndrome. Sleep 33:A22717, 2010

Inoue Y: Sleep-related eating disorder and its associated conditions. Psychiatry Clin Neurosci 69(6):309–320, 2015

Irfan M, Schenck C, Howell M, et al: Non-rapid eye movement sleep and overlap parasomnias. Continuum 23(4):1035–1050, 2017 28777175

Joncas S, Zadra A, Paquet J, et al: The value of sleep deprivation as a diagnostic tool in adult sleepwalkers. Neurology 58(6):936–940, 2002

Kushida CA, Littner MR, Morgenthaler T, et al: Practice parameters for the indications for polysomnography and related procedures: an update for 2005. Sleep 28(4):499–521, 2005

Licis AK, Desruisseau D, Yamada KA, et al: Novel genetic findings in an extended family pedigree with sleepwalking. Neurology 76(1):49–52, 2011

Lopez R, Jaussent I, Dauvilliers Y: Pain in sleepwalking: a clinical enigma. Sleep 38(11):1693–1698, 2015

Lopez R, Shen Y, Chenini S, et al: Diagnostic criteria for disorders of arousal: a video-polysomnographic assessment. Ann Neurol 83(2):341–351, 2018 29360192

Mahowald MW, Schenck CH: Status dissociates: a perspective on states of being. Sleep 14(1):69–79, 1991

Manni R, Toscano G, Terzaghi M: Therapeutic symptomatic strategies in the parasomnias. Curr Treat Options Neurol 20(7):26, 2018 29869076

Muza R, Lawrence M, Drakatos P: The reality of sexsomnia. Curr Opin Pulm Med 22(6):576–582, 2016 27607155

Petit D, Pennestri M, Paquet J, et al: Childhood sleepwalking and sleep terrors: a longitudinal study of prevalence and familial aggregation. JAMA Pediatr 169(7):653–658, 2015

Pressman MR: Factors that predispose, prime and precipitate NREM parasomnias in adults: clinical and forensic implications. Sleep Med Rev 11(1):5–33, 2007

Proserpio P, Terzaghi M, Manni R, et al: Drugs used in parasomnia. Sleep Med Clin 13(2):191–202, 2018 29759270

Provini F, Albani F, Vetrugno R, et al: A pilot double-blind placebo-controlled trial of low-dose pramipexole in sleep-related eating disorder. Eur J Neurol 12(6):432–436, 2005

Schenck CH: Update on sexsomnia, sleep related sexual seizures, and forensic implications. NeuroQuantology 13(4):518–541, 2015

Schenck CH, Mahowald MW: Long-term, nightly benzodiazepine treatment of injurious parasomnias and other disorders of disrupted nocturnal sleep in 170 adults. Am J Med 100(3):333–337, 1996

Schenck CH, Mahowald MW: Topiramate therapy of sleep related eating disorder (SRED). Sleep 29(suppl):A268, 2006

Schenck CH, Milner DM, Hurwitz TD, et al: A polysomnographic and clinical report on sleep-related injury in 100 adult patients. Am J Psychiatry 146(9):1166–1173, 1989 2764174

Schenck CH, Hurwitz TD, Bundlie SR, et al: Sleep-related eating disorders: polysomnographic correlates of a heterogeneous syndrome distinct from daytime eating disorders. Sleep 14(5):419–431, 1991

Schenck CH, Hurwitz TD, O'Connor KA, et al: Additional categories of sleep-related eating disorders and the current status of treatment. Sleep 16(5):457–466, 1993

Schenck CH, Arnulf I, Mahowald MW: Sleep and sex: what can go wrong? A review of the literature on sleep related disorders and abnormal sexual behaviors and experiences. Sleep 30(6):683–702, 2007

Terzano MG, Parrino L, Smerieri A, et al: Atlas, rules, and recording techniques for the scoring of cyclic alternating pattern (CAP) in human sleep. Sleep Med 3(2):187–199, 2002 14592244

Wills L, Garcia J: Parasomnias: epidemiology and management. CNS Drugs 16(12):803–810, 2002

Wilson SJ, Lillywhite AR, Potokar JP, et al: Adult night terrors and paroxetine. Lancet 350(9072):185, 1997 9250190

Winkelman JW: Efficacy and tolerability of open-label topiramate in the treatment of sleep-related eating disorder: a retrospective case series. J Clin Psychiatry 67(11):1729–1734, 2006

Winkelman JW, Herzog DB, Fava M: The prevalence of sleep-related eating disorder in psychiatric and non-psychiatric populations. Psychol Med 29(6):1461–1466, 1999

Winkelman JW, Wipper B, Purks J, et al: Topiramate reduces nocturnal eating in sleep-related eating disorder. Sleep 2020 Epub ahead of print

CHAPTER 15

REM Sleep Behavior Disorder

Muna Irfan, M.D.

Carlos H. Schenck, M.D.

REM sleep behavior disorder (RBD) is a parasomnia (sleep behavioral and experiential disorder) that consists of abnormal behavioral release during REM sleep with loss of the mammalian generalized skeletal muscle paralysis ("REM-atonia") (Schenck and Mahowald 2002). The current definition of RBD therefore requires both a history of dream enactment during REM sleep and electrophysiological evidence of loss of REM-atonia on video polysomnography (vPSG) (American Academy of Sleep Medicine 2014).

RBD was first identified in humans in a series of five patients in 1986 that closely matched findings from an experimental animal model first reported in 1965 in cats with pontine tegmental lesions (Schenck and Mahowald 2002). RBD represents how one of the core features of mammalian REM sleep, REM-atonia, can become compromised, resulting in clinically consequential behavioral release during REM sleep. Individuals with RBD move with their eyes closed while attending to inner dream action and are unaware of the actual bedside surroundings. This is a highly vulnerable state that often results in injury (Schenck and Mahowald 2002). Behavioral release during REM sleep often involves the acting-out of confrontational, aggressive, and violent dreams (Schenck et al. 2009), usually involving unfamiliar people and animals. Dreamers are rarely the primary aggressor and often are defending themselves or a partner. The reported dream action closely matches the observed behaviors during polysomnographic evaluation. RBD is a dream disorder almost as much as a sleep behavioral disorder. A recent review article summarized current knowledge on RBD (Dauvilliers et al. 2018), and the first textbook on RBD was published in 2018 (Schenck et al. 2018).

Pathophysiology

Multiple scientists have focused their efforts on unraveling the complex neuronal network that leads to abnormal behavior in REM sleep, which is facilitated through increased skeletal muscle tone and the enacting of energetic dream content. Lesioning of the dorsal pontine tegmentum (noradrenergic neurons in the locus coeruleus and cholinergic neurons of the laterodorsal tegmental nucleus) in feline models resulted in physically active "paradoxical sleep" (synonym of REM sleep), with presumed dream-enacting behaviors (Jouvet and Delorme 1965).

Neurons in the sublaterodorsal tegmental nucleus (SLD) were subsequently identified to be involved in the generation of skeletal muscle atonia in REM sleep. Neuromelanin-sensitive imaging techniques have demonstrated reduced signals in the locus coeruleus and SLD in patients with RBD, which suggests that degeneration of SLD glutamatergic neurons leads to RBD. Neurons in the SLD directly project to GABA- and glycine-containing neurons in the nucleus magnocellularis located in the ventral medulla. Their inhibitory projections to spinal cord anterior horn cells synapsing on skeletal muscle cells induce REM-atonia. Thus, structural or functional lesions of the ventral medulla cause a decrease or loss of GABAergic and glycinergic inhibitory output, resulting in the motor release of RBD (Dauvilliers et al. 2018). The violent movements of RBD are proposed to be mediated by glutamatergic phasic excitation of motor neurons in the (relative) absence of tonic inhibition.

The role of other brain regions in RBD is still under investigation. Single-photon emission computed tomography of patients with RBD has localized the supplementary motor area as the generator of violent motoric dream-enacting behavior. The emotional undertone of RBD-related dreams might suggest involvement of the cortical limbic areas. Overall, the neuronal circuitry of REM sleep motor regulation and motor dysregulation in RBD is complex and heterogenous (Dauvilliers et al. 2018). A simplified neuronal pathway mediating skeletal muscle tone release is illustrated in Figure 15–1.

Epidemiology

The traditional clinical profile of patients with RBD is middle-aged and older men with violent and injurious dream-enacting behaviors (Schenck and Mahowald 2002). More than 80% of these patients eventually develop a parkinsonian (α-synucleinopathy) neurodegenerative disorder,

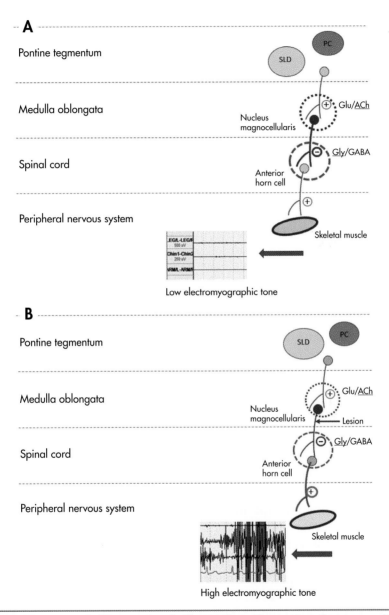

FIGURE 15–1. *A,* **Diagrammatic illustration of neural pathways mediating normal muscle atonia in REM sleep.** *B,* **Diagrammatic illustration of disruption of the pathway leading to loss of REM-associated atonia and thus increased electromyographic tone.**

Note. +=excitatory neurotransmitter; –=inhibitory neurotransmitter; ACh=acetylcholine; Glu=glutamate; Gly=glycine; PC=perilocus coeruleus; SLD=sublaterodorsal tegmental nucleus.

usually Parkinson's disease or dementia with Lewy bodies (DLB), with a mean interval from RBD onset to overt neurodegeneration of approximately 10 years (Galbiati et al. 2018). These striking findings have forced a reconsideration in current thinking. RBD should now be considered prodromal parkinsonism, and thus what originally was called "idiopathic RBD" should now be called "isolated RBD," which implies the eventual transformation of the isolated clinical RBD state into overt parkinsonism with RBD (Högl et al. 2018). This close association has spurred major research efforts to develop and test neuroprotective/disease-modifying agents in patients with isolated RBD in an effort to slow or halt progression to overt neurodegeneration.

A recent population-based study of middle-aged to older adults with polysomnographically confirmed RBD found a 1.06% prevalence of RBD and gender parity. Thus, the traditional clinical profile of RBD needs to be reconsidered (Haba-Rubio et al. 2018). Because women generally have less aggressive and less injurious RBD, they present for medical attention much less frequently than men. Therefore, the traditional RBD profile reflects a clinical referral bias on account of the more aggressive and more injurious sleep behaviors among men with RBD. However, once a promising neuroprotective agent becomes available, a concerted effort must be initiated to identify women with RBD who have not sought medical attention (as well as men with mild RBD), because it is the *presence* of REM sleep without atonia (RSWA) or RBD, and not the *severity*, that carries the strong risk for future parkinsonism. This effort would entail collaboration with geriatric medicine, geriatric psychiatry, primary care, and neurology clinics. Also, the 1.06% prevalence of RBD found in this study is the first prevalence rate of this condition in the general population to be polysomnographically confirmed (Haba-Rubio et al. 2018); thus, RBD is not an uncommon disease.

The phenotype of RBD in patients younger than 50 years has recently been recognized to differ from that of middle-aged and older men with aggressive RBD behaviors (Ju 2018). Younger patients have greater gender parity, less severe RBD, and a greater association with narcolepsy-cataplexy (narcolepsy type 1), psychiatric disorders and antidepressant use, and parasomnia overlap disorder (defined by the presence of both RBD and non-REM [NREM] sleep parasomnia [sleepwalking or sleep terrors] in the same individual) (American Academy of Sleep Medicine 2014; Schenck et al. 1997). RBD in children and adolescents, although rare, is usually associated with narcolepsy type 1, parasomnia overlap disorder, brain stem tumors, and antidepressant use (Schenck and Mahowald 2002). Most antidepressant medications (especially the selective serotonin reuptake inhibitors [SSRIs], venlafaxine, and the tricyclic antidepressants [TCAs]) can trigger or aggravate RBD, with the exception of bupropion, which is a dopaminergic-noradrenergic agent (Li et al. 2018). Finally, acute RBD exists and emerges in the context of acute toxic-metabolic disturbances and acute drug withdrawal (Provini and Tachibana 2018; Schenck and Mahowald 2002).

Regarding the genetic basis of the disorder, familial RBD has recently been reported in one family, with autosomal transmission and altered GABAergic circuits implicated (Mateo-Montero et al. 2018). A recent large-scale, familial case-control study involved patients with idiopathic RBD (iRBD) and their first-degree relatives (Liu et al. 2019). Subjects were interviewed and underwent vPSG studies and other clinical assessments. The authors found that iRBD has a familial aggregation, ranging from isolated features of RSWA to full-blown RBD; also, first-degree relatives of patients with iRBD carry an increased risk of α-synucleinopathy (Parkinson's disease and dementia), thus suggesting a familial aggregation and staging pathology of α-synucleinopathy (Liu et al. 2019). Moreover, unaffected first-degree relatives also demonstrated an increased risk for prodromal Parkinson's disease (Liu et al. 2019). A strong research effort is being undertaken on the genetics of RBD (Gan-Or and Rouleau 2018), particularly in light of its strong link with Parkinson's disease and related α-synucleinopathy neurodegenerative disorders, DLB, and multiple system atrophy (MSA). Of the two genes most associated with Parkinson's, *GBA* and *LRRK2*, mutations in *GBA* are clearly important risk factors for RBD, whereas mutations in *LRRK2* probably have no pathogenic role in RBD.

Individuals with RBD who develop Parkinson's disease often represent a specific subtype, with typical clinical features. The progression to Parkinson's, DLB, or MSA from RBD is variable, ranging from immediate to decades after onset of RBD, and it is not apparent which factors determine the rate and type of progression. Genetic studies of RBD, therefore, can help clarify these critical issues. Genetic studies of Parkinson's disease include all the different phenotypes, including those without RBD, although specific genetic factors might be associated with RBD. Furthermore, studying RBD may help identify genetic factors associated with the age at onset, future risk of synucleinopathies, and rate of progression. Understanding the genetic background of RBD and its progression to the different synucleinopathies may facilitate future prognosis, genetic counseling, patient stratification for clinical trials, and precision medicine.

To properly map the genetic risk loci in RBD, two approaches could be taken (Gan-Or and Rouleau 2018): 1) performing genome-wide association studies on idiopathic, vPSG-documented, and properly phenotyped RBD cohorts, or 2) reanalyzing data from the Parkinson's disease genome-wide association studies only for patients with the disease who also have RBD or those who had RBD prior to developing overt Parkinson's. Once the genetic factors that affect either the rate of progression from RBD to synucleinopathies or the specific type of synucleinopathy (i.e., markers that predict conversion to Parkinson's disease, DLB, or MSA specifically) are identified, better prognosis and genetic counseling could be given. Finally, drugs are in development and in clinical trials that target a specific gene or its protein product, such as *GBA*. Identifying patients with RBD who have variants of this and other genes, as well as identifying future novel genes that may be associated specifically with RBD, may bring us one step closer to precision medicine, tailored for each patient based on his or her genetic background and the biological process responsible for the disease.

IDIOPATHIC REM SLEEP BEHAVIOR DISORDER

Idiopathic RBD refers to the occurrence of RBD in healthy patients without any associated neurological disorder. Although this term is still used in the literature, many propose the use of "isolated RBD" because it appears that most patients with iRBD will go on to develop neurodegenerative disorder and hence it is considered a prodromal symptom of α-synuclein disorders and not truly idiopathic.

SECONDARY REM SLEEP BEHAVIOR DISORDER

RBD is "secondary" when it is present in association with neurological disorders, such as α-synucleinopathies, narcolepsy, and paraneoplastic disorders. The term "symptomatic RBD" is also used synonymously by some experts in the field.

Alpha-Synucleinopathies

The association between RBD and neurodegenerative disorders has been illustrated by several longitudinal studies. It is now well established as a prodromal symptom of α-synuclein disorders (Galbiati et al. 2018; Högl et al. 2018; Schenck and Mahowald 2002), a group of neurodegenerative disorders (Parkinson's disease, DLB, MSA) characterized by pathological accumulation of α-synuclein protein aggregates in the neurons and glial cells. Lewy bodies are aggregates of α-synuclein and other proteins, including ubiquitin and neurofilament, and mark the neurodegeneration in these disorders (Hu et al. 2015). The brain stem regions involved in REM-atonia generation are affected by Lewy body accumulation much earlier than the cortical areas, which explains the emergence of RBD decades before clinical phenoconversion to a neurological disorder. On longitudinal follow-up of a cohort >13 years from onset of RBD, 81% of patients had developed neurodegenerative disorders (Schenck et al. 2018). When the cohort was assessed by another clinical group >14 years from onset of RBD, this number rose to 91%. The International RBD Study Group combined data from 12 different centers and demonstrated an average 8% annual risk of phenoconversion to α-synucleinopathy (Postuma et al. 2015). This signifies that RBD is much more than a parasomnia because it heralds a high risk for future development of a neurodegenerative disorder in persons older than 50 years and hence warrants serial monitoring for early diagnosis and proper management.

Other Neurological Disorders

RBD is also seen in other neurological disorders in which the pontine pathways involved in REM-atonia generation may be disrupted by various pathological processes. In such conditions, it may occur concurrently with or subsequent to the other neurological symptoms. These include amyloidopathies, tauopathies, TAR DNA binding protein 43 proteinopathies, tri- and tetranucleotide repeat disorders, and genetic, congenital, and some developmental conditions associated with RBD at a lower frequency.

Narcolepsy, especially type 1, also has a strong association (60%) with RBD but phenotypically is different, occurring at a younger age, with less aggressive manifestations, no sex predilection, and no identified increased risk for parkinsonism (Dauvilliers et al. 2013).

Lesional REM Sleep Behavior Disorder

Cases of RBD with vascular, neoplastic, demyelinating, vasculitic, and traumatic insults have also been reported. In such instances, the structural lesion can frequently be localized to the pontine areas governing REM sleep atonia by imaging techniques.

Autoimmune REM Sleep Behavior Disorder

RBD can also occur in certain autoimmune and inflammatory encephalitides without identifiable structural lesions. These include voltage-gated potassium antibody encephalitis (limbic encephalitis and Morvan's syndrome) and other encephalitides such as Ma-2 encephalitis and paraneoplastic cerebellar degeneration. Reciprocal neural connections between limbic system and brain stem regions are presumed to affect REM sleep muscle tone in such cases. Most respond favorably to immunotherapy, except the IgLON5 parasomnia that is part of a fatal syndrome comprising NREM and REM parasomnias, sleep-related breathing dysfunction,

TABLE 15–1.   Disorders associated with REM sleep behavior disorder

α-Synucleinopathy

   Dementia with Lewy bodies

   Multiple system atrophy

   Parkinson's disease

   Pure autonomic failure

Amyloidopathy

   Alzheimer's disease

Tauopathy

   Amyotrophic lateral sclerosis

   Guadeloupean parkinsonism

   Frontotemporal dementia

   Progressive supranuclear palsy

Trinucleotide/Tetranucleotide repeat disorders

   Huntington's disease

   Myotonic dystrophy type 2

   Spinocerebellar ataxia type 3

Immune-mediated/Inflammatory disorders

   Guillain-Barré syndrome

   IgLON5 parasomnia

   Limbic encephalitis

   Ma2 encephalitis

   Paraneoplastic cerebellar degeneration

   Voltage-gated K antibody encephalitis

Other neurological disorders

   Narcolepsy type 1

Genetic disorders

   Pantothenate kinase-associated neurodegeneration

   Wilson's disease

Congenital/Developmental disorders

   Autism

   Moebius syndrome

   Smith-Magenis syndrome

   Tourette's disorder

Structural lesions

   Acoustic neuroma

   Astrocytoma

   CNS vasculitis

   Infarct

   Multiple sclerosis

   Vascular malformations

Medication-induced

   Bisoprolol

   Monoamine oxidase inhibitors

   Selective serotonin reuptake inhibitors

   Serotonin and norepinephrine reuptake inhibitors

   Tricyclic and tetracyclic antidepressants

Drug withdrawal

   Alcohol

   Barbiturate

   Amphetamine

   Cocaine

dysautonomia, bulbar or neurological dysfunction, and pathological features suggesting a tauopathy refractory to immunosuppressive agents (Sabater et al. 2014). Table 15–1 lists the conditions associated with RBD.

Medication-Induced REM Sleep Behavior Disorder

In a population younger than 50 years, psychotropic medication is the most common cause of RBD induction, especially SSRIs and serotonin-norepinephrine reuptake inhibitors (SNRIs), particularly venlafaxine.

Also, TCAs and tetracyclic antidepressants, monoamine oxidase inhibitors (MAOIs), tramadol, and acetylcholinesterase inhibitors have been incriminated. Drug-induced RBD tends to manifest as increased phasic tone in tibial leads (Ju 2018).

Although antidepressants are assumed to induce increase REM tone, evidence has shown that they unmask subclinical neurodegeneration rather than inducing it de novo. This is supported by a study demonstrating the presence of other prodromal symptoms such as hyposmia, constipation, and subtle visual and motor findings in such patients (Postuma et al. 2013). Reduced striatal dopamine uptake, as measured by ^{18}F-DOPA PET imaging in patients with medication-induced RBD, suggests that antidepressant-induced RBD may be considered a prodromal symptom of synuclein degeneration (Wu et al. 2014). Further investigation is warranted in this area.

Diagnosis

CLINICAL PRESENTATION

RBD is characterized by physically active motor behaviors and vocalizations representing dream enactment in REM sleep. The motor activity ranges from subtle upper-extremity movements (often referred to as hand babbling) to more aggressive, violent, rapid, jerky, and apparently purposeful oneiric behaviors such as punching, kicking, running, or jumping. These actions can be potentially injurious to the patient and bed partner, compromising safety.

Vocalizations are typically loud, in the form of screaming, yelling, or hollering, and are often profanity laced, contradictory to the person's usual demeanor. Dream content typically involves emotionally charged fearful and hostile situations, such as unfamiliar people or animals chasing the patient or loved ones, wherein the dreamer assumes the role of defender and thus may engage in combative behavior that can lead to self-injury or pose inadvertent threat to the bed partner. The dreams, when recalled, are quite vivid and tend to happen in the latter part of the night as REM episodes become prolonged, with greater phasic activity. Frequency of the dreams and dream-enactment behaviors can vary from several times per night to once a month or even less. Dream recall may be inconsistent, with >40% of patients being unaware of RBD episodes (Fernández-Arcos et al. 2016).

The diagnostic criteria for RBD according to the *International Classification of Sleep Disorders*, 3rd Edition (American Academy of Sleep Medicine 2014), are listed in Table 15–2.

TABLE 15–2.   **American Academy of Sleep Medicine diagnostic criteria for REM sleep behavior disorder**

1. Repeated sleep-related vocalization and/or complex motor behavior

2. Documented on polysomnography to occur in REM sleep OR presumed to occur in REM sleep clinically

3. Polysomnography demonstrates evidence of REM sleep without atonia (Frauscher et al. 2012) in at least 27% of REM sleep epochs using a combination of chin and finger flexor electromyography

4. Not attributed to other conditions, disorders, or medications/substances

Source.   American Academy of Sleep Medicine 2014.

QUESTIONNAIRES

Several clinical screening surveys and questionnaires are available to help identify RBD (Li et al. 2018). They comprise questions aimed at inquiring about dream-enactment behaviors. Collateral historians can greatly improve the yield of these questionnaires. The RBD Questionnaire–Hong Kong is a 13-item questionnaire; the REM Sleep Behavior Disorder Screening Questionnaire is a 10-item screen; and the Innsbruck RBD inventory is a 5-item survey. The Mayo Sleep Questionnaire and RBD Single-Question are 1-question measures. The sensitivity and specificity of the latter are 93.8% and 87.2%, respectively. It consists of a single question: "Have you ever been told, or suspected yourself, that you seem to 'act out your dreams' while asleep (e.g., punching, flailing your arms in the air, making running movement)?" (Postuma et al. 2012).

POLYSOMNOGRAPHIC CHARACTERISTICS

RBD is the only parasomnia that requires objective vPSG confirmation to establish the diagnosis (American Academy of Sleep Medicine 2014). The polysomnographic hallmark of RBD consists of electromyographic abnormalities during REM sleep, called "loss of REM atonia" or RSWA, with increased muscle tone or increased phasic muscle twitching. Other polysomnographic features of RBD include excessive tonic activity in REM sleep on chin electromyography and phasic activity in REM sleep activity on chin or limb electromyography.

Tonic activity (sustained muscle activity) is characterized by an increase in submental electromyographic amplitude in REM sleep for at least 50% of a 30-second epoch. A polysomnographic recording with increased tonic activity in the chin is shown in Figure 15–2A. *Phasic activity* (excessive transient muscle activity) is assessed when a 30-second epoch divided into 10 sequential 3-second mini-epochs has at least 5 (50% of the total duration) mini-epoch bursts of transient muscle activity. These

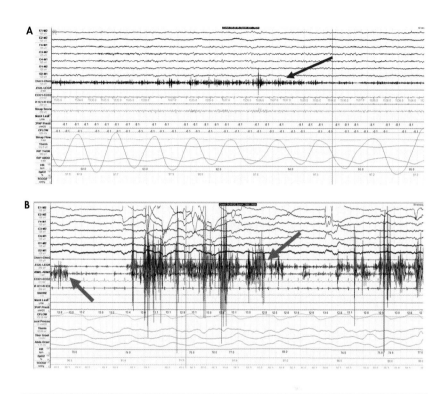

FIGURE 15–2.   Tonic and phasic electromyographic activity.

A, Polysomnographic recording of REM tonic activity (*arrow*) on a chin electromyography lead for more than half of the 30-second epoch. **B,** A 30-second epoch on polysomnogram showing increased phasic activity in the upper (*left arrow*) and lower limbs (*right arrow*).

bursts must be at least four times greater in amplitude than background electromyography and 0.1–5.0 seconds in duration. Thus, for proper evaluation, extra limb leads should be added to the vPSG to be able to assess REM tone. Current recommendations require the presence of at least 27% RSWA on electromyography using a combination of finger flexor and chin leads (American Academy of Sleep Medicine 2014; Frauscher et al. 2012). Figure 15–2B demonstrates the neurophysiological recording of phasic activity in REM sleep on polysomnography.

Differential Diagnosis

A meticulously obtained historical account and carefully monitored vPSG facilitate the exclusion of other diagnoses such as obstructive sleep apnea (OSA), periodic limb movements (PLMs), sleepwalking, sleep talking, con-

TABLE 15–3.   Differential diagnosis for RBD

Sleepwalking	Rhythmic movement disorder
Sleep talking	PTSD/trauma-associated sleep disorder
Sleep terrors	Sleep-related hypermotor epilepsy
Confusional arousals	Sleep-related dissociative disorder
Pseudo-RBD (OSA)	Pseudo-RBD (PLMs)

Note.   OSA=obstructive sleep apnea; PLM=periodic limb movement; RBD=REM sleep behavior disorder.

fusional arousals, night terrors (NREM parasomnias) and nightmares (Irfan and Howell 2016; Schenck and Mahowald 2002). Sleep-related hypermotor seizures can also mimic RBD. Table 15–3 lists the differential diagnosis in detail.

NON-REM PARASOMNIAS

The bed partner's detailed account can be very revealing in terms of observational details. NREM parasomnias typically occur in first part of the night and can involve prolonged ambulation with little or no recollection of the episode or dream content, such as in sleepwalking. The nocturnal episodes in RBD differ from NREM parasomnias (see Chapter 14) because RBD episodes tend to occur in the latter part of the night and are associated mostly with vivid dream recollection (when dreams are recalled at all); the patient's eyes remain closed and his or her movements are rapid, jerky, and sometimes purposeful but are shorter in duration and can be abolished if the patient is aroused, with quick return to wakefulness and intact orientation. Walking during RBD episodes is very rare.

PERIODIC LIMB MOVEMENTS

High-magnitude PLMs may be mistaken for thrashing about in sleep, but polysomnography can clearly delineate movements occurring mainly in NREM sleep (Gaig et al. 2017), with preserved REM-atonia and with response to the standard treatment of PLM disorder with dopaminergic agents (see Chapter 17).

PSEUDO-RBD RELATED TO OBSTRUCTIVE SLEEP APNEA

OSA pseudo-RBD is a term used for arousals that occur in sleep due to increased respiratory effort at the end of OSA events (see Chapter 8) (Iranzo and Santamaría 2002).

SEIZURES

Sleep-related hypermotor epilepsy presents with bizarre sleep-related behaviors with unusual ictal semiology, but the highly stereotypical nature of these behaviors points to their epileptic origin. An extended electroencephalogram should be added to polysomnographic monitoring to capture any rhythmic electrocerebral activity suggestive of seizures, especially in conjunction with abnormal sleep-related behaviors (American Academy of Sleep Medicine 2014).

PTSD AND OTHER MIMICS

Other differential diagnoses include rhythmic movement disorder and psychogenic dissociative disorders. Behaviors that emerge with PTSD-related nightmares pose a clinical presentation similar to RBD, but the pathophysiological mechanism is not yet fully understood as to whether they represent increased muscle tone in REM sleep or increased arousals from REM due to hypervigilance (Mysliwiec et al. 2014). Also, the response to prazosin in the few reported cases of "trauma-associated sleep disorder" is a (non-absolute) distinguishing feature from RBD.

Treatment

The main goal of RBD management is reducing disruptive nightmares to prevent injuries to the patient and bed partner and to improve quality of life by reducing interruptions in sleep. The patient's violent, jerky movements during REM sleep to "defend" against a dream assailant can lead to injuries, and many times bed partners are forced to move into a separate room for safety. In one study, all of the bed partners of patients with RBD reported impaired quality of life due to disturbance of sleep attributed to the patient's disruptive nocturnal movements. Physical injuries from aggressive movements had been reported by 62.5% of the bed partners (Jung and St Louis 2016; Lam et al. 2016).

ENVIRONMENTAL MODIFICATIONS

Environmental accommodations to ensure safety are the mainstay of treatment (level A evidence) according to standard guidelines (Aurora et al. 2010). The patient and bed partner should be advised to remove sharp objects, furniture, and weapons from the immediate sleeping environment to avoid any injuries. For those patients with demonstrated potential to jump out of bed, a soft padding or mattress should be placed on the floor. A low-height bed is preferable, and the bed should be placed away from windows, which should be secured and thickly curtained to prevent defenestration. Any factors that might interrupt sleep, such as sleep deprivation or insufficient sleep, should be addressed.

NONPHARMACOLOGICAL THERAPIES

Comorbid OSA should be treated to reduce the arousals from increased respiratory effort that can occur more frequently during REM sleep. A pressurized bed alarm with a prerecorded calming message in a familiar voice that gently prompts the patient to return to sleep has been shown to help (Howell et al. 2011) but is still not widely used. Hypnosis has been attempted to treat parasomnia, including RBD, with some success but is not standard practice (Hauri et al. 2007). If feasible, drugs that aggravate or unmask RBD symptoms, such as SSRIs, SNRIs, TCAs, and MAOIs, should be reduced or replaced with agents that do not cause dream enactment, such as bupropion. Such an adjustment should be attempted very judiciously and in consultation with any treating psychiatrist or other clinician.

PHARMACOTHERAPY

Clonazepam

Clonazepam historically has been used successfully as first-line therapy at dosages of 0.5–1 mg or more at bedtime, with a reduction in nighttime behaviors in most cases (level B evidence) (Aurora et al. 2010). A recent randomized controlled trial (RCT) comparing clonazepam 0.5 mg with placebo was unable to show benefit, but case series and clinical experience suggest a dose-dependent response, indicating that the dose used in the trial may have been subtherapeutic (Shin et al. 2019). Although the mechanism of action is not clear, one study posited that clonazepam reduces phasic activity in REM, although RSWA and mild abnormal behavior are not altered much (Aurora et al. 2010). Adverse effects are dose related and include respiratory depression, somnolence, gait trouble, altered cognition, dizziness, and falls. Thus, caution should be exercised in patients with cognitive impairment and OSA (Li et al. 2016).

Melatonin

Due to its preferable side effect profile, melatonin has been increasingly used as a first-line agent (level B evidence) at doses ranging from 2 mg to 15 mg, especially in elderly patients with cognitive impairment (McGrane et al. 2015). Melatonin has been shown to reduce the number of REM epochs with RSWA and to decrease excessive tonic and phasic motor activity. Side effects include headache, mild sedation, and delusions/

hallucinations. Its exact mechanism of action is not clear, but it has been shown to decrease REM phase shifts and has a direct impact on restoring REM sleep modulation. Another theory proposed that melatonin enhances the action of GABA on GABA$_A$ receptors on the spinal motor neurons, leading to reduced RSWA in RBD (Dauvilliers et al. 2018; McGrane et al. 2015). Outcome data on patients with RBD treated with melatonin are few compared with the larger number of reported patients treated with clonazepam. A small RCT showed improvement with melatonin 3 mg on both polysomnographic epochs with RSWA and Clinical Global Impression Scale scores (Kunz and Mahlberg 2010), whereas another failed to show benefit of prolonged-release melatonin in doses of 2 mg and 6 mg (Jun et al. 2019). Thus, further RCTs to evaluate the true efficacy and optimal dosing and formulation of melatonin are needed. A combination of clonazepam and melatonin may be needed if single therapy is not efficacious or when use at lower doses may reduce the risk of side effects.

Other Drugs

If these drugs fail, dopamine agonists (pramipexole, rotigotine) have also been used to treat RBD, especially if PLMs are present. Rivastigmine has shown efficacy in two small RCTs in patients with treatment-refractory RBD (Brunetti et al. 2014; Di Giacopo et al. 2012). Other agents used, based on limited case reports and series, include cholinesterase inhibitors (donepezil), anticonvulsants (carbamazepine), other benzodiazepines (triazolam), antipsychotics (clozapine, quetiapine), levodopa, sodium oxybate, and ramelteon.

COUNSELING

Patients with iRBD, particularly those older than 50 years of age, should be appropriately counseled about the risk of future development of α-synucleinopathies. Yearly surveillance with detailed clinical evaluation should be performed, for early detection and proper management of the clinical syndrome. This is especially relevant in current times, when neuroprotective trials are soon to be under way under the guidance of the North American Preclinical Synucleinopathy (NAPS) Consortium.

Conclusion

RBD represents an intriguing parasomnia with forensic and clinical implications that is still worthy of concerted research efforts decades after its original description in animals and humans. In the search for neuroprotective agents, RBD provides a perfect substrate for investigational studies. Although the nocturnal behaviors should be addressed symptomatically, continued yearly surveillance of these patients is of prime importance in order to diagnose them as early as possible during phenoconversion to α-synuclein disorders. Early detection and management of patients can help reduce morbidity and improve quality of life while empowering them to make informed clinical decisions.

KEY CLINICAL POINTS

- REM sleep behavior disorder (RBD) is characterized by abnormal vocalizations and motoric behaviors in REM sleep represented by potentially injurious dream-enacting episodes.
- REM sleep without atonia is the neurophysiological marker of RBD.
- According to the American Academy of Sleep Medicine, RBD is the only parasomnia that warrants video polysomnography as a part of the evaluation to confirm diagnosis.
- RBD in patients older than 50 years of age has a strong association with the risk of phenoconversion to α-synuclein neurodegenerative disorders.
- Environmental safety is the mainstay of treatment, with melatonin and clonazepam used as pharmacological agents as needed.
- Patients with RBD should undergo yearly neurological surveillance.

References

American Academy of Sleep Medicine: International Classification of Sleep Disorders, 3rd Edition. Darien, IL, American Academy of Sleep Medicine, 2014

Aurora RN, Zak RS, Maganti RK, et al: Best practice guide for the treatment of REM sleep behavior disorder (RBD). J Clin Sleep Med 6(1):85–95, 2010 20191945

Brunetti V, Losurdo A, Testani E, et al: Rivastigmine for refractory REM behavior disorder in mild cognitive impairment. Curr Alzheimer Res 11(3):267–273, 2014 24597506

Dauvilliers Y, Jennum P, Plazzi G: Rapid eye movement sleep behavior disorder and rapid eye movement sleep without atonia in narcolepsy. Sleep Med 14(8):775–781, 2013 23219054

Dauvilliers Y, Schenck CH, Postuma RB, et al: REM sleep behaviour disorder. Nat Rev Dis Primers 4(1):19, 2018 30166532

Di Giacopo R, Fasano A, Quaranta D, et al: Rivastigmine as alternative treatment for refractory REM behavior disorder in Parkinson's disease. Mov Disord 27(4):559–561, 2012 22290743

Fernández-Arcos A, Iranzo A, Serradell M, et al: The clinical phenotype of idiopathic rapid eye movement sleep behavior disorder at presentation: a study in 203 consecutive patients. Sleep 39(1):121–132, 2016 26940460

Frauscher B, Iranzo A, Gaig C, et al: Normative EMG values during REM sleep for the diagnosis of REM sleep behavior disorder. Sleep 35(6):835–847, 2012 22654203

Gaig C, Iranzo A, Pujol M, et al: Periodic limb movements during sleep mimicking REM sleep behavior disorder: a new form of periodic limb movement disorder. Sleep 40(3), 2017 28364416

Galbiati A, Verga L, Giora E, et al: The risk of neurodegeneration in REM sleep behavior disorder: a systematic review and meta-analysis of longitudinal studies. Sleep Med Rev 43:37–46, 2018 30503716

Gan-Or Z, Rouleau GA: Genetics of REM sleep behavior disorder, in Rapid-Eye-Movement Sleep Behavior Disorder. Edited by Schenck CH, Högl B, Videnovic A. Cham, Switzerland, Springer Nature, 2018, pp 589–609

Haba-Rubio J, Frauscher B, Marques-Vidal P, et al: Prevalence and determinants of REM sleep behavior disorder in the general population. Sleep 41(2), 2018 29216391

Hauri P, Silber M, Boeve B: The treatment of parasomnias with hypnosis: a 5-year follow-up study. J Clin Sleep Med 3:369–373, 2007 17694725

Högl B, Stefani A, Videnovic A: Idiopathic REM sleep behaviour disorder and neurodegeneration: an update. Nat Rev 14(1):40–55, 2018 29170501

Howell MJ, Arneson PA, Schenck CH: A novel therapy for REM sleep behavior disorder (RBD). J Clin Sleep Med 7(6):639–644, 2011 22171203

Hu Y, Yu SY, Zuo LJ, et al: Parkinson disease with REM sleep behavior disorder: features, alpha-synuclein, and inflammation. Neurology 84(9):888–894, 2015 25663225

Iranzo A, Santamaría J: Severe obstructive sleep apnea/hypopnea mimicking REM sleep behavior disorder. Sleep 28(2):203–206, 2002 16171244

Irfan M, Howell MJ: Rapid eye movement sleep behavior disorder: overview and current perspective. Curr Sleep Med Rep 2(2):64–73, 2016

Jouvet M, Delorme F: Locus coeruleus et sommeil paradoxal. Comptes Rendus des Séances de la Société de Biologie 159:895–899, 1965

Ju Y-ES: RBD in adults under 50 years old, in Rapid-Eye-Movement Sleep Behavior Disorder. Edited by Schenck CH, Högl B, Videnovic A. Cham, Switzerland, Springer Nature, 2018, pp 201–214

Jun J, Kim R, Byun J, et al: Prolonged-release melatonin in patients with idiopathic REM sleep behavior disorder. Ann Clin Transl Neurol 6(4):716–722, 2019 31560845

Jung Y, St Louis EK: Treatment of REM sleep behavior disorder. Curr Treat Opt Neurol 18(11):50, 2016 27752878

Kunz D, Mahlberg R: A two-part, double-blind, placebo-controlled trial of exogenous melatonin in REM sleep behaviour disorder. J Sleep Res 19(4):591–596, 2010 20561180

Lam SP, Wong CC, Li SX, et al: Caring burden of REM sleep behavior disorder—spouses' health and marital relationship. Sleep Med 24:40–43, 2016 27810184

Li SX, Lam SP, Zhang J, et al: A prospective, naturalistic follow-up study of treatment outcomes with clonazepam in rapid eye movement sleep behavior disorder. Sleep Med 21:114–120, 2016 27448481

Li SX, Lam SP, Zhang J, et al: Instruments for screening, diagnosis and assessment of RBD severity and monitoring treatment outcome, in Rapid-Eye-Movement Sleep Behavior Disorder. Edited by Schenck CH, Högl B, Videnovic A. Cham, Switzerland, Springer Nature, 2018, pp 255–270

Liu Y, Zhang J, Lam SP, et al: A case-control-family study of idiopathic rapid eye movement sleep behavior disorder. Ann Neurol 85(4):582–592, 2019 30761606

Mateo-Montero RC, Pedrera-Mazarro A, Martín-Palomeque G, et al: Clinical and genetical study of a familial form of REM sleep behavior disorder. Clin Neurol Neurosurg 175:130–133, 2018 30419424

McGrane IR, Leung JG, St Louis EK, et al: Melatonin therapy for REM sleep behavior disorder: a critical review of evidence. Sleep Med 16(1):19–26, 2015 25454845

Mysliwiec V, O'Reilly B, Polchinski J, et al: Trauma associated sleep disorder: a proposed parasomnia encompassing disruptive nocturnal behaviors, nightmares, and REM without atonia in trauma survivors. J Clin Sleep Med 10(10):1143–1148, 2014 25317096

Postuma RB, Arnulf I, Hogl B, et al: A single-question screen for rapid eye movement sleep behavior disorder: a multicenter validation study. Mov Disord 27(7):913–916, 2012

Postuma RB, Gagnon JF, Tuineaig M, et al: Antidepressants and REM sleep behavior disorder: isolated side effect or neurodegenerative signal? Sleep 36(11):1579–1585, 2013 24179289

Postuma RB, Iranzo A, Hogl B, et al: Risk factors for neurodegeneration in idiopathic rapid eye movement sleep behavior disorder: a multicenter study. Ann Neurol 77(5):830–839, 2015 25767079

Provini F, Tachibana N: Acute REM sleep behavior disorder, in Rapid-Eye-Movement Sleep Behavior Disorder. Edited by Schenck CH, Högl B, Videnovic A. Cham, Switzerland, Springer Nature, 2018, pp 153–172

Sabater L, Gaig C, Gelpi E, et al: A novel non-rapid-eye movement and rapid-eye-movement parasomnia with sleep disordered breathing associated with antibodies to IgLON5: a case series, characterization of the antigen, and post-mortem study. Lancet Neurol 13:575–586, 2014 24703753

Schenck CH, Mahowald MW: REM sleep behavior disorder: clinical, developmental, and neuroscience perspectives 16 years after its formal identification in SLEEP. Sleep 25(2):120–138, 2002 11902423

Schenck CH, Boyd JL, Mahowald MW: A parasomnia overlap disorder involving sleepwalking, sleep terrors, and REM sleep behavior disorder in 33 polysomnographically confirmed cases. Sleep 20(11):972–981, 1997 9456462

Schenck CH, Lee SA, Cramer Bornemann MA, et al: Potentially lethal behaviors associated with rapid eye movement sleep behavior disorder (RBD): review of the literature and forensic implications. J Forensic Sci 54(6):1475–1484, 2009 19788703

Schenck CH, Högl B, Videnovic A (eds): Rapid-Eye-Movement Sleep Behavior Disorder. Cham, Switzerland, Springer Nature, 2018

Shin C, Park H, Lee WW, et al: Clonazepam for probable REM sleep behavior disorder in Parkinson's disease: a randomized placebo-controlled trial. J Neurol Sci 401:81–86, 2019 31035190

Wu P, Yu H, Peng S, et al: Consistent abnormalities in metabolic network activity in idiopathic rapid eye movement sleep behavior disorder. Brain 137(pt 12):3122–3128, 2014 25338949

CHAPTER 16

Other Parasomnias

NIGHTMARE DISORDER, RECURRENT ISOLATED SLEEP PARALYSIS, SLEEP-RELATED HALLUCINATIONS, EXPLODING HEAD SYNDROME, SLEEP ENURESIS

Joss Cohen, M.D.

Alon Y. Avidan, M.D., M.P.H.

Parasomnias are undesirable sensorimotor or verbal phenomena arising from the sleep-to-wake transition. Parasomnias are fairly heterogeneous, ranging from sensory phenomena to abnormal emotions and autonomic activity to complex and sometimes aggressive motor activity (Broughton 1998). They exemplify a sleep-stage admixture in which the intrusion of one sleep state into another results in an abnormal behaviors (Mahowald et al. 2004). Parasomnias are typically explainable, diagnosable, and treatable (Broughton 1998; Mahowald et al. 2004). They may occur in response to internal factors such as sleep-disordered breathing, an agent that induces CNS depression, fever, or external stimuli. The *International Classification of Sleep Disorders*, 3rd Edition (ICSD-3; American Academy of Sleep Medicine 2014), classifies parasomnias based on the sleep stage in which they occur: disorders of arousal, which are associated with non-REM (NREM) sleep; parasomnias, usually associated with REM sleep; and other parasomnias.

This chapter covers two REM parasomnias, REM nightmare and recurrent isolated sleep paralysis (RISP), as well as three conditions classified as "other parasomnias": sleep-related hallucinations (SRH), exploding head syndrome (EHS), and sleep enuresis. These conditions are grouped in this chapter because they share an abnormal behavioral manifestation during sleep or the wake-to-sleep transition as a fundamental feature. Each condition is defined and its epidemiology, underlying pathophysiology, and clinical presentation are highlighted, as are diagnostic and management approaches. NREM parasomnias (disorders of arousal) and REM sleep behavior disorder (RBD) are covered in Chapters 14 and 15, respectively.

Nightmare Disorder

DIAGNOSTIC CRITERIA

Nightmares are a universal phenomenon of REM sleep commonly experienced during childhood and throughout adulthood, often related to anxiety, stress, and trauma. A *nightmare* is typically defined as a vivid and frightening dream sequence that awakens the dreamer, with generally good immediate recall of the dream content eliciting a dysphoric emotional response that usually, but not necessarily, involves fear. The person is immediately and fully alert upon awakening. ICSD-3 classifies nightmares as a disorder when recurrent episodes are frequent enough to impair emotional or physical well-being in domains relating to sleep, mood, cognition, family, behavior, daytime sleepiness, fatigue, and occupational or social functioning (American Academy of Sleep Medicine 2014). Common causes include stress, negative life events, and depression. Nightmares may be encountered following use of benzodiazepines, dopamine agonists, or antihypertensives (β-blockers); in the setting of rapid withdrawal from REM sleep-suppressing medications, such as selective serotonin reuptake inhibitors (SSRIs); and following alcohol ingestion or sudden withdrawal from barbiturates, in which case they are classified as "secondary nightmares."

PATHOPHYSIOLOGY

Although the attribution of nightmares as comorbid with various pathological states implies they are symptomatic, the ubiquity of the phenomenon may suggest a functional purpose as an "adaptive modification of emotional response over time" (Nielsen and Carr 2017). The exact explanation for nightmares is not well understood, but current theories include emotional memory regulation and consolidation, fear extinction, and threat simulation, although opinion remains divided given limited and controversial evidence. Physically stressed animals demonstrate heightened activation within the secondary somatosensory and primary auditory cortices and the amygdala (Yu et al. 2015).

Nightmares are believed to be a dreaming disturbance that involves a perturbation of emotional expression typically arising during REM sleep, although they may occur in NREM sleep (Fisher et al. 1968). They occur more frequently in the latter third of the night, which is when REM sleep predominates, but may occur earlier during sleep when associated with PTSD. Patients with frequent nightmares exhibit an electroencephalographic pattern of alpha-frequency oscillations. This represents more propensity toward wakefulness, with high alpha activity during REM sleep and low alpha activity during NREM sleep when compared with control subjects, reflective of sleep instability (Simor et al. 2013). Other studies have shown enhanced arousal during sleep supported by elevated sympathetic activation (Nielsen et al. 2010) and an increase in periodic leg movements in both REM and NREM sleep seen in both those with PTSD and those with idiopathic forms of nightmares (Germain and Nielsen 2003). Smaller studies on idiopathic nightmares reported more global sleep disturbances, such as decreased total sleep time, increased number of nocturnal awakenings, and increased or unchanged REM sleep, as well as decreased slow-wave sleep (Newell et al. 1992).

EPIDEMIOLOGY

Nightmares are normal phenomena that occur in up to half of children, beginning at ages 3–5 years but decreasing in frequency with maturation. Recurring nightmares (more than one per week) are rare (<1%) but have a strong association with various psychiatric conditions including PTSD, borderline personality disorder, schizophrenia, stress, anxiety, and substance abuse. Special attention must be given to patients with PTSD, because nightmares are highly prevalent in this population at a rate of around 60% (Roth et al. 1997).

Although the specific lifetime prevalence for a nightmare experience is unknown, the condition is a universal feature of human sleep. The prevalence of recurrent nightmares varies between 3% per week and 10% per month (Hublin et al. 1999; Spoormaker et al. 2006). A large cross-sectional study (consisting of 69,813 Finnish participants) reported a predominance of nightmares in young women that narrowed between the sexes after the age of 60 years (Sandman et al. 2013). Sex difference may be attributed to a higher dream recall frequency in women but does not explain why men report more nightmares as they age.

CLINICAL FEATURES

Dream content is generally vivid and involves threats to survival, security, or self-esteem. Common themes include being chased by another person, accidents, physical aggression, risk of failure, and helplessness. Upon awakening, the dream is remembered and may be associated with feelings of fear, sadness, anger, or anxiety. A nightmare as a "disorder" requires quality-of-life impairment in at least one of the following domains: sleep, mood, cognition, behavior, daytime sleepiness, fatigue, occupational or social functioning, or caregiver or family functioning. The consequences of recurring nightmares include sleep avoidance and deprivation, which in turn increase the intensity and frequency of nightmares. They may also exacerbate underlying psychiatric disorders.

DIAGNOSIS

Nightmare disorder is a clinical diagnosis based on history taking but requires that ICSD-3 criteria be met. Components of the clinical history should include a description of the nightmares (including frequency, duration, and severity), assessment of sleep quality and quantity, and adverse consequences on sleep and daytime function. When clinically appropriate, care should be taken to assess for history of a stressful or traumatic life event (PTSD), depression, and use of or rapid withdrawal from any pharmacological agent or substances temporally related to the nightmares. A diagnostic nocturnal polysomnogram is not required but may be indicated if the clinician suspects an underlying history of sleep apnea that might trigger episodes and when differentiation from RBD is essential (see Chapters 8 and 15).

DIFFERENTIAL DIAGNOSIS

Nightmares should be differentiated from sleep terrors. Although both awaken the patient from sleep, the latter usually arises from NREM slow-wave sleep, with amnesia for the event, and is accompanied by screams, heightened sympathetic activity, relative confusion, and disorientation following the event. Nightmares should also be distinguished from "bad dreams," which do not awaken the sleeper. If the nightmares are associated with motor activity, including dream enactment behavior, then the clinician may consider RBD or sleep-related epilepsy as well as sleep terrors. Nightmares should also be differentiated from brief hallucinatory experiences at sleep onset (hypnagogic hallucinations) or sleep offset (hypnopompic hallucinations), which are typical in narcolepsy and sleep deprivation.

Nightmares are common in patients with PTSD and represent a cardinal feature of the disorder along with symptoms such as flashbacks, hypervigilance, and intrusive thoughts. The underlying traumas experienced may include war and combat, mass conflict and displacement, severe medical illnesses or injuries, or sexual violence (Koffel et al. 2016; Mohsenin and Mohsenin 2014). One important distinction, however, is that dream experiences in PTSD occur not only during REM sleep but also at sleep onset, contributing to significant insomnia.

TREATMENT

Management of nightmare disorder includes the use of medications and behavioral therapies. Most studies evaluating the efficacy of medications were conducted in patients with PTSD, so their effectiveness in idiopathic nightmares is unknown. Several medications are aimed at reducing CNS adrenergic activity, which is hypothesized to be an underlying mechanism. As discussed earlier, numerous other drugs may induce nightmares and vivid dreams in the absence of CNS activation, such as SSRIs, serotonin-norepinephrine reuptake inhibitors, β-blockers, barbiturates, dopaminergic agents, macrolide antibiotics, and alcohol (Proserpio et al. 2018).

At this writing, a level A ("strong") recommendation exists for prazosin, a generally well-tolerated centrally acting α_1 antagonist that has been shown to reduce trauma-related nightmares. Treatment should last 3–9 weeks, and patients should be screened for relapse if the medication is discontinued (Aurora et al. 2010). However, this recommendation may change because a recent large, multicenter randomized trial failed to show benefit of prazosin over placebo in reducing the frequency or intensity of PTSD-related nightmares (Raskind et al. 2018). Clonidine, an α_2 agonist, has a therapeutic rationale similar to prazosin but a less robust level of evidence for recommendation (level C, an "option"). Clonidine is reported to increase REM sleep and decrease NREM sleep at low doses but to decrease REM sleep and increase N2 sleep at higher doses. The presumed activity at low doses is believed to exist at the level of the locus coeruleus norepinephrine neurons presynaptically, reducing the release of norepinephrine, while medium-dose clonidine acts more postsynaptically (Miyazaki et al. 2004).

Other medications to consider that have low-grade or sparse data include trazodone, atypical antipsychotics, topiramate, low-dose cortisol, fluvoxamine, triazolam, nitrazepam, phenelzine, gabapentin, cyproheptadine, and tricyclic antidepressants (TCAs). Synthetic cannabinoids have been shown to reduce the frequency and intensity of nightmares with improved sleep quality when used in an "add-on" fashion in those with PTSD (Fraser 2009). Combination of these medications may be required for treatment of patients with more refractory illness, giving careful consideration to treatment-emergent side effects.

Nonpharmacological treatment options include cognitive-behavioral therapy, which encompasses a broad range of techniques such as image rehearsal therapy, lucid dreaming, and systemic desensitization. Image rehearsal therapy may be delivered at successive sessions individually or in groups. The initial sessions target nightmares as a learned behavior:

patients are asked to focus on recognizing the impact of nightmares on sleep and how nightmares promote learned (conditioned) insomnia. Subsequent sessions engage the patient in the human imagery system: appreciating the connections between daytime imagery and dreams. Patients are asked to identify a nightmare, change the nightmare into a new dream, and rehearse the new dream while generating pleasant images (Krakow and Zadra 2006). Other nonpharmacological therapies include progressive deep muscle relaxation for idiopathic nightmares and hypnosis and eye movement desensitization and reprocessing for PTSD-associated nightmares (Aurora et al. 2010).

Recurrent Isolated Sleep Paralysis

DIAGNOSTIC CRITERIA

Sleep paralysis is a rather peculiar phenomenon that arises during transitions between sleep and wakefulness in which an individual lays in bed fully conscious but paralyzed—with loss of most skeletal muscle control but retaining diaphragmatic function and eye movements—creating a level of severe anxiety. Sleep paralysis occurs with high frequency in narcolepsy; however, it can occur in the absence of narcolepsy and is in this case considered isolated. According to the ICSD-3 criteria, RISP consists of multiple episodes of isolated sleep paralysis that are associated with clinically significant distress; no specific frequency or clinical impairment thresholds have been stated (American Academy of Sleep Medicine 2014). Sleep paralysis can also be associated with other sleep disorders, such as narcolepsy, but would no longer be defined as isolated. The cause of this often-frightening experience is presumed to be a dissociation of REM-associated muscle atonia from sleep into the waking state. Episodes typically last only seconds to minutes and are often associated with preservation of multisensory dream activity in the patient, who is temporarily conscious but paralyzed.

EPIDEMIOLOGY

Isolated sleep paralysis is surprisingly common. It is suspected that approximately 7.6% of the general population has experienced at least one episode during their lifetime, with higher rates of approximately 30% in students and psychiatric patients (Sharpless and Barber 2011). Determining precise rates of RISP is difficult, because it is not routinely assessed in clinical practice.

PATHOPHYSIOLOGY

RISP is thought to be caused by a dissociation of REM-based atonia from sleep into the waking state. It has occurred in non-narcoleptic cases in the context of significant sleep deprivation/restriction, sleep interruptions, or substance use disorder as well as in untreated obstructive sleep apnea. Stress and social anxiety may be indirectly associated with sleep paralysis via poor sleep habits or a propensity toward hypervigilance during sleep (Takeuchi et al. 2002). Sleeping in the supine position tends to increase risk of sleep paralysis (Cheyne 2002), and RISP has a slight preponderance in females and nonwhite individuals (Sharpless 2016). Familial forms of isolated sleep paralysis have been reported (Roth et al. 1968).

CLINICAL FEATURES

Uninformed patients may initially describe the loss of voluntary bodily control and dream activity into the waking state and attempt to explain these, occasionally attributing them to supernatural forces or to alien abduction. Sleep paralysis is usually, but not necessarily, accompanied by vivid, often unpleasant auditory or visual hypnagogic hallucinations. The skeletal muscles that control extraocular movements and the diaphragm are preserved; however, patients may describe sensations of choking, suffocating, or an excessive weight being placed on their chest, likely reflective of the sensation associated with the REM-related atonia of accessory muscles of respiration. The episodes are harmless in themselves and last from seconds to minutes but can be quite distressing given the bizarre and frightening quality of the hallucinations in the setting of paralysis. Common associated sensory phenomena described usually fall into three distinct categories (Cheyne 2002): incubus experiences involving the aforementioned sensation of breathing difficulties or choking; intruder experiences often involving a threatening visual, auditory, or tactile presence (e.g., a shadowy demonic creature lurking in the corner of the room, sounds of whispering or buzzing); and spatial, temporal, and orientational experiences that include out-of-body experiences or feelings of floating, flying, or being dragged out of bed.

DIAGNOSIS

The diagnosis of RISP is based on the clinical history rather than any formal polysomnography. The ICSD-3 criteria do not specify frequency of episodes but require multiple episodes associated with clinically significant distress. Distress can take the form of catastrophic worrying about the implications of these episodes, avoidance behaviors, and other neg-ative sequelae such as daytime sleepiness or embarrassment.

DIFFERENTIAL DIAGNOSIS

Other competing diagnoses should be ruled out, such as focal or atonic seizures, periodic hyper- or hypokalemic paralysis, dissociative states, and psychotic disorders. Careful attention should be paid to discerning RISP from narcolepsy, because sleep paralysis is also a core feature of the latter. The presence of hypersomnolence in the absence of sleep depriva-tion and symptoms of cataplexy may also indicate narcolepsy. Polysom-nography can be used if diagnostic uncertainty remains.

MANAGEMENT

Management is usually patient education and reassurance, because most patients do not experience clinically significant distress. Sleep depriva-tion must be corrected, as should other attributes relating to inadequate sleep hygiene or considerable stress at bedtime. One may also consider the use of focused-attention meditation combined with muscle relax-ation therapy (Jalal 2016, 2017; Sharpless and Doghramji 2017). How-ever, if the patient and clinician believe the benefits of pharmacological treatment outweigh the risks, then TCAs (clomipramine, imipramine, desmethylimipramine) and SSRIs (fluoxetine, femoxetine, and vilox-azine) may be considered. The mechanism of action of these medications is hypothesized to be related to suppression of REM sleep (Snyder and Hams 1982). Sodium oxybate has been shown to reduce sleep paralysis in narcolepsy but has not been tested or approved in the setting of RISP. Well-established data for medical management are considerably lacking, and most of the existing data are based on isolated case studies or extrap-olated from narcolepsy.

Sleep-Related Hallucinations

DIAGNOSTIC CRITERIA

Hallucinations are perceived sensory phenomena that arise from the mind itself without an objective correlate in the real world. SRH occur around sleep and are classified as hypnagogic if they occur just prior to sleep on-set and hypnopompic if they occur immediately upon awakening, with the experience typically lasting a few seconds. The perceived sensations are predominantly visual but may also include auditory or tactile hallu-cinations. Diagnosis by ICSD-3 criteria requires that the hallucinations not otherwise be explained by an alternative sleep disorder, mental disorder, medication-related side effect, or substance use (American Academy of Sleep Medicine 2014). Another distinct entity of hallucinations, complex nocturnal visual hallucinations (CNVH), involves intricate and vivid visual hallucinations that occur at night surrounding sleep onset or awakening. These hallucinations generally persist longer, up to several minutes, and disappear once ambient light is increased.

PATHOPHYSIOLOGY

The exact pathophysiology of SRH is unknown, but it is believed to be due to an intrusion of REM-sleep dream activity into wakefulness. An alternative theory implicates a mechanism involving a cortical release phenomenon that may occur in the setting of decreased input from the ascending reticular activating system. Polysomnographic data for CNVH are limited; however, one small study found that the hallucinations all arose from NREM sleep (Silber et al. 2005).

EPIDEMIOLOGY

SRH are highly prevalent in the general population. According to two large telephone survey studies, hypnagogic hallucinations are more common than hypnopompic hallucinations (25%–37% vs. 6%–12.5%) in the general population, without relation to a specific pathology (i.e., mental disorder) in more than half the cases (Ohayon 2000; Ohayon et al. 1996). The prevalence of hallucinations occurring on at least a weekly basis is 1.8% and 0.8% for hypnagogic and hypnopompic hallucinations, respectively; however, this increases to 18% and 4.6%, respectively, at the rate of less than once per month. They tend to occur more frequently in the young (ages 15–44) and in women. Risk factors include the presence of coexisting sleep disorders (e.g., insomnia, excessive daytime sleepiness, narcolepsy), CNS drug use (especially sedative-hypnotics), alcohol use, and psychiatric disorders (anxiety and mood disorders).

CNVH may occur in association with a range of neurological disorders, such as ophthalmological conditions (e.g., macular degeneration) or neurodegenerative diseases (particularly the α-synucleinopathies [Parkinson's disease, dementia with Lewy bodies]), or it may occur idiopathically. The prevalence of CNVH is unknown but is probably rare. No familial or genetic patterns have been identified (Ohayon et al. 1996).

CLINICAL FEATURES

Hallucinations can take virtually any form—visual, auditory, tactile, kinetic, and olfactory. Visual hallucinations can range from seeing spots of light to seeing complex images, including human figures and animals. Examples of auditory hallucinations include hearing one's name being called, neologisms, a doorbell ringing, and both sensical and nonsensical sentences. Other commonly reported hallucinatory phenomena include the sensation of falling in space or of being attacked. Often, the hallucination may be a component of other parasomnias, such as auditory perceptions associated with EHS (discussed later) or ominous shadowy presences experienced in sleep paralysis. The nature of the hallucinations in CNVH is similar, with imagery that is usually more vivid, multicolor, or distorted. Patients may retain insight into the fact that they are hallucinating in CNVH but lack insight in SRH. Both variants of hallucination will usually disappear once ambient light is increased; however, CNVH may persist for several minutes and in rare circumstances up to 1 hour (Silber et al. 2005). The content of these perceptions is often frightening and distressing.

DIAGNOSIS

Diagnosis of SRH is mainly through clinical history. A detailed past medical, neurological, and psychiatric history should be obtained. Polysomnography and multiple sleep latency tests are not necessary but may be helpful if narcolepsy is suspected. If substance use is suspected, a toxicology screen may be helpful. Electroencephalography may be obtained if a history of seizure is suspected. Appropriate neuroimaging may be helpful for evaluating spells in the context of diagnosing other neurological causes of hallucinations.

DIFFERENTIAL DIAGNOSIS

The diagnosis of SRH by ICSD-3 criteria requires the disturbance not be better explained by another sleep disorder. The following are disorders that may be considered by the clinician in the context of the patient's history and likely comorbidities (Mahowald et al. 1998).

Narcolepsy

Narcolepsy is known to be associated with both hypnagogic and hypnopompic hallucinations, especially in type 1 narcolepsy (see Chapter 6).

Charles-Bonnet Syndrome

Charles-Bonnet syndrome involves visual hallucinations in those who have lost vision. It is thought to be a cortical release phenomenon that occurs in the absence of external visual stimuli (Coltheart 2018).

Neurodegenerative Disorders

Neurodegenerative disorders are associated with sleep disturbances. The α-synucleinopathies (Parkinson's disease and Lewy body dementia) may cause hallucinations due to side effects of medications (dopaminergic or anticholinergic drugs) or deposition of Lewy bodies in brain stem formations that regulate the sleep-wake transition and neocortical structures. Patients with parkinsonism can also develop RBD with dream enactment during sleep but often have no recollection of this. Patients with Alzheimer's disease or other related dementias may also develop hallucinatory behavior as evidenced by the phenomenon of "sundowning," defined as a state characterized by restlessness, confusion, anxiety, and disorientation late in the day, often as the sun sets.

Peduncular Hallucinosis

Peduncular hallucinosis involves waking hallucinations that occur in the setting of brain stem, thalamic, and hypothalamic lesions and can last a few minutes to several hours.

Epilepsy

Epilepsy can produce a wide array of hallucinatory phenomena that manifest with sleep. The hallucinations are usually brief but are likely stereotyped and may be associated with an altered state of consciousness.

Migraine With Aura

Migraine with aura can manifest predominantly in the form a peripheral scotoma; however, this can usually be distinguished from SRH by the association of headache. The aura may consist of nonvisual sensory modalities.

Drug-Induced Hallucinations

Hallucinations may be caused by use of sedative-hypnotics, β-blockers, amiodarone, ergot derivatives, alcohol, and recreational drugs (e.g., lysergic acid diethylamide [LSD], mescaline).

Nightmares

Nightmares can also involve frightening auditory and visual content, but they do not protrude into wakefulness, and the dreamer will retain insight.

MANAGEMENT

Little evidence has been found for specific treatment interventions. Reassurance and education may be all that is required for termination of episodes in otherwise healthy individuals. Treatment should be directed at managing any associated underlying disorders (e.g., epilepsy, migraines, narcolepsy). Withdrawal of potentially offending medication (such as β-blockers) may be helpful. Some clinicians have had success using melatonin for complex nocturnal visual hallucinations (Lysenko and Bhat 2018).

Exploding Head Syndrome

DIAGNOSTIC CRITERIA

EHS is characterized by the painless perception of a sudden loud noise in the head during any stage of sleep, followed by an immediate arousal with a sense of fright (American Academy of Sleep Medicine 2014).

PATHOPHYSIOLOGY

The mechanism underlying EHS is unknown; however, the most popular theory is that it is a sensory variant of sleep starts or hypnic jerks (see Chapter 18) that manifest during the wake-to-sleep transition (American Academy of Sleep Medicine 2014). As the brain stem reticular formation switches off high cortical functions around sleep onset, a desynchrony is presumed to arise, resulting in a burst of neuronal activity to cerebral hemispheres that causes the perceived sensation (Sharpless 2014). Furthermore, polysomnographic evidence supports the observation that this particular auditory phenomenon is a separate entity from hypnagogic phenomena because those events have only been observed to occur in the awake and relaxed state (Sachs and Svanborg 1991).

EPIDEMIOLOGY

The prevalence of EHS is unknown. It generally occurs in patients older than 50 years, and no risk factors have been identified. Some clinicians have noted increased attacks associated with personal stress (Pearce 1989). EHS has been reported to occur within the same family, but evidence supporting a truly familial pattern is insufficient.

CLINICAL PRESENTATION

In EHS, the noise perceived is brief, lasting only seconds, and may be described in various ways beyond an explosion, such as a snap, door slam, fireworks, cymbals, crash of lightning, or electric shocks (Pearce 1989). A simultaneous flash of light and a myoclonic jerk may be associated with the sound. The frequency of the attacks is variable, occurring from only sporadically over the course of months to multiple times a week, with several episodes during the course of a night. The patient may initially believe the sensation is painful, but upon further investigation will admit the absence of pain. The episode is benign but can induce panic with momentary tachycardia and palpitations. In most cases the syndrome resolves spontaneously.

DIAGNOSIS

Diagnosis is based on clinical history. Polysomnography is not required but in a small sample of patients revealed a sleep-stage-predominant alpha rhythm suggestive of sleep-state instability with interspersed theta activity but no epileptic abnormalities (Sachs and Svanborg 1991). Interestingly, although patients may report being awakened from sleep, data demonstrate that the patients were actually awake when the episodes occurred, which may highlight the propensity toward sleep-state misperception. Some patients with EHS undergo needless neuroimaging and lumbar puncture because clinicians often incorrectly fixate on the "snapping" sensation out of concern for a vascular event (e.g., subarachnoid hemorrhage, reversible cerebral vasoconstriction syndrome).

DIFFERENTIAL DIAGNOSIS

EHS should be distinguished from other headache disorders. Hypnic headaches, sleep-related migraines, cluster headaches, and nocturnal paroxysmal hemicrania can all occur at night and awaken the patient from sleep; however, these are readily differentiated from EHS by the presence of pain, longer duration of symptoms (minutes to hours rather seconds), and other clinical manifestations common in migraine phenomena (e.g., nausea, autonomic symptoms). Primary stabbing headache ("ice pick" headache) is characterized by brief transient painful stabs to the head that may occur at sleep onset but more often occur during wakefulness. A thunderclap headache, which also has a sudden onset, can indicate a subarachnoid hemorrhage; however, this is usually painful and does not usually occur during sleep onset. Those with nightmare disorder may report hearing loud noises during sleep, but these episodes are differentiated by their association with more complex dream content, which is lacking with EHS. Sleep starts occur during the wake-to-sleep transition but have a myoclonic motor pattern and are devoid of sensory symptoms. Lastly, simple partial seizures in the setting of sleep-related epilepsy should be considered, but these are stereotyped and more frequent.

MANAGEMENT

The treatment of EHS is based on several cases studies that have shown TCAs (clomipramine) to be helpful (Sachs and Svanborg 1991). Additional agents that may be effective include the calcium channel blockers (slow-release nifedipine) and carbamazepine (Jacome 2001). Topiramate reduced the intensity of the auditory component but did not impact the frequency (Palikh and Vaughn 2010). Counseling is the mainstay of treatment because reassurance about the benign nature of the phenomenon leads to remission in most cases.

Sleep Enuresis

DIAGNOSTIC CRITERIA

Sleep or nocturnal enuresis, colloquially known as "bedwetting," is a heterogeneous disorder involving involuntary voiding during sleep. It is clinically significant due to the detrimental psychosocial effects. The disorder is common among children and tends to wane into adulthood as one's neurobehavioral and micturition systems mature. Treatment modalities are tailored to behavioral modifications as opposed to the use of medications. Enuresis is differentiated as primary sleep enuresis (PSE) if the patient has never been consistently dry and as secondary sleep enuresis (SSE) if the patient was previously dry for ≥6 months (Wolfish 2002). Clinically, SSE does not differ significantly from PSE and is thought to be due to a maturational lag but may also be associated with another disease process. To meet the diagnostic criteria as defined by ICSD-3 (American Academy of Sleep Medicine 2014), the patient must be older than 5 years of age and experience at least two involuntary voiding episodes during sleep per week, persisting for ≥3 months.

PATHOPHYSIOLOGY

Several theories have been proposed to explain the mechanism behind sleep enuresis, and this is dependent on the form of enuresis. The basic principle has three essential components: 1) failure of conscious arousal to a full bladder that results from 2) a mismatch between nocturnal urine production and 3) anomalous or insufficient bladder capacity (Wolfish 2002). Any condition that affects one or more of these components can result in sleep enuresis.

Likely mechanisms contributing to PSE include elevated arousal thresholds or uninhibited bladder contributions, which is theorized to be partly due to brain stem dysfunction (Ornitz et al. 1999). Additionally, some patients may have an anomalous circadian rhythm–mediated secretion of antidiuretic hormone or other hormones that leads to an overproduction of urine (Yeung 2003).

SSE may be caused by a variety of disease processes or substances. Any factor that increases urine production or decreases the ability of the kidneys to concentrate urine, such as diabetes insipidus, diabetes mellitus, sickle cell disease, hyperthyroidism, diuretics, and caffeine, may induce enuresis. Nocturnal enuresis may also be induced by obstructive sleep apnea (see Chapters 8 and 9), especially in the pediatric population, through increased secretion of atrial natriuretic peptide as an evoked response to raised intrathoracic pressure combined with an increased arousal threshold (Umlauf and Chasens 2003). Other inciting disorders to consider include pathology of the urinary tract (e.g., urinary tract infections and congenital abnormalities), encopresis (fecal incontinence or soiling), seizures, neurogenic bladder, and psychosocial stressors (e.g., sexual abuse, neglect, and parental divorce).

EPIDEMIOLOGY

Until about age 18 months, voiding is a spinal reflex that occurs automatically. Between ages 18 months and 3 years, children become able to control voiding during the day, progressing to gradual control of voiding during sleep as developmental maturation continues. A somewhat arbitrary cutoff age of 5 years is set as a criterion for PSE, with a spontaneous resolution rate of about 15% per year (Forsythe and Redmond 1974). According to a questionnaire-based survey (Yeung et al. 2006), the approximate prevalence of PSE is 16% at 5 years of age, 3% at 9 years of age, and 2.2% at 19 years of age, as opposed to SSE, which can manifest at any age. This study demonstrated male predilection and a concurrent daytime incontinence in 20%. Although the prevalence of PSE decreases with age, the severity worsens, with nightly bedwetting occurring in 48% of adolescents (age 19) with the disorder compared with 14% of children (age 5). A follow-up study of patients 40 years of age or younger showed that the prevalence remained static at roughly 2% after age 10, with half of those experiencing symptoms at least three times per week and 25% experiencing symptoms nightly (Yeung et al. 2004).

A hereditary component is suspected to play a role in PSE, with an autosomal dominant pattern of inheritance and high penetrance; however, environmental factors have a major modulatory effect (von Gontard et al. 2001).

Parents of children with PSE have noted that their children are fairly "heavy" sleepers, which is further corroborated by polysomnographic data that show a high incidence of associated periodic limb movements. This leads some to implicate an impaired arousal system (Dhondt et al. 2009; Nevéus et al. 1999). A proposed model for the maintenance of nocturnal enuresis is that children who wet their beds have more nighttime awakenings as a result, leading to sleep deprivation and subsequently to increased arousal threshold, which in turn leads to a failure to respond to signals from a full bladder and enuresis (Cohen-Zrubavel et al. 2011).

The primary complication of PSE is impaired self-esteem, which may impact a child's normal activities and can evolve into anxiety or depression that extends to other family members, especially if it is not mediated by the parents or primary caregiver. Adverse effects have been shown to resolve once the child becomes dry, indicating that the psychological issues are more likely a result of the disorder rather than a cause (Hägglöf et al. 1997).

DIAGNOSIS

Clinicians must distinguish between PSE and SSE. The mainstay of evaluation consists of reviewing the patient's clinical history, including fluid intake and voiding diary (frequency and timing of episodes). Care should be taken to gather a thorough medical, psychological, and social history.

Workup for secondary etiologies is tailored to each case at the discretion of the clinician. Routine laboratory tests to consider include—but are not limited to—a basic metabolic panel, complete blood count, urinalysis, urine solutes, and thyroid studies evaluating for hyperthyroidism. Urological imaging should be considered if the patient has daytime episodes, which may indicate an anatomical anomaly. Neuroimaging (brain and spine) can be useful if other focal neurological abnormalities are found on examination. Polysomnography is indicated if comorbid sleep disorders are suspected, especially sleep-disordered breathing. Referral to subspecialty clinics (i.e., neurology, endocrinology, nephrology, urology, psychiatry) should be considered if a high suspicion remains for secondary enuresis.

MANAGEMENT

PSE almost always resolves spontaneously over time, and treatment should be delayed until a child is able to participate in a program. Behavioral therapy is the first-line treatment and includes several strategies, including use of an enuresis alarm that wakes the child in response to a wet bed as well as biofeedback, bladder training, dry-bed training, and motivational therapy (Ramakrishnan 2008). Other lifestyle modifications include refraining from drinking large volumes of fluid prior to bed, emptying the bladder prior to sleep, and eating a low-sodium diet. It may take up to 6–8 weeks for these therapies to demonstrate efficacy.

Pharmacological therapy is rarely indicated in children younger than 7 years of age and should be used only if behavioral therapies have failed and enuresis continues to be distressing. One medication option is vasopressin (also called antidiuretic hormone), which has had favorable response rates of >60% (defined as >50% reduction in wet nights); however, relapse is common upon cessation (Hjälmås et al. 1998). Vasopressin is generally well tolerated, but hyponatremia can result if the patient is simultaneously drinking large volumes of water. Other medication options include antimuscarinic agents, such as oxybutynin, and TCAs, such as imipramine; however, these carry adverse side effect profiles such as dry mouth, blurry vision, and grogginess that may not be tolerated. When selecting a treatment modality, the clinician should remember that spontaneous resolution will occur in about 15% of patients annually.

Treatment of SSE entails addressing the underlying pathology—disimpaction for constipation, blood glucose control for diabetes, and psychotherapy if psychogenically induced. If obstructive sleep apnea is suspected, surgical correction of the airway obstruction may be considered. If a reduction in nocturnal bladder capacity is suspected, as indicated by episodes of daytime incontinence, then bladder dysfunction is "almost invariably" the most common etiology and will likely improve with anticholinergics in addition to behavioral therapies (Yeung 2003).

Conclusion

Recent neurophysiological data support the notion that parasomnias represent intermediate states of dissociation between wakefulness, REM sleep, and NREM sleep and are characterized by dysfunctional arousal. Patients may simultaneously retain elements of dream mentation such as hallucinations and motor paralysis while awake, leading to severe anxiety. Differentiation of NREM from REM parasomnias, sleep-related epilepsy, and sleep-related movement disorders is occasionally challenging. Diagnostic workup focuses on careful evaluation of presentation, timing, duration, clinical semiology, and associated features; polysomnography also may help shed light on conditions that may contribute to sleep instability. Management is typically focused on patient education, improvement of sleep duration, cognitive restructuring, and relaxation techniques. Treatment may occasionally also include CNS-acting medications in severe or refractory cases.

KEY CLINICAL POINTS

- Nightmares are common, particularly in children, but may be related to certain medications and substances, stress, and anxiety in adult patients.

- Polysomnography is rarely indicated to confirm the diagnosis but may be useful when a primary sleep disorder is suspected, such as REM sleep behavior disorder or obstructive sleep apnea.

- Cognitive-behavioral therapy, relaxation techniques, and lifestyle modifications tend to improve the frequency and severity of nightmares. Nightmares often improve with successful treatment of the primary psychiatric disorder (e.g., anxiety, depression, PTSD).

- Complex nocturnal visual hallucinations are rare but may be encountered in the setting of narcolepsy, Parkinson's disease, or Lewy body dementia and with certain medications, such as β-blockers.

- Exploding head syndrome should be differentiated from migraine headache syndromes, cluster headache, thunderclap headaches, hypnic headaches, and nocturnal seizures.

- Recurrent isolated sleep paralysis is characterized by persistence of REM sleep–related muscle atonia into wakefulness. Episodes may be accompanied by an intense sense of impending doom, a sensation of difficult breathing, or an urgency to flee.

- Difficulty arousing from sleep is an important factor in primary enuresis, whereas bladder overactivity is more important in secondary enuresis.

References

American Academy of Sleep Medicine: International Classification of Sleep Disorders, 3rd Edition. Darien, IL, American Academy of Sleep Medicine, 2014

Aurora RN, Zak RS, Auerbach SH, et al: Best practice guide for the treatment of nightmare disorder in adults. J Clin Sleep Med 6(4):389–401, 2010 20726290

Broughton R: Behavioral Parasomnias. Boston, MA, Butterworth-Heinemann, 1998

Cheyne JA: Situational factors affecting sleep paralysis and associated hallucinations: position and timing effects. J Sleep Res 11(2):169–177, 2002

Cohen-Zrubavel V, Kushnir B, Kushnir J, et al: Sleep and sleepiness in children with nocturnal enuresis. Sleep (Basel) 34(2):191–194, 2011 21286252

Coltheart M: Charles Bonnet syndrome: cortical hyperexcitability and visual hallucination. Curr Biol 28(21):R1253–R1254, 2018 30399348

Dhondt K, Raes A, Hoebeke P, et al: Abnormal sleep architecture and refractory nocturnal enuresis. J Urol 182(4 suppl):1961–1965, 2009 19695632

Fisher C, Byrne JV, Edwards A: NREM and REM nightmares. Psychophysiology 5(2): 221–222, 1968

Forsythe WI, Redmond A: Enuresis and spontaneous cure rate. Study of 1129 enuretis. Arch Dis Child 49(4):259–263, 1974 4830115

Fraser GA: The use of a synthetic cannabinoid in the management of treatment-resistant nightmares in posttraumatic stress disorder (PTSD). CNS Neurosci Ther 15(1):84–88, 2009 19228182

Germain A, Nielsen TA: Sleep pathophysiology in posttraumatic stress disorder and idiopathic nightmare sufferers. Biol Psychiatry 54(10):1092–1098, 2003 14625152

Hägglöf B, Andrén O, Bergström E, et al: Self-esteem before and after treatment in children with nocturnal enuresis and urinary incontinence. Scand J Urol Nephrol Suppl 183:79–82, 1997 9165615

Hjälmås K, Hanson E, Hellström AL, et al: Long-term treatment with desmopressin in children with primary monosymptomatic nocturnal enuresis: an open multicentre study. Br J Urol 82(5):704–709, 1998 9839587

Hublin C, Kaprio J, Partinen M, et al: Nightmares: familial aggregation and association with psychiatric disorders in a nationwide twin cohort. Am J Med Genet 88(4):329–336, 1999 10402498

Jacome DE: Exploding head syndrome and idiopathic stabbing headache relieved by nifedipine. Cephalalgia 21(5):617–618, 2001 11472389

Jalal B: How to make the ghosts in my bedroom disappear? Focused-attention meditation combined with muscle relaxation (MR therapy)-a direct treatment intervention for sleep paralysis. Front Psychol 7:28, 2016 26858675

Jalal B: Response: commentary: how to make the ghosts in my bedroom disappear? Focused-attention meditation combined with muscle relaxation (MR therapy): a direct treatment intervention for sleep paralysis. Front Psychol 8:760, 2017 28559867

Koffel E, Khawaja IS, Germain A: Sleep disturbances in posttraumatic stress disorder: updated review and implications for treatment. Psychiatr Ann 46(3):173–176, 2016 27773950

Krakow B, Zadra A: Clinical management of chronic nightmares: imagery rehearsal therapy. Behav Sleep Med 4(1):45–70, 2006 16390284

Lysenko L, Bhat S: Melatonin-responsive complex nocturnal visual hallucinations. J Clin Sleep Med 14(4):687–691, 2018 29609711

Mahowald MW, Woods SR, Schenck CH: Sleeping dreams, waking hallucinations, and the central nervous system. Dreaming 8(2):89–102, 1998

Mahowald MW, Bornemann MC, Schenck CH: Parasomnias. Semin Neurol 24(3):283–292, 2004 15449221

Miyazaki S, Uchida S, Mukai J, et al: Clonidine effects on all-night human sleep: opposite action of low- and medium-dose clonidine on human NREM-REM sleep proportion. Psychiatry Clin Neurosci 58(2):138–144, 2004 15009817

Mohsenin S, Mohsenin V: Diagnosis and management of sleep disorders in posttraumatic stress disorder: a review of the literature. Prim Care Companion CNS Disord 16(6), 2014 25834768

Nevéus T, Hetta J, Cnattingius S, et al: Depth of sleep and sleep habits among enuretic and incontinent children. Acta Paediatr 88(7):748–752, 1999 10447134

Newell SA, Padamadan H, Drake ME Jr: Neurophysiologic studies in nightmare sufferers. Clin Electroencephalogr 23(4):203–206, 1992 1395059

Nielsen T, Carr M: Nightmares and nightmare function, in Principles and Practice of Sleep Medicine. Edited by Kryger MH, Roth T, Dement WC. Philadelphia, PA, Elsevier, 2017, pp 546–554

Nielsen T, Paquette T, Solomonova E, et al: Changes in cardiac variability after REM sleep deprivation in recurrent nightmares. Sleep 33(1):113–122, 2010 20120628

Ohayon MM: Prevalence of hallucinations and their pathological associations in the general population. Psychiatry Res 97(2–3):153–164, 2000 11166087

Ohayon MM, Priest RG, Caulet M, et al: Hypnagogic and hypnopompic hallucinations: pathological phenomena? Br J Psychiatry 169(4):459–467, 1996 8894197

Ornitz EM, Russell AT, Hanna GL, et al: Prepulse inhibition of startle and the neurobiology of primary nocturnal enuresis. Biol Psychiatry 45(11):1455–1466, 1999 10356628

Palikh GM, Vaughn BV: Topiramate responsive exploding head syndrome. J Clin Sleep Med 6(4):382–383, 2010 20726288

Pearce JM: Clinical features of the exploding head syndrome. J Neurol Neurosurg Psychiatry 52(7):907–910, 1989 2769286

Proserpio P, Terzaghi M, Manni R, et al: Drugs used in parasomnia. Sleep Med Clin 13(2):191–202, 2018 29759270

Ramakrishnan K: Evaluation and treatment of enuresis. Am Fam Physician 78(4):489–496, 498, 2008 18756657

Raskind MA, Peskind ER, Chow B, et al: Trial of prazosin for post-traumatic stress disorder in military veterans. N Engl J Med 378(6):507–517, 2018 29414272

Roth B, Buuhová S, Berkova L: Familial sleep paralysis. Schweiz Arch Neurol Neurochir Psychiatr 102(2):321–330, 1968 5734594

Roth S, Newman E, Pelcovitz D, et al: Complex PTSD in victims exposed to sexual and physical abuse: results from the DSM-IV Field Trial for Posttraumatic Stress Disorder. J Trauma Stress 10(4):539–555, 1997 9391940

Sachs C, Svanborg E: The exploding head syndrome: polysomnographic recordings and therapeutic suggestions. Sleep 14(3):263–266, 1991 1896728

Sandman N, Valli K, Kronholm E, et al: Nightmares: prevalence among the Finnish general adult population and war veterans during 1972–2007. Sleep (Basel) 36(7):1041–1050, 2013 23814341

Sharpless BA: Exploding head syndrome. Sleep Med Rev 18(6):489–493, 2014 24703829

Sharpless BA: A clinician's guide to recurrent isolated sleep paralysis. Neuropsychiatr Dis Treat 12:1761–1767, 2016 27486325

Sharpless BA, Barber JP: Lifetime prevalence rates of sleep paralysis: a systematic review. Sleep Med Rev 15(5):311–315, 2011 21571556

Sharpless BA, Doghramji K: Commentary: how to make the ghosts in my bedroom disappear? Focused-attention meditation combined with muscle relaxation (MR therapy)—a direct treatment intervention for sleep paralysis. Front Psychol 8:506, 2017 28421022

Silber MH, Hansen MR, Girish M: Complex nocturnal visual hallucinations. Sleep Med 6(4):363–366, 2005 15946898

Simor P, Horváth K, Ujma PP, et al: Fluctuations between sleep and wakefulness: wake-like features indicated by increased EEG alpha power during different sleep stages in nightmare disorder. Biol Psychol 94(3):592–600, 2013 23831546

Snyder S, Hams G: Serotoninergic agents in the treatment of isolated sleep paralysis. Am J Psychiatry 139(9):1202–1203, 1982 7114320

Spoormaker VI, Schredl M, van den Bout J: Nightmares: from anxiety symptom to sleep disorder. Sleep Med Rev 10(1):19–31, 2006 16377217

Takeuchi T, Fukuda K, Sasaki Y, et al: Factors related to the occurrence of isolated sleep paralysis elicited during a multi-phasic sleep-wake schedule. Sleep 25(1):89–96, 2002 11833865

Umlauf MG, Chasens ER: Sleep disordered breathing and nocturnal polyuria: nocturia and enuresis. Sleep Med Rev 7(5):403–411, 2003 14573376

von Gontard A, Schaumburg H, Hollmann E, et al: The genetics of enuresis: a review. J Urol 166(6):2438–2443, 2001 11696807

Wolfish NM: Enuresis: a maturational lag. Paediatr Child Health 7(8):521–523, 2002 20046463

Yeung CK: Nocturnal enuresis (bedwetting). Curr Opin Urol 13(4):337–343, 2003 12811299

Yeung CK, Sihoe JD, Sit FK, et al: Characteristics of primary nocturnal enuresis in adults: an epidemiological study. BJU Int 93(3):341–345, 2004 14764133

Yeung CK, Sreedhar B, Sihoe JD, et al: Differences in characteristics of nocturnal enuresis between children and adolescents: a critical appraisal from a large epidemiological study. BJU Int 97(5):1069–1073, 2006 16643494

Yu B, Cui S-Y, Zhang X-Q, et al: Different neural circuitry is involved in physiological and psychological stress-induced PTSD-like "nightmares" in rats. Sci Rep 5:15976, 2015 26530305

CHAPTER 17

Restless Legs Syndrome and Periodic Limb Movements

Julia Buchfuhrer, D.O.

Mark Buchfuhrer, M.D.

Restless legs syndrome (RLS) is a sensorimotor disorder that, despite being a common disorder, is very often underdiagnosed or misdiagnosed (Allen et al. 2005). RLS causes an almost irresistible urge to move the legs or other affected body parts, often associated with sensations that are hard to describe, occur at rest, are improved by movement, and worsen at bedtime. The term *restless legs syndrome* was first coined by Dr. Karl-Axel Ekbom in 1945; more recently, the term *Willis-Ekbom disease* was proposed. Patients may have mild, intermittent symptoms that need no treatment or severe, disruptive symptoms that need significant medical intervention. This chapter should enable physicians to identify RLS, choose which patients need medical treatment, and guide them to the appropriate therapies.

Periodic limb movements (PLMs) are highly stereotyped repetitive limb movements that usually involve the lower extremities (but may include the arms). They consisting of extension of the big toe and flexion of the ankle, knee, and hip (triple flexion) in sequences of four or more movements, each lasting 0.5–10 seconds and separated by intervals of 5–90 seconds. Periodic limb movement disorder (PLMD) results when the PLMs result in disturbed sleep such that next-day symptoms of sleepiness occur that cannot be explained by another disorder.

Pathophysiology

The pathophysiology of RLS is not fully understood. Clearly, dopamine transmission is involved, because drugs that block the dopamine receptors (metoclopramide) worsen RLS symptoms, whereas drugs that bind

TABLE 17–1.   Dopamine agonists

Drug	Half-life, hours	Route metabolized or eliminated	FDA approved for RLS	Individual dose range, mg	Average daily dose, mg
Pramipexole	8–12	Kidneys	Yes	0.125–0.5	0.125–0.375
Ropinirole	6	Liver	Yes	0.25–4	0.5–2
Transdermal rotigotine	NA	Kidneys	Yes	1–3	2
Pramipexole ER	NA	Kidneys	No	0.375–0.75	0.375
Ropinirole ER	NA	Liver	No	2–4	2

Note.   ER=extended release; NA=not available; RLS=restless legs syndrome.

to dopamine receptors (Table 17–1) relieve symptoms. Dopamine agonist drugs that target the dopamine D_3 subreceptors are the most effective for treating RLS, indicating that activation of the D_3 receptors is responsible for this therapeutic response. However, long-term treatment with D_3 receptor agonists may cause upregulation of D_1 subreceptors (Dinkins et al. 2017); this, in turn, causes an increase in RLS symptoms, a commonly observed phenomenon called *augmentation*. Furthermore, D_1 receptors—but not D_3 receptors—tend to increase with aging, which likely explains the worsening of RLS when patients reach their 50s and 60s.

Iron deficiency, especially in the brain as demonstrated on autopsy and in vivo cerebrospinal fluid and brain imaging studies, has been associated with increased RLS symptoms. At first it was thought that the iron effect was due to dampening of tyrosine hydroxylase, an enzyme that catalyzes the rate limiting step for dopamine formation. However, unlike the dopamine-depleted brains of patients with Parkinson's disease, the brains of patients with RLS have normal dopamine levels. How brain iron deficiency results in worsening RLS symptoms is still not clear, but interactions with the dopamine system or even the glutamate or adenosine system may occur, as detailed in the following discussion.

Studies (Allen et al. 2013) have demonstrated increased glutamate in the thalamus of patients with RLS, and the increase in glutamate is thought to be responsible for the hyperarousal found in these patients. $\alpha_2\delta$ Ligands (Table 17–2) decrease glutamate and decrease the hyperarousal, thus diminishing RLS-related insomnia.

Newer studies (Ferré et al. 2018) have also implicated the adenosine system in RLS. Iron deficiency causes downregulation of the inhibitory adenosine A_1 receptors in the brain (Rivera-Oliver et al. 2019), which in turn results in an increase in brain glutamate release and a presynaptic

TABLE 17–2. a₂δ Drug dosing

Drug	Initial dose up to age 65, *mg*	Initial dose after age 65, *mg*	Maximum dose, *mg*
Gabapentin enacarbil	600	300	1,200–1,800
Gabapentin	300	100	900–1,200 per dose
Pregabalin	75	50	300–450

hyperdopaminergic response. This sets up an imbalance in the interaction among the adenosine, glutamate, and dopamine systems that may result in the clinical manifestations of RLS. In fact, studies employing dipyridamole, an inhibitor of adenosine transport that increases extracellular adenosine availability and A_1 receptor activation, improves RLS symptoms (Garcia-Borreguero et al. 2018). Thus, the decrease in brain iron may result in a decrease in the adenosine system, which in turn creates an imbalance of the glutamate and dopaminergic systems in the brain. This may be the pivotal neurotransmitter cause of RLS symptoms.

Although opioids are very potent drugs for relieving RLS symptoms, the mechanism for their action on RLS is not understood. Issues with opioid binding or downregulation/internalization of opioid receptors may be involved, or opioids may act through activation of the dopamine system, as demonstrated by dopamine antagonists blocking the beneficial effects of opioids on RLS (Silber et al. 2018).

Epidemiology

PREVALENCE

Most physicians are not aware of how common RLS is in Western populations. Studies (Ohayon et al. 2012) have found the prevalence of RLS in the adult general population ranges between 5% and 8.8% based on the International RLS Study Group (IRLSSTG) criteria. Clinically significant RLS (at least twice-weekly symptoms that are moderately distressing) occurs in 2%–3% of the population (Allen et al. 2005). The prevalence of RLS is much lower in Asian and African populations, with estimates typically below 1%–3%. However, African Americans have prevalence rates approaching those of white Americans.

The prevalence of RLS in children (Picchietti et al. 2007) is also higher than previously thought, with a prevalence of 2% (often misdiagnosed as "growing pains"). Furthermore, 0.5% of children reported their RLS symptoms as moderately or severely distressing, whereas 1% reported that their symptoms occurred two or more times per week.

The prevalence of RLS in adults older than 30 years has been reported as being twice as high in women as compared with men. However, this difference is valid only for women who have had at least one pregnancy; otherwise, the prevalence is equal. Interestingly, the prevalence of RLS in women does not increase with additional pregnancies.

RISK FACTORS AND COMORBID DISEASE

Many risk factors and comorbid diseases increase the likelihood of patients developing RLS. The original classification of primary and secondary RLS is probably not valid, because all patients with RLS have similar symptoms, and treatment options are equally efficacious. Comorbid diseases or other triggers may provoke RLS symptoms by causing an imbalance of the dopamine-glutamate-adenosine system described earlier.

Demographic Factors

AGE.   As noted, even children have a significant incidence of RLS (2%), but the prevalence increases with age; symptoms typically peak in the 50s and 60s. However, the incidence of RLS decreases after age 70.

FEMALE SEX.   Females are twice as likely to have RLS as males. However, this relationship is only valid for females who have had one or more pregnancies.

LIVING AT HIGHER ALTITUDES.   Studies have found a higher prevalence of RLS in people living at high altitudes. One study (Gupta et al. 2017) found a fivefold increase in RLS (12% vs. 2.5%) among Himalayan people living at high altitudes (1,900–3,200 m) compared with those living at lower altitudes (400 m). This altitude effect may result from hypoxia, which causes increased erythropoiesis, resulting in the production of more hemoglobin to carry oxygen. This production of hemoglobin depletes iron from the blood and brain, thus creating an imbalance in the dopamine-glutamate-adenosine system.

Lifestyle Factors

A study that followed two large cohorts found that healthy lifestyle factors reduced the incidence of RLS (Batool-Anwar et al. 2016). People with normal weight, regular physical activity, and some alcohol intake had less risk than those who were obese, did not exercise, and consumed no alcohol. However, significant alcohol intake before bedtime most often exacerbates RLS symptoms, and vigorous exercise (as opposed to mild to moderate exercise) may trigger severe symptoms. Smoking increases RLS risk in women but not in men. Contrary to previous claims, no link has been found between RLS and heavy consumption of caffeine.

Changes in work or daily activities from an active lifestyle to a more sedentary one often exacerbates RLS, and patients will request an increase in treatment. Adequate sleep is essential to help control RLS. Sleep deprivation, often caused by RLS, results in increased daytime sleepiness, which in turn increases RLS, resulting in a vicious circle of worsening RLS and insomnia.

Comorbid Conditions

The three most important comorbid conditions associated with RLS are iron deficiency anemia, renal failure, and pregnancy. The role of iron deficiency was discussed in detail in the "Pathophysiology" section earlier in the chapter. An increased RLS prevalence of 25%–80% has been found in patients on dialysis and 20%–25% in pregnant women, especially in the third trimester. The cause of this marked increase in RLS in these populations is not known. Interestingly, kidney transplantation (but not dialysis) in end-stage renal disease and delivery in pregnant patients often improve RLS.

A long list of medical conditions/diseases have been associated with RLS, but the studies linking them have been limited in their methodologies. Conditions with possible but weak associations with RLS include polyneuropathies, diabetes mellitus, Parkinson's disease, multiple sclerosis, hypothyroidism, gastric resection, vitamin B_{12} and folate deficiencies, lung transplantation, magnesium deficiency, spinocerebellar ataxia type 3, hypertension, rheumatological diseases, small intestinal bacterial overgrowth, headache/migraine, and chronic obstructive pulmonary disease. Whether treating any of these comorbid conditions improves RLS symptoms is unclear. About 25%–40% of children with RLS also have ADHD, and about 25% of children with ADHD also have RLS.

Increased depression and anxiety are very commonly associated with RLS. Whether they are present as a result of poorly controlled RLS or of primary problems that enhance RLS is not clear. It is not uncommon for the depression and anxiety to resolve once the RLS is controlled. In patients with RLS, suicidal ideation and behavior are very prevalent, and the likelihood of suicide is strongly correlated with RLS severity and depression history (Para et al. 2019).

Medications That Worsen Restless Legs Syndrome

Many medications, including over-the-counter (OTC) and most psychiatric medications, tend to worsen or trigger RLS symptoms. Therefore, a complete medication reconciliation should be done every visit to make sure that patients are not taking one of the drugs listed here.

- **Sedating antihistamines:** First-generation antihistamines (H_1 receptor blockers) include diphenhydramine and doxylamine, both of which are the main ingredients in the OTC sleep aids often used by patients to self-treat insomnia. Others include chloropyramine, carbinoxamine, orphenadrine, bromazine, clemastine, and dimenhydrinate. The newer, nonsedating second-generation antihistamines (e.g., loratadine, fexofenadine, and cetirizine) do not worsen RLS.
- **Antihistamines to treat nausea and motion sickness ("zine drugs"):** These include meclizine, hydroxyzine, cyclizine, chlorcyclizine, promethazine, and trimeprazine. Alternatives that should not worsen RLS include granisetron, ondansetron for nausea, and transdermal scopolamine for motion sickness.
- **Other antinausea drugs or dopamine antagonists:** Metoclopramide usually markedly worsens RLS symptoms.
- **Antidepressants:** Due to their serotonergic action, all of the selective serotonin reuptake inhibitors (SSRIs) and serotonin-norepinephrine reuptake inhibitors (SNRIs), except nefazodone (which may cause massive hepatic injury), tend to worsen RLS and should be used with caution in these patients. Older tricyclic antidepressants (TCAs) also exacerbate RLS, with the possible exception of desipramine. Bupropion and trazodone are alternative choices that do not affect RLS.
- **Antipsychotics:** Most antipsychotics block dopamine receptors and thus tend to worsen RLS. Aripiprazole, brexpiprazole, and cariprazine, which are partial dopamine agonists, may have a more neutral effect.

The risks and benefits of using RLS-exacerbating drugs should be discussed with patients. In some situations, alternative drugs may not be appropriate or available, especially in serious conditions such as depression, anxiety, and psychosis.

Genetics

RLS is highly familial, with estimates of heritability between 54% and 83% in twin studies. Familial studies suggest an autosomal dominant inheritance with variable penetrance. An interplay most likely occurs between genetic and environmental factors and iron deficiency, including all the comorbid diseases and risk factors mentioned. In families who have one child with RLS, siblings are 3.6 times more likely to also have RLS. Genome-wide association studies have found 19 loci associated with RLS. Of those 19, the *MEIS1* locus on chromosome 2 is the strongest genetic risk factor for RLS, with almost 50% increased odds of having the disorder. *MEIS1* has been implicated in neurogenesis, specification of neuronal cell type, and establishing connectivity between neurons and their target field. This risk allele may also be involved in the iron system and with neurological developmental changes in the fetus.

Diagnosis

RLS is diagnosed by obtaining the patient's clinical history of symptoms. No tests (including sleep studies) are indicated to establish the diagnosis in adults. The patient must fulfill the five diagnostic criteria updated by the IRLSSG in 2014 (Allen et al. 2014b), detailed in Table 17–3. These criteria can easily be remembered by the acronym "URGES."

TABLE 17–3. **URGES criteria for diagnosing restless legs syndrome**

Urge to move the legs associated with unpleasant leg sensations

Rest induces symptoms

Gets better with activity

Evening and nighttime worsening

Not **S**olely accounted for by another medical or behavioral condition

It should be noted that the *International Classification of Sleep Disorders*, 3rd Edition (ICSD-3; American Academy of Sleep Medicine 2014), criteria for diagnosing RLS are similar to the IRLSSG criteria, except for the proviso that the symptoms of RLS cause concern, distress, sleep disturbance, or impairment in mental, physical, social, occupational, educational, behavioral, or other important areas of daily functioning. This additional qualifier for diagnosing RLS ensures that the disease is a true clinical disorder and thus has adverse consequences. However, the ICSD-3 criteria allow for excluding significant clinical issues for research purposes. The IRLSSG criteria add a specifier for the clinical significance of RLS, which is identical to the ICSD-3 qualifier for diagnosing RLS as a disease state. However, for the IRLSSG criteria, this specifier is not necessary to establish the diagnosis of RLS.

URGE TO MOVE THE LEGS ASSOCIATED WITH UNPLEASANT LEG SENSATIONS

The first and most important criterion often helps differentiate RLS from other conditions that may mimic its symptoms. Patients with RLS feel an irresistible urge to move their legs, often associated with hard-to-describe, uncomfortable sensations. This urge is specific to the affected limb and not generalized, as with akathisia. The actual sensations are usually not painful—such as being tickled for a few seconds is not painful—but when they persist, patients often describe them as painful—similar to being tickled for a prolonged time. Although many patients describe the abnormal sensations as "bugs crawling deep in my legs," "water, electricity, or worms moving in my legs," "tingling in my legs," or even "aching legs," most patients have considerable difficulty finding the words to articulate their experience. The sensations are felt deep in the legs and are rarely superficial. A significant percentage of patients can only describe the sensation as an irresistible urge to move their legs.

RLS always starts with symptoms in the legs (occasionally in the feet) and then may progress to the arms and any other body parts, especially when symptoms become severe. With time, some patients may experience symptoms only in their arms, but they *must* have had symptoms in their legs prior to this migration. Although most patients complain of the RLS symptoms in both legs, many patients may experience symptoms in only one leg at a time, which may alternate over time.

REST INDUCES SYMPTOMS

RLS symptoms are evoked by rest, independent of position, and occur equally with sitting or lying down (sometimes even when standing and leaning against a wall). The rest state involves a decrease in both motor activity and mental alertness. One of the most frequent triggers of RLS is being confined to a seat while on an airplane; symptoms worsen markedly while watching an inflight movie but can be relieved with mental activity, such as doing a crossword puzzle, playing a video or chess game, or playing solitaire. As RLS progresses and becomes more severe, the interval of rest that provokes symptoms decreases. Patients may try to resist the urge to move, but this only heightens symptoms, ultimately requiring the patient to move.

GETS BETTER WITH ACTIVITY

Patients with RLS who have the urge to move when at rest typically get significant relief with movement. Walking tends to be the movement of choice, but if walking is not possible (e.g., when confined to a seat on an airplane), stretching, flexing, rubbing or massaging, shaking, or even pounding the affected limb may provide relief. The more vigorous the activity, the greater the relief. The improvement in symptoms tends to be minimal for severe cases and complete with milder RLS. Symptoms will remain improved for the duration of the activity but can return fairly quickly once the patient rests again. Once back at rest, the duration of relief depends on the severity of the RLS (relief may last less than a few minutes for severely affected patients) and may last longer with activities of higher intensity and longer duration.

EVENING AND NIGHTTIME WORSENING

Most RLS symptoms follow a patient's circadian rhythm, typically peaking in the evening and sleep period. Insomnia often occurs in patients with significant disease. RLS symptoms are usually least troublesome between 8 A.M. and 12 P.M. Symptoms often occur in the daytime but need much longer periods at rest (e.g., an airplane trip or movie) to become active in the daytime compared with the evening. However, in patients with severe RLS, especially those with augmentation, symptoms may become equally severe around the clock, without any circadian variation, although nighttime-only worsening was present earlier in their disease.

NOT SOLELY ACCOUNTED BY ANOTHER MEDICAL OR BEHAVIORAL CONDITION

Although RLS is often underdiagnosed or misdiagnosed, overdiagnosing RLS and missing another disease state must be avoided. As such, conditions that mimic RLS should be ruled out so that the symptoms are clearly not being caused by another condition. Common mimics include peripheral neuropathy, arthritis, habitual foot tapping, akathisia, claudication, varicose veins, hypnic jerks, leg cramps, and anxiety (Table 17–4).

Clinical Presentation and Features

The clinical presentation of RLS follows the first four diagnostic criteria, remembered by the URGES acronym (see Table 17–3). Patients will notice sensations in their legs, which are difficult to describe, and an urge to move their legs when at rest. Initially, the symptoms arise briefly in the late evening or just after getting into bed, are quite mild, and may not require movement for relief. Approximately one-quarter of adult patients developed RLS as children (RLS can be diagnosed in patients as young as 3 years), but most often this diagnosis is made retrospectively because complaints are typically labeled as "growing pains" in youth. RLS tends to be a chronic disease with a variable but slowly progressive course over decades. Symptoms become severe enough for patients to seek treatment on average by age 40–60. However, it is common to see younger patients with severe RLS symptoms requiring treatment. A small percentage of patients may have spontaneous remissions that may last for years to decades, but many will eventually have a reemergence of symptoms.

TABLE 17–4.   Common mimics of RLS

Mimic	How to differentiate
Neuroleptic-induced akathisia	Does not follow the circadian rhythm; inner general restlessness as opposed to RLS that occurs only in the limbs; not associated with PLM
Peripheral neuropathy	May fulfill most of the RLS diagnostic criteria, but patient has no urge to move and symptoms do not improve with movement
Leg muscle cramps	May fulfill first four diagnostic criteria, but severe pain is most prominent feature, typically localized to one muscle group with muscle tightening
Arthritis	Localized to affected joints; worsens with movement and improves with rest
Vascular claudication (arterial insufficiency)	May occur at rest but is more severe with movement
Habitual foot tapping	Can easily be stopped without causing discomfort; no real urge to move
Hypnic jerks	Only occur at sleep onset, with a jerk of limbs and feeling of falling
Varicose veins	Unless thrombosed, no associated symptoms except edema
Anxiety	No associated discomfort in the legs

Note.   PLM=periodic limb movement; RLS=restless legs syndrome.

Symptoms *must* initially appear in the lower extremities but can spread to other body parts with time or other provocation. Typically, the arms are the first area of symptom expansion, followed by the trunk, but sensations can extend to any body part, including the head. As the disease progresses, symptoms become more intense, are provoked by shorter periods of rest, and occur earlier in the day. Patients with severe RLS may have symptoms that occur all day, and the intensity does not vary with the circadian rhythm. he IRLSSG diagnostic criteria divide RLS into two categories based on severity and frequency of the disease: intermittent and chronic persistent (Allen et al. 2014b).

INTERMITTENT RESTLESS LEGS SYNDROME

Patients with untreated intermittent RLS have experienced symptoms less than twice weekly for the past year, on average, with at least five lifetime events. Symptoms tend to be milder and less bothersome in this group, most often needing little to no treatment, and tend to occur in certain predictable situations, such as when taking a long airplane flight. According to the large RLS Epidemiology, Symptoms, and Treatment (REST) epidemiological study (Allen et al. 2005), 30% of subjects with RLS had symptoms less than once per week, and 13% had symptoms once per week.

CHRONIC-PERSISTENT RESTLESS LEGS SYNDROME

Patients with chronic-persistent RLS, when not treated, have symptoms at least twice weekly for the past year. This group comprises patients with more severe RLS symptoms that often need treatment. In the REST study, 55% of the patients (Allen et al. 2005) had symptoms twice a week or more, placing them in this category. Of those patients, 66% reported their symptoms as moderate to severely disturbing and were referred to as "RLS sufferers."

In addition to being a sensorimotor disorder, RLS often becomes a sleep disorder, with >75% of patients reporting at least one sleep-related symptom (Allen et al. 2005). Because symptoms worsen with rest and at bedtime, one of the most frequent and bothersome complaints is insomnia. As the disease progresses, it may be several hours before the patient can fall asleep. To add to the misery of the severe insomnia, patients most often cannot relax in bed while awake and must move or rub their legs, get up and walk, take hot baths, or perform other rituals to abate the RLS symptoms sufficiently to fall asleep. Sir Thomas Willis, who first described the disease in 1685, wrote that individuals with RLS "are no more able to sleep than if they were in a place of the greatest torture."

Patients with chronic-persistent RLS experience reduced quality of life. Significantly reduced Short Form–36 Health Survey scores were found among this group, comparable with those of patients with other chronic medical conditions such as type 2 diabetes mellitus, osteoarthritis, and depression (Allen et al. 2005). Additionally, patients with RLS have increased prevalence rates of anxiety and depression (Li et al. 2012; Picchietti and Winkelman 2005; Winkelmann et al. 2005). This may be due in part to the chronic insomnia with resultant daytime fatigue and in part to the anxiety engendered by anticipating these adverse effects and RLS symptoms. Furthermore, treatment with antidepressant medication most often worsens RLS symptoms, which may in turn increase the depression and anxiety levels, prompting further increases in RLS-exacerbating treatment.

Many social and occupational consequences arise from uncontrolled chronic-persistent RLS. Sedentary activities, such as going to the theater, religious services, or lectures or even spending an evening with family or friends, are often avoided. Intimate relationships are difficult to establish due to the associated PLMs while asleep and conscious movements while awake in bed to relieve the RLS symptoms. Airplane or long car trips may be so challenging that patients will avoid traveling, which may impair both social and work-related functions. Sedentary jobs that require prolonged desk work, meeting with clients, or working as a receptionist may be impossible for severely affected patients. In addition, due to the lack of sleep, cognitive dysfunction is common, which further decreases work productivity.

Periodic Limb Movements

As described at the beginning of this chapter, PLMs are highly stereotyped repetitive limb movements that usually involve the lower extremities, consisting of extension of the big toe and flexion of the ankle, knee, and hip, also known as "triple flexion" (Figure 17–1). The upper extremities may also be involved. PLMs consist of sequences of four or more movements, each lasting 0.5–10 seconds and separated by intervals of between 5 and 90 seconds (see criterion A, Table 17–5). They mostly occur during sleep, and typically only the bed partner is aware of them. Therefore, it is important to obtain a history from the patient's sleep partner. PLMs during wakefulness tend to occur exclusively in patients with RLS.

Although >85% of patients with RLS experience PLMs, the movements are not diagnostic of RLS because many other disorders have frequent PLMs as well. Increased PLMs are noted in sleep apnea, end-stage renal disease, heart failure, spinal cord injury, multiple sclerosis, narcolepsy, REM behavior disorder, Parkinson's disease, and multiple system atrophy. PLMs also increase with age. PLMs and RLS share the same pathophysiology. This includes common genetic factors, a central role of brain (and serum) iron deficiency, and a significant susceptibility to antidepressants, especially SSRIs, SNRIs, and TCAs.

Periodic Limb Movement Disorder

PLMD is generally considered to be very rare, and some controversy exists about how often it may occur (see Table 17–5). To establish a diagnosis of PLMD, other disorders (discussed in the previous paragraph) must be ruled out, because the PLMs cannot be secondary to another underlying disorder or cause. Furthermore, a relationship between frequent PLMs (>15 per hour in adults) and a resultant sleep disorder (hypersom-

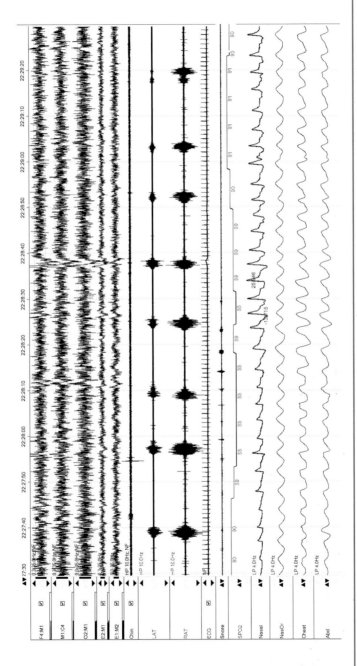

FIGURE 17–1. **A 2-minute polysomnography window showing PLMs in right and left legs during stage N2 sleep.**

LAT = left anterior tibialis muscle; PLMs = periodic limb movements; RAT = right anterior tibialis muscle.

TABLE 17–5.   Periodic limb movement and periodic limb movement disorder criteria

A. Polysomnography demonstrates repetitive, highly stereotyped limb movements that

- Are 0.5–10 seconds in duration
- Exceed the baseline electromyographic voltage by 8 μV
- Occur in a sequence of four or more movements
- Are separated by an interval of 5–90 seconds (onset to onset; typically these movements recur at intervals of 15–40 seconds)

B. The periodic limb movement index exceeds 5 per hour in children and 15 per hour in adults

C. Clinical sleep disturbance or a complaint of daytime fatigue is present

D. Related symptoms are not better explained by another concurrent sleep disorder, medical or neurological disorder, mental disorder, or medication or substance use disorder

Source.   American Academy of Sleep Medicine 2014.

nia, insomnia, or unrefreshing sleep) must be established. Most studies evaluating PLMs have not been able to determine a connection between increased PLMs and sleep disturbance causing next-day consequences. Therefore, linking increased PLMs and true PLMD is very difficult.

Diagnostic Procedures, Tests, and Questionnaires

The diagnosis of RLS is based primarily on the five diagnostic criteria discussed in Table 17–3. However, due to patient communication difficulties or existing comorbid conditions, such as neuropathy or other confounding issues, the diagnosis may at times be difficult to establish. A sleep study is not usually necessary to diagnose RLS unless sleep apnea is suspected and needs to be ruled out. However, if patients have frequent PLMs (>15 per hour) on a sleep study or their bed partner reports frequent PLMs, this evidence can be supportive in borderline cases (as long as other possible causes of PLM are ruled out, including medication). Frequent PLMs noted on a sleep study do not establish a diagnosis of RLS, but if other causes of PLM are ruled out, it should trigger a strong suspicion of RLS. Additionally, as noted in the "Genetics" discussion earlier, a family history of RLS significantly increases the likelihood of the patient having RLS. In cases that are difficult to diagnose, a short trial of levodopa or a dopamine agonist can be helpful to confirm a diagnosis of

RLS because about 90% of patients will respond to a dopamine class of drug (Stiasny-Kolster et al. 2006).

Although currently used more for research to evaluate the effect of treatments on RLS, the Suggested Immobilization Test can help confirm the diagnosis of RLS and assess its severity (Garcia-Borreguero et al. 2013). During this test, patients relax comfortably in a recliner for 1 hour and complete a 10-level severity rating every 10 minutes while being monitored for PLMs during wakefulness.

One of the most commonly used RLS questionnaires to assess severity, for both office and research use, is the International RLS Study Group Rating Scale, which consists of 10 questions rated from 0 to 4 that cover the severity of RLS symptoms and consequences (Walters et al. 2003).

Every patient with RLS should undergo a thorough history and physical examination, with special attention to neurological (e.g., neuropathy) and psychiatric disorders. General laboratory tests should be included to rule out significant renal disease and anemia. In addition, even in the absence of anemia, a serum ferritin and an iron and transferrin level should be included; this should be drawn after an overnight fast with no iron products for 24 hours.

Differential Diagnosis

The differential diagnosis includes the various mimics, as described by the fifth RLS diagnostic criterion (see Table 17–3). Common mimics that are easily confused with RLS are listed in Table 17–4, with details that help differentiate them from RLS. In addition, none of the mimics includes a family history of RLS, increased PLMs, or response to dopaminergics. One aspect that often makes RLS difficult to diagnose and treat is that patients often have RLS concurrently with one or more of its mimics. Treatment with a dopamine drug may help differentiate which symptoms are due to RLS and which are associated with a mimic.

Management

Not all patients with RLS need treatment. Many patients have mild intermittent symptoms that are not bothersome enough to require intervention. When mild symptoms occur at bedtime, they may only delay sleep by a few minutes, not warranting medication. However, with time (often decades), the symptoms may progress and require additional measures. Treatment strategies should be instituted based on the classification of patients into intermittent or chronic-persistent RLS as determined by the

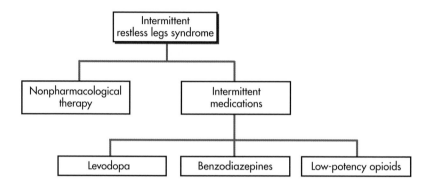

FIGURE 17–2.   Algorithm for treating intermittent restless legs syndrome.

Source.   Adapted from Silber et al. 2013.

frequency and severity of symptoms, per the IRLSSG (see "Clinical Presentation and Features").

INTERMITTENT RESTLESS LEGS SYNDROME

The management of intermittent RLS (symptoms less than twice weekly) is based on the algorithm in Figure 17–2 (Silber et al. 2013).

Nonpharmacological Therapy

When possible, drug treatment should be avoided for patients with intermittent RLS. Several measures can be taken that do not require medications.

ALERTING ACTIVITIES.   One of the most predictable triggers of RLS is confinement to a seat, such as in an airplane. However, RLS occurs with both physical and mental rest or inactivity. Watching the in-flight movie only makes symptoms worse, whereas playing a video game or chess, solving a crossword puzzle, or playing solitaire can completely resolve bothersome symptoms.

ABSTINENCE FROM SUBSTANCES.   Alcohol consumption often triggers RLS symptoms and thus should be avoided or kept to a minimum. Caffeine, which is an adenosine receptor antagonist, has been implicated in causing RLS symptoms; it is likely that symptoms only occur upon withdrawal from caffeine, as sleepiness increases.

AVOIDANCE OF EXACERBATING DRUGS.   Drugs that trigger RLS and alternatives were discussed earlier (see "Medications That Worsen Restless

Legs Syndrome"). Classes of drugs to be avoided include sedating antihistamines, antinausea/motion sickness drugs, antidepressants, and antipsychotics.

IRON THERAPY. Patients with relatively low serum iron levels (transferrin saturation <20%, serum ferritin <50–75 µg/L) should receive oral iron supplementation on an empty stomach with 200 mg of vitamin C *only once daily* (Allen et al. 2018). Taking oral iron more than once daily triggers an increase in hepcidin production, leading to decreased iron absorption and a smaller increase in iron than with once-daily supplementation. Furthermore, due to this feedback loop, most patients will have difficulty achieving adequate iron levels with oral supplementation and will require an iron infusion. Therefore, intravenous iron therapy should be considered for patients with RLS, using 1,000 mg of low-molecular-weight iron dextran or ferric carboxymaltose (other iron products do not work as well), with a target ferritin level between 200 and 300 µg/L. It is still not clear why patients with RLS are iron depleted or why they may need repeat infusions on an average of once per year. Significant benefit from intravenous iron is noted in about 60% of patients, and failure of this therapy may be due to not driving enough peripheral iron into the brain.

MECHANICAL DEVICES. Two FDA-cleared devices are currently available for treating RLS. The first is the Relaxis vibration pad (Burbank et al. 2013), which is placed under the legs when the patient goes to bed. A remote handheld unit starts the vibration process; this acts as a counter stimulation similar to the patient rubbing the legs and may diminish RLS symptoms enough to permit the patient to fall asleep. The second device is the Restiffic foot wrap (Kuhn et al. 2016), which is wrapped around both forefeet when going to bed.

SLEEP HYGIENE AND BEHAVIORAL OR LIFESTYLE THERAPY. RLS symptoms occur more readily when patients are sleepy. Therefore, getting adequate sleep is important. As such, shift work often presents a challenge. Because RLS follows the circadian rhythm and is worse later in the day, patients can plan sedentary activities earlier in the day and perform more active ones (e.g., shopping, house cleaning, laundry) later in the day. Sedentary jobs must often be avoided, but adjustable/standing desks are one possible workaround. Mild to moderate regular exercise may diminish RLS symptoms, whereas vigorous exercise may provoke symptoms. At bedtime, many patients find that measures such as hot or cold baths, stretching exercises, deep knee bends, massages, and other physical activities may provide enough relief that they can go to bed and fall asleep before the RLS symptoms recur. Separate beds or a memory foam mattress may be helpful for couples, to preserve harmony in light of the RLS patient's sleep-disturbing leg kicks.

Drug Therapy

When nonpharmacological therapy is insufficient, drugs may be needed to help control RLS symptoms. Symptoms may be predictable, such as when the patient goes to the movies or travels by airplane, but often occur unpredictably and may be quite bothersome. Two types of medication are used for intermittent RLS: those that directly relieve the symptoms and those that instead indirectly treat by helping the patient sleep.

RELIEVING MEDICATIONS.   Medications that relieve RLS include carbidopa/levodopa or low-potency opioids. Carbidopa/levodopa at 25 mg/100 mg can be extremely effective and quick acting (within 15 minutes on an empty stomach) for either predictable daytime RLS symptoms or unexpected bedtime exacerbations. It can be used up to three times a week without raising concerns of augmentation (see "Dopamine Agonists"). Low-potency opioids such as tramadol 50 mg or codeine 30 mg may also be effective for both predictable and unexpected RLS symptoms. Their onset of action (about 30 minutes) is somewhat slower than that of carbidopa/levodopa, but they tend to act longer (4–6 hours for low-potency opioids compared with 2–4 hours with carbidopa/levodopa).

SLEEPING PILLS OR SEDATIVES.   Sleeping pills and sedatives do not decrease RLS symptoms unless anxiety is a significant component. The first such drug described was clonazepam, but with its ≥40-hour half-life, next-day sedation is common. Shorter-acting benzodiazepines (alprazolam, lorazepam, temazepam, or triazolam) or selective benzodiazepine receptor drugs (zolpidem, eszopiclone, or zaleplon) may be more appropriate. This class of drug should be used exclusively for bedtime RLS symptoms. Caution should be used when prescribing hypnotics in patients with RLS, however, due to an increased risk of parasomnia, particularly sleep-related eating disorder (Howell and Schenck 2012).

CHRONIC-PERSISTENT RESTLESS LEGS SYNDROME

Patients with more frequent symptoms often require additional treatment (Figure 17–3). Nonpharmacological therapy should be tried first, but these patients typically need medication for optimal control. Although first-line choices have historically included dopamine agonists in addition to $\alpha_2\delta$ ligands, using short-acting dopamine agonists on a daily basis raises important concerns.

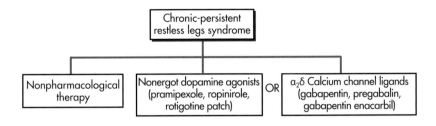

FIGURE 17–3. **Algorithm for treating chronic-persistent restless legs syndrome.**

Source. Adapted from Silber et al. 2013.

Dopamine Agonists

Three of the five drugs (the two short-acting versions of pramipexole and ropinirole and the rotigotine patch) in the dopamine agonist category are FDA approved to treat RLS (Figure 17–4) and considered first-line therapy. Initially, most patients get dramatic relief with dopamine agonists. Early side effects of these drugs are similar and include nausea, orthostatic hypotension, dizziness, sleepiness (including next-day sleep attacks), insomnia, headache, and fatigue. Short-acting dopamine drugs should be started at their lowest doses and increased every 5–7 days until the lowest effective dose is achieved. The rotigotine patch is started at 1 mg/day and increased weekly if needed to a maximum of 3 mg/day. The maximum approved doses (Figure 17–4) should not be exceeded, and some experts suggest a safer upper limit of 0.25 mg for pramipexole and 1 mg for ropinirole.

Although dopamine agonists provide dramatic relief initially, their long-term daily use raises grave concerns. Two long-term side effects of dopamine drugs include impulse-control disorders and augmentation. Impulse-control disorders include compulsive gambling, shopping, eating, and medication use; hypersexuality; internet addiction; and punding. These dose-related adverse effects often progress insidiously and may become so severe that patients lose hundreds of thousands of dollars or end up losing family and friends. Diagnosing the behavior as abnormal is difficult because patients enjoy their impulsivity, often do not link it to their dopaminergic drugs, and try to hide their actions until disastrous consequences ensue. The best treatment is stopping the dopamine drug. The frequency of this problem is not fully known but may be as high as 10% of patients taking these drugs.

Currently, the short-acting dopamine agonists are the most frequently prescribed drugs for treating RLS, which is fueling the most common iat-

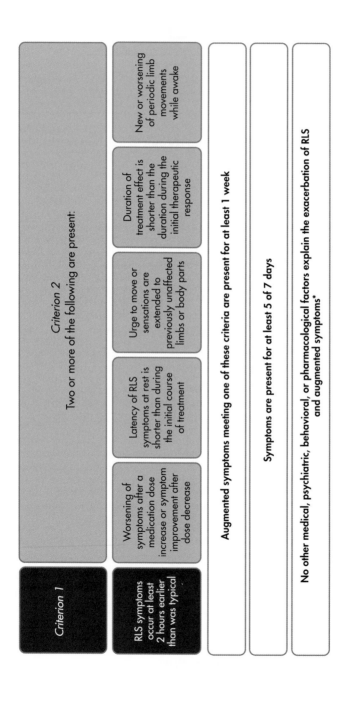

FIGURE 17–4.   Augmentation criteria.

*Medical, psychiatric, and pharmacological factors considered alternate explanations for symptom augmentation include significant decrease in physical activity, introduction of antihistamines, SSRIs, SNRIs, frequent blood donations (≥3 times per year), substantial blood loss (e.g., due to an accident), and iron deficiency/anemia diagnosis.

RLS=restless legs syndrome; SNRI=serotonin-norepinephrine reuptake inhibitor; SSRI=selective serotonin reuptake inhibitor.

Source.   Reprinted from Allen RP, Ondo WG, Ball E, et al: "Restless Legs Syndrome (RLS) Augmentation Associated With Dopamine Agonist and Levodopa Usage in a Community Sample." *Sleep Medicine* 12(5):431–439, 2011. Copyright © 2011 Elsevier. Used with permission.

rogenic complication, known as RLS augmentation. Patients with RLS augmentation most often have the worst symptoms and are among the most miserable patients with RLS. First described in 1996 (Allen and Earley 1996), augmentation is a worsening of RLS symptoms due to taking dopamine drugs (levodopa or dopamine agonists) or tramadol. Initially, these drugs markedly improve RLS symptoms, but with time, symptoms dramatically worsen. The best criteria for diagnosing augmentation in patients presenting in doctors' offices are based on the 2003 National Institutes of Health criteria (Allen et al. 2003), summarized in Figure 17–4 (Allen et al. 2011). The key sign that should trigger suspicion of augmentation is an earlier onset of symptoms by >2 hours compared with before starting the medication. Symptoms become more intense, less rest time is needed to evoke symptoms, the effective treatment duration shortens, symptoms may spread to other body parts, and PLMs while awake may occur for the first time or worsen. A simpler and easier rule is that augmentation is present whenever a patient who has been on stable treatment for at least 6 months requests more medication.

The rate of augmentation is about 7%–8% per year in patients receiving pramipexole or ropinirole (Allen et al. 2014a). Thus, the vast majority of patients need to change therapy within 10 years of starting these short-acting dopamine agonists. Augmentation rates are lower with long-acting dopamine agonists, such as the rotigotine patch (1% per year), so these are a much better option when a dopamine drug needs to be prescribed. Treatment of augmentation is outlined in Figure 17–5 (Garcia-Borreguero et al. 2016) but is complex; patients should be referred to a specialist who has experience treating it. Preventing augmentation is much easier than treating it. Daily therapy with short-acting dopamine agonists should not be physicians' first line of therapy, because many safer and equally effective alternative treatments are available. When alternative drugs are not available or effective, short-acting dopamine agonists should be started at the lowest dose (even half a tablet) and should not exceed the maximum recommended dose, and once a stable dose has been achieved, further increases should be made with extreme caution.

Alpha-2-Delta Ligands

The $\alpha_2\delta$ ligands, which include gabapentin, gabapentin enacarbil, and pregabalin, are often very effective for treating RLS, and many experts consider them first-line therapy in lieu of dopaminergic drugs. The $\alpha_2\delta$ ligands bind to $\alpha_2\delta$ subunits of voltage-gated calcium channels on presynaptic neurons in the CNS. They reduce glutamate release into the syn-

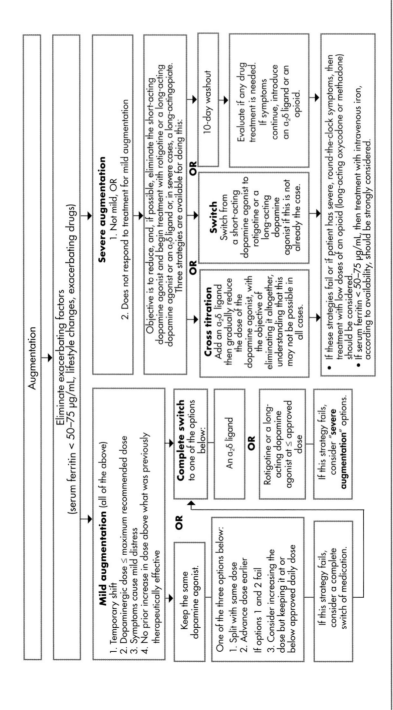

FIGURE 17–5. Treatment of augmentation algorithm.

Source. Reprinted from Garcia-Borreguero D, Silber MH, Winkelman JW, et al: "Guidelines for the First-Line Treatment of Restless Legs Syndrome/Willis-Ekbom Disease, Prevention and Treatment of Dopaminergic Augmentation: a Combined Task Force of the IRLSSG, EURLSSG, and the RLS-Foundation. *Sleep Medicine* 21:1–11, 2016. Copyright © 2016 Elsevier. Used with permission.

apse, which is likely how they improve RLS symptoms and insomnia. Only gabapentin enacarbil is FDA approved for RLS. These drugs relieve painful RLS symptoms and have the added benefit of improving insomnia (often a separate feature of RLS not improved with dopamine drugs), anxiety, PLMs resulting in arousals, and any associated neuropathy symptoms. The $\alpha_2\delta$ ligands are equally as effective as dopamine drugs but do not cause augmentation or impulse-control disorders. The most common side effects involve CNS sedation (sleepiness, dizziness, difficulty concentrating), weight gain, and edema (especially at higher doses). In some patients, these drugs could be associated with depression and suicidal thoughts.

Gabapentin should be taken 2–3 hours before onset of symptoms, whereas pregabalin should be dosed about 1 hour before onset, at the starting doses detailed in Table 17–2. The starting dose may be increased every 5–7 days if needed until adequate relief is achieved. Earlier doses may be necessary for daytime symptoms, but sedation can be limiting. Gabapentin has limited bowel absorption, so higher doses may not provide much additional efficacy. Gabapentin enacarbil, a prodrug of gabapentin, should be taken once daily with dinner because it is a slow-release product that lasts about 12 hours and is better absorbed with food. It is well absorbed at all dose levels and thus may be effective when gabapentin has failed. Although the maximum FDA-approved dose for gabapentin enacarbil is 600 mg, some patients benefit from doses up to 1,800 mg. Pregabalin is absorbed well at all doses, with 90% bioavailability and peak action at 1 hour, but otherwise has similar pharmacokinetics to gabapentin. All $\alpha_2\delta$ drugs are eliminated through the kidneys, so dose adjustments are required for patients with renal impairment.

REFRACTORY RESTLESS LEGS SYNDROME

RLS becomes refractory (Silber et al. 2013) when it is not resolved with first-line therapy as described earlier for chronic-persistent RLS. The most common culprit is augmentation, but other causes include intolerance and lack of effectiveness of first-line medications. If all nonpharmacological issues have been addressed and iron stores are adequate, combination therapy with lower doses of previously tried drugs including low-potency opioids (e.g., tramadol or codeine) may often be effective. However, many of these patients—especially patients with severe augmentation—may need high-potency opioids to achieve acceptable control of their RLS symptoms.

The most commonly used opioids to treat refractory RLS are methadone and oxycodone, although most of the other potent opioids may be used when necessary. When properly prescribed and monitored (Silber et al. 2018), these drugs can be very safe and extremely effective, even for severe refractory RLS. Patients should be seen on a regular basis and opioid contracts instituted with periodic drug testing. Following the recommended guidelines should prevent issues with tolerance, dependence, and addiction. Opioids should not be prescribed to patients with a history of drug abuse, and the lowest effective dose should be sought, not to exceed a morphine-equivalent dose of 60–90 mg. Once an effective dose is found, most patients have sustained relief for decades or longer with little or no increase in the opioid dose. The most common side effects are constipation and nausea, but physicians should watch out for the more severe adverse opioid effects such as respiratory depression (increase in obstructive and especially central sleep apnea; caution is advised in patients with chronic obstructive pulmonary disease who are more prone to respiratory depression), CNS issues such as sedation and dizziness, and tolerance or dependence. Due to concerns with QT interval prolongation, patients taking methadone should have a baseline electrocardiogram, and other drugs that prolong QT intervals should be used with caution.

TREATMENT OF PERIODIC LIMB MOVEMENTS

Because true PLMD is quite rare, management of this disorder is not often required. Although the most effective therapy for reducing PLMs are the dopamine agonists, many patients with PLMD may actually have an early form of RLS and thus are prone to develop both RLS and PLM augmentation. When needed, $\alpha_2\delta$ ligands may not reduce the total PLMs as much as dopamine agonists, but they produce comparable reductions of the PLMs associated with arousals.

The most common complaint about the PLMs come from the patient's bed partner. As such, a better remedy is separate beds, with an inch or so between them, or a king-size bed with a memory foam mattress.

Conclusion

Most of the psychotropic drugs tend to worsen RLS symptoms. Doctors treating depression, anxiety, and other psychiatric disorders should be keenly aware of the diagnosis and treatment of RLS. Currently available treatments should control RLS symptoms in the vast majority of patients, even with concurrent use of exacerbating psychiatric medications. Some experts consider RLS to be a disorder of insufficient iron in the brain; therefore iron therapy, including intravenous iron, can be a very effective tool for treating even difficult RLS cases. Research is being done to determine the cause of decreased brain iron levels in patients with RLS and how to deliver iron more effectively to the brain. Current research in RLS treatment involves interacting with the adenosine system using drugs such as dipyridamole to help decrease the need for dopamine agonist or opioid drugs.

KEY CLINICAL POINTS

- If significant depression or anxiety presents after the onset of moderate to severe restless legs syndrome (RLS) symptoms, it is likely that successful treatment of RLS will lead to complete remission of the depression/anxiety without the need for any antidepressant or anxiolytic drugs.

- If significant depression or anxiety precedes the onset of RLS symptoms, the medications used to treat these disorders should be maintained at their lowest effective dose even if they exacerbate the RLS, with the knowledge that more aggressive RLS treatment may be needed.

- Check iron and ferritin levels in all patients with RLS, even if they have normal hemoglobin levels, because low iron or ferritin levels is a common finding in RLS. Iron supplementation, especially intravenously, may dramatically improve RLS symptoms. Oral iron should be taken only once daily.

- Consider augmentation whenever a patient who has been on stable dopamine agonist treatment for at least 6 months requests more medication.

- When initiating daily therapy for patients with chronic-persistent RLS, consider first-line therapy with an $\alpha_2\delta$ drug or the rotigotine patch rather than short-acting dopamine agonists.

- When prescribing short-acting dopamine agonists, do not exceed FDA limits and, even better, consider lower maximum doses of pramipexole at 0.25 mg and ropinirole at 1 mg.

- Remember to question patients taking dopamine agonists diligently and repeatedly about impulse-control disorders, because these are often hard to diagnose and can result in disastrous consequences.

- Although RLS should be ruled out whenever increased periodic limb movements are found on a sleep study, these are not diagnostic of RLS and are more likely due to another disorder or medication.

References

Allen RP, Earley CJ: Augmentation of the restless legs syndrome with carbidopa/levodopa. Sleep 19(3):205–213, 1996 8723377

Allen RP, Picchietti D, Hening WA, et al: Restless legs syndrome: diagnostic criteria, special considerations, and epidemiology. Sleep Med 4(2):101–119, 2003 14592341

Allen RP, Walters AS, Montplaisir J, et al: Restless legs syndrome prevalence and impact: REST general population study. Arch Intern Med 165(11):1286–1292, 2005 15956009

Allen RP, Ondo WG, Ball E, et al: Restless legs syndrome (RLS) augmentation associated with dopamine agonist and levodopa usage in a community sample. Sleep Med 12(5):431–439, 2011 21493132

Allen RP, Barker PB, Horská A, Earley CJ: Thalamic glutamate/glutamine in restless legs syndrome: increased and related to disturbed sleep. Neurology 80(22):2028–2034, 2013 23624560

Allen RP, Chen C, Garcia-Borreguero D, et al: Comparison of pregabalin with pramipexole for restless legs syndrome. N Engl J Med 370(7):621–631, 2014a 24521108

Allen RP, Picchietti DL, Garcia-Borreguero D, et al: Restless legs syndrome/Willis-Ekbom disease diagnostic criteria: updated International Restless Legs Syndrome Study Group (IRLSSG) consensus criteria—history, rationale, description, and significance. Sleep Med 15(8):860–873, 2014b 25023924

Allen RP, Picchietti DL, Auerbach M, et al: Evidence-based and consensus clinical practice guidelines for the iron treatment of restless legs syndrome/Willis-Ekbom disease in adults and children: an IRLSSG task force report. Sleep Med 41:27–44, 2018 29425576

American Academy of Sleep Medicine: International Classification of Sleep Disorders, 3rd Edition. Darien, IL, American Academy of Sleep Medicine, 2014

Batool-Anwar S, Li Y, De Vito K, et al: Lifestyle factors and risk of restless legs syndrome: prospective cohort study. J Clin Sleep Med 12(2):187–194, 2016 26446243

Burbank F, Buchfuhrer MJ, Kopjar B: Sleep improvement for restless legs syndrome patients. Part 1: pooled analysis of two prospective, double-blind, sham-controlled, multi-center, randomized clinical studies of the effects of vibrating pads on RLS symptoms. J Parkinsonism Restless Legs Syndrome 13(3):1–10, 2013

Dinkins ML, Lallemand P, Clemens S: Long-term treatment with dopamine D_3 receptor agonists induces a behavioral switch that can be rescued by blocking the dopamine D_1 receptor. Sleep Med 40:47–52, 2017 29221778

Ferré S, Quiroz C, Guitart X, et al: Pivotal role of adenosine neurotransmission in restless legs syndrome. Front Neurosci 11:722, 2018 29358902

Garcia-Borreguero D, Kohnen R, Boothby L, et al: Validation of the multiple suggested immobilization test: a test for the assessment of severity of restless legs syndrome (Willis-Ekbom disease). Sleep (Basel) 36(7):1101–1109, 2013 23814348

Garcia-Borreguero D, Silber MH, Winkelman JW, et al: Guidelines for the first-line treatment of restless legs syndrome/Willis-Ekbom disease, prevention and treatment of dopaminergic augmentation: a combined task force of the IRLSSG, EURLSSG, and the RLS-foundation. Sleep Med 21:1–11, 2016 27448465

Garcia-Borreguero D, Guitart X, Garcia Malo C, et al: Treatment of restless legs syndrome/Willis-Ekbom disease with the non-selective ENT1/ENT2 inhibitor dipyridamole: testing the adenosine hypothesis. Sleep Med 45:94–97, 2018 29680437

Gupta R, Ulfberg J, Allen RP, et al: High prevalence of restless legs syndrome/Willis Ekbom disease (RLS/WED) among people living at high altitude in the Indian Himalaya. Sleep Med 35:7–11, 2017 28619185

Howell MJ, Schenck CH: Restless nocturnal eating: a common feature of Willis-Ekbom syndrome (RLS). J Clin Sleep Med 8(4):413–419, 2012 22893772

Kuhn PJ, Olson DJ, Sullivan JP: Targeted pressure on abductor hallucis and flexor hallucis brevis muscles to manage moderate to severe primary restless legs syndrome. J Am Osteopath Assoc 116(7):440–450, 2016 27367949

Li Y, Mirzaei F, O'Reilly EJ, et al: Prospective study of restless legs syndrome and risk of depression in women. Am J Epidemiol 176(4):279–288, 2012 22805376

Ohayon MM, O'Hara R, Vitiello MV: Epidemiology of restless legs syndrome: a synthesis of the literature. Sleep Med Rev 16(4):283–295, 2012 21795081

Para KS, Chow CA, Nalamada K, et al: Suicidal thought and behavior in individuals with restless legs syndrome. Sleep Med 54:1–7, 2019 30529070

Picchietti D, Winkelman JW: Restless legs syndrome, periodic limb movements in sleep, and depression. Sleep 28(7):891–898, 2005 16124671

Picchietti D, Allen RP, Walters AS, et al: Restless legs syndrome: prevalence and impact in children and adolescents—the Peds REST study. Pediatrics 120(2):253–266, 2007 17671050

Rivera-Oliver M, Moreno E, Álvarez-Bagnarol Y, et al: Adenosine A_1-dopamine D_1 receptor heteromers control the excitability of the spinal motoneuron. Mol Neurobiol 56(2):797–811, 2019 29797183

Silber MH, Becker PM, Earley C, et al: Willis-Ekbom Disease Foundation revised consensus statement on the management of restless legs syndrome. Mayo Clin Proc 88(9):977–986, 2013 24001490

Silber MH, Becker PM, Buchfuhrer MJ, et al: The appropriate use of opioids in the treatment of refractory restless legs syndrome. Mayo Clin Proc 93(1):59–67, 2018 29304922

Stiasny-Kolster K, Kohnen R, Möller JC, et al: Validation of the "L-DOPA test" for diagnosis of restless legs syndrome. Mov Disord 21(9):1333–1339, 2006 16705685

Walters AS, LeBrocq C, Dhar A, et al: Validation of the International Restless Legs Syndrome Study Group rating scale for restless legs syndrome. Sleep Med 4(2):121–132, 2003 14592342

Winkelmann J, Prager M, Lieb R, et al: "Anxietas tibiarum." Depression and anxiety disorders in patients with restless legs syndrome. J Neurol 252(1):67–71, 2005 15654556

CHAPTER 18

Other Sleep-Related Movement Disorders

Ambra Stefani, M.D.

Birgit Högl, M.D.

This chapter discusses sleep-related movement disorders other than restless legs syndrome (RLS) and periodic limb movements, which are presented in Chapter 17. Sleep-related movement disorders are a heterogeneous group of disorders including sleep-related leg cramps (SRLC), sleep-related bruxism (SRB), sleep-related rhythmic movement disorder (SRRMD), and propriospinal myoclonus (PSM) at sleep onset. In addition, some entities currently listed as "isolated symptoms and normal variants" within the section on sleep-related movement disorders in the *International Classification of Sleep Disorders*, 3rd Edition (ICSD-3; American Academy of Sleep Medicine 2014b), such as excessive fragmentary myoclonus (EFM), hypnagogic foot tremor, and alternating leg muscle activation, as well as hypnic jerks, are briefly covered here. Finally, some other sleep-related movement variants, often either accidental findings during polysomnography or of unknown significance and not currently listed in the ICSD-3, are briefly mentioned, namely, neck myoclonus (head jerks) during REM sleep and high-frequency leg movements.

Sleep-Related Leg Cramps

SRLC, also known as nocturnal leg cramps, are a frequent sleep-related movement disorder characterized by painful contractions of the small muscles of the calves and minor foot muscles.

DIAGNOSTIC CRITERIA

According to ICSD-3, a positive diagnosis of SRLC requires all three of the following criteria to be met:

1. Painful sensation in the leg or foot and sudden, involuntary muscle hardness or tightness, indicating a strong muscle contraction.
2. Painful muscle contractions occur during time in bed, although they may arise from either wakefulness or sleep.
3. Pain is relieved by forceful stretching of affected muscles, thus releasing the contraction.

PATHOPHYSIOLOGY

The pathophysiology of SRLC is mostly unknown. Electromyography undertaken during SRLC shows high-frequency discharges of up to 300 per second. SRLC can occur spontaneously or be triggered by certain conditions such as physical exhaustion, dehydration, pregnancy, or prediabetic metabolism (American Academy of Sleep Medicine 2014a). Family patterns or genetic risk factors are not known.

EPIDEMIOLOGY

SRLC have a reported prevalence of approximately 7% in children that increases with age to about 30%–50% in those older than 60 years (American Academy of Sleep Medicine 2014b). Most affected individuals report only occasional leg cramps, but in those 60 years of age and older, the prevalence of cramps occurring every night or even several times during the same night can be as high as 6% (American Academy of Sleep Medicine 2014a). Some studies have reported a seasonal variability, with increased SRLC during the summer (Garrison et al. 2015). No sex prevalence has been reported, and geographical differences have not been adequately studied. A cross-sectional epidemiological study in the United States found no racial differences in the two cohorts they investigated. Interestingly, in one cohort, Hispanic/Latino ethnicity was found to be protective (OR 0.65, 95% CI 0.46–0.91, $P=0.013$) after full adjustments for health and demographic variables (Grandner and Winkelman 2017).

CLINICAL PRESENTATION, COURSE, AND COMPLICATIONS

The typical clinical presentation of SRLC is a sudden and very painful contraction of the calf or small foot muscles, with onset during self-perceived wakefulness or sleep and a visible and palpable hardening of the affected muscles and abnormal positioning due to the muscle contraction. Cessation of an individual muscle cramp is often spontaneous or can be achieved with passive extension of the affected muscles. Cramps can last for up to several minutes and are sometimes followed by prolonged wakefulness. SRLC can cause frequent awakenings because they require the person to get out of bed and stand in order to use the affected muscles or to apply hot or warm water. It ensues, therefore, that leg cramps can be associated with severe insomnia (Grandner and Winkelman 2017). When leg cramps are very frequent and lead to sleep impairment, quality of life may be severely impaired.

DIFFERENTIAL DIAGNOSIS

Primary SRLC can usually be diagnosed by presenting clinical features alone; however, in patients who have a language barrier with the physician or a speech or cognitive impairment, history taking may be difficult. RLS and myopathies, myotonic dystrophy, and peripheral neuropathies need to be considered in the differential diagnosis, but SRLC can also occur in association with these disorders and in that case need to be investigated in more detail. RLS has typical clinical features that allow differentiation from SRLC, and a painful muscle contraction is not present in RLS (see Chapter 17).

Dystonia (e.g., early morning dystonia in Parkinson's disease), stiff-person syndrome, and painful legs and moving toes are also part of the differential diagnosis. Muscle contraction of dystonia is sustained or repetitive, whereas SRLC usually cease spontaneously and do not last more than several minutes. Early morning dystonia typically occurs upon awakening and not during sleep.

Stiff-person syndrome is characterized by severe muscle stiffness and painful spasms involving more muscle groups, usually the trunk and limbs, which lead to an impairment of daily activities.

Painful legs and moving toes is a syndrome characterized by pain in the legs and spontaneous movements of the toes. The involuntary movements of the toes, as well as the occurrence of other symptoms, also happens during the daytime, allowing distinction from SRLC.

If SRLC worsen following physical effort, cramp fasciculation syndrome should be considered.

TREATMENT

In most cases, SRLC will cease spontaneously or with passive physical stretching. Although magnesium has been used in the past to relieve muscle cramps, no quality evidence supports this. A recent double-blind, randomized controlled treatment study failed to find magnesium efficacious (Roguin Maor et al. 2017).

Quinine sulfate treatment has been reported to be efficacious, but the FDA does not recommend treatment with quinine sulfate because of the risk of cardiac arrhythmias and hematological adverse effects (El-Tawil et al. 2015; Rabbitt et al. 2016; Roguin Maor et al. 2017). Regarding non-pharmacological approaches, prophylactic stretching has been reported to prevent nocturnal leg cramps, but evidence is conflicting (Blyton et al. 2012; Hallegraeff et al. 2012).

Sleep-Related Bruxism

DIAGNOSTIC CRITERIA

ICSD-3 lists the following diagnostic criteria for SRB, all of which must be met:

1. Presence of regular or frequent tooth grinding sounds occurring during sleep
2. Presence of one or both of the following clinical signs:
   - Abnormal tooth wear consistent with reports of teeth grinding during sleep
   - Transient morning jaw muscle pain or fatigue or temporal headache or jaw locking upon awakening consistent with reports of teeth grinding during sleep

PATHOPHYSIOLOGY

In the historical literature, malocclusion, psychosocial components, and genetic predisposing factors have been discussed as contributing to the pathophysiology of bruxism. However, for malocclusion such an association has yet to be proven.

What has been established is the fact that SRB episodes occur mostly during non-REM (NREM) stages 1 and 2 and are temporally associated with arousals (American Academy of Sleep Medicine 2014b). This is not only true for arousals due to sleep-disordered breathing but also for arousals related to gastroesophageal reflux (Cruz-Fierro et al. 2018). Along these lines, experimental esophageal acidification was shown to induce SRB in these cases (Ohmure et al. 2011).

EPIDEMIOLOGY

The prevalence of SRB has been reported to be highest during childhood (between 14% and 17%; American Academy of Sleep Medicine 2014b) and to decrease thereafter with age. Nevertheless, the reported prevalence in the general population needs to be interpreted with caution, because only a few prevalence studies have performed polysomnography, and prevalence rates reported based on questionnaire alone differ greatly from those reported following confirmation by polysomnogram (12% vs. 5.5%, respectively; Maluly et al. 2013). A recent online survey of a large sample of 6,357 individuals that assessed the prevalence of SRB in Quebec, Canada, reported a prevalence of 8.6% in the general population, a decrease with age, and no sex differences (Khoury et al. 2016). Clinically, SRB was associated with disorders of sleep maintenance in almost one-half of the individuals, and one-third reported pain associated with SRB.

Among schoolchildren in Brazil, the prevalence of probable SRB was reported to be higher in older children with mixed dentition than in those with primary dentition (Massignan et al. 2019). Interestingly, a study comparing parent-reported SRB among 7- to 12-year-olds from the Netherlands, Armenia, and Indonesia found that the overall prevalence of parent-reported SRB was significantly higher in Armenia compared with the Netherlands and Indonesia (van Selms et al. 2019). However, the use of different questionnaires or interviews to evaluate SRB and lack of polysomnography somewhat limit the comparability of results from the large number of studies carried out in different parts of the world.

RISK FACTORS

Among risk factors that can induce or aggravate SRB, both drug use and abuse have been reported (Bertazzo-Silveira et al. 2016). SRB has been associated with methamphetamine and stimulant use or abuse (in the context of "methamphetamine mouth," SRB is concomitant with damage to mucosa and teeth) as well as with the use of dopaminergic drugs (Mukherjee et al. 2018). The mechanism behind the association of SRB with these drugs could be arousals during sleep. Furthermore, an association with obstructive sleep apnea has been reported (see Chapters 8 and 9) (Ferreira et al. 2015), and an association with malocclusion is still under debate (Flores-Mir et al. 2013).

Craniocervical dystonia is not only in the differential diagnosis but also can be associated with SRB (Borie et al. 2016).

FAMILIAL PATTERNS AND GENETICS

Individuals with SRB have a 2.5 risk ratio of having a first-degree family member with SRB (diagnosed via questionnaire and reported by the individuals themselves); an even higher 4.6 relative risk ratio was found in individuals with SRB who underwent polysomnographic validation (Khoury et al. 2016).

A review of the literature on SRB and genetics retrieves mostly family studies, a few twin studies, and only one study that includes genetic analysis (Lobbezoo et al. 2014). Thus, despite family studies pointing toward genetic contributions, the exact genes, genetic variants, or other factors have not been fully elucidated. However, studies have shown that the C allele carrier of the serotonin 2A receptor (*HTR2A*) single nucleotide polymorphism rs6313 is associated with an increased risk of SRB (Abe et al. 2012; Hoashi et al. 2017). Interestingly, the G allele of *DRD2* rs1800497 is associated with risk reduction of awake and sleep bruxism, the C allele of *DRD3* rs6280 with increased risk of SRB, and the C allele of *DRD5* rs6283 with decreased risk of awake bruxism (Oporto et al. 2018). This is particularly interesting in light of circadian variations in dopamine, which are relevant also in other sleep-related movement disorders such as RLS (see Chapter 17). A possible role of epigenetics has also been considered (Calic and Peterlin 2015).

CLINICAL PRESENTATION, COURSE, AND COMPLICATIONS

In this chapter we only discuss *sleep* bruxism, not *awake* bruxism, which is a distinct circadian manifestation. SRB can manifest as repetitive grinding or sustained jaw clenching. A bed partner disturbed by the grinding sounds or a dentist noting abnormal tooth wear is usually the first to notice or suspect SRB. Although it can accompany sleep maintenance and other disorders, SRB often goes unnoticed by the patients themselves unless dental wear, jaw joint problems or evaluation of morning jaw, or headache problems lead to a polysomnographic evaluation.

Isolated SRB is not a progressive disorder, and prevalence decreases with age. Nevertheless, tooth damage, jaw problems, and morning headaches can be associated with SRB.

Severe dental and oral complications, such as dental fractures and mucosal damage, are very rare in primary bruxism but can be present in bruxism-associated drug abuse, such as "methamphetamine mouth."

DIAGNOSTIC PROCEDURES, TESTS, AND QUESTIONNAIRES

Any history taking in SRB is usually straightforward but relies on proxy reports. Patients are asked about whether they have ever been told they make grinding sounds while sleeping. Additionally, home smartphone recording with a sound-activated recording app can be useful. Although polysomnography is not obligatory, it is recommended to definitively confirm the diagnosis and to evaluate or rule out any associated sleep-disordered breathing or sleep fragmentation. In addition to the standard recording, in which SRB can often be recognized by electromyographic activation in the mental/submental muscles or rhythmic movement artifacts in the electroencephalographic leads, for specific diagnosis of SRB, additional surface electromyographic leads over the masseter and temporalis muscles as well as time-synchronized video and audio recording are recommended (American Academy of Sleep Medicine 2014b, 2018). Dental status should involve investigation and documentation of any damage, such as dental fractures.

DIFFERENTIAL DIAGNOSIS

SRB needs to be differentiated from epileptic seizures as well as other disorders, such as dystonic syndromes, Meige syndrome, or faciomandibular dyskinesias in patients with Parkinson's disease.

TREATMENT

The most important treatment approach in SRB is use of an individually crafted dental splint to protect the teeth from abnormal wear and damage, because the force the teeth are exposed to in SRB can lead to tooth cracking and fractures. Evidence on the efficacy of most other treatment approaches used for bruxism is limited, including antidepressants, dopaminergic treatment, and clonazepam. Also, evidence of the usefulness of other potential treatment approaches, such as contingent electrical stimulation of the upper lip and botulinum toxin injections into the masseter muscles, is also very limited (De la Torre Canales et al. 2017; Guaita and Högl 2016), although a recent randomized, placebo-controlled, parallel-design trial reported subjective improvement with botulinum injections into the masseter and temporalis muscles (Ondo et al. 2018).

SRB has been reported as an adverse event of certain medications, including the selective serotonin reuptake inhibitors, selective serotonin-norepinephrine reuptake inhibitors, and antipsychotics (Guaita and Högl 2016), and if such an association is suspected, these medications should be withdrawn if possible. In cases of SRB associated with gastroesophageal reflux, a preliminary pilot study showed that a proton pump inhibitor can be efficacious (Ohmure et al. 2016).

Sleep-Related Rhythmic Movement Disorder

SRRMD is also well known by its alternate names: body rocking, body rolling, head banging, head rolling, and *jactatio capitis nocturna*. The following diagnostic criteria must be met for a positive diagnosis (American Academy of Sleep Medicine 2014b):

1. Patient exhibits repetitive, stereotyped, and rhythmic motor behaviors involving large muscle groups.
2. Movements are predominantly sleep-related, occurring near nap or bedtime or when individual appears drowsy or sleepy.
3. Movement behaviors result in significant complaints that are manifest by at least one of the following:

   - Interference with normal sleep
   - Significant impairment in daytime function
   - Self-inflicted body injury or likelihood of injury if preventive measures are not used

4. Rhythmic movements are not better explained by another movement disorder or epilepsy.

ICSD-3 further notes that when the rhythmic movements have no clinical consequences, they are noted but the term *rhythmic movement disorder* is not employed.

EPIDEMIOLOGY

Rhythmic movements during sleep are highly prevalent in infants until the age of 9 months and in one-third of toddlers at 18 months. At the age of 5 years, only 5% of children still exhibit rhythmic movement during sleep, but the phenomenon is not considered a disorder. The term *rhythmic movement disorder* is used only when clinical consequences arise or movements persist into adulthood. The prevalence of rhythmic movements in adulthood is not known. Because of the ubiquity of rhythmic movements in infants and toddlers, a soothing effect of the movement or its contribution to the maturation of the vestibular system has been discussed (Cogen and Loghmanee 2014). A recent study in children found a lower prevalence (maximum 2.87%) when a standardized clinical questionnaire and 3 nights of home video polysomnography were used. This study also reported a male-to-female ratio of 5:3 in cases of confirmed SRRMD (Gogo et al. 2019). A male preponderance has been reported in adults as well (Mayer et al. 2007). Prevalence decreases from childhood to adulthood. A progressive course has not been reported.

RISK FACTORS

SRRMD has been reported in association with obstructive sleep apnea (Chiaro et al. 2017; Chirakalwasan et al. 2009; Mayer et al. 2007), REM sleep behavior disorder (Manni and Terzaghi 2007; Yeh and Schenck 2012), RLS (Lombardi et al. 2003; Walters et al. 1988), insomnia (Attarian et al. 2009), and ADHD (Walters et al. 2008).

FAMILIAL PATTERNS AND GENETICS

In at least a few cases, a genetic predisposition to SRRMD has been suggested (Attarian et al. 2009; Hayward-Koennecke et al. 2019). However, the potential contribution of genetic factors still needs to be investigated.

CLINICAL PRESENTATION, COURSE, AND COMPLICATIONS

The clinical presentation of SRRMD can manifest as head banging, body rocking, or body rolling. Involvement of large muscle groups is a common aspect of all these, as is the repetitiveness of the movements (often involving the trunk or neck muscles), with a slow repetitive movement frequency of approximately 0.5–2 Hz per second. The movement sequences appear during wakefulness or in the transition from wakefulness to sleep or reappear during short awakenings or arousals from sleep. Complications have been rarely reported, ranging from subdural hematoma to carotid artery dissection.

DIAGNOSTIC PROCEDURES, TESTS, AND QUESTIONNAIRES

Because the classical diagnostic criteria are quite characteristic, short video documentation of the SRRMD in question may be useful. Specific telephone interviews have been used, and standardized clinical questionnaires have also been developed (Gogo et al. 2019).

DIFFERENTIAL DIAGNOSIS

All other types of sleep-related movement disorders and parasomnias, as well as epilepsy and stereotypies or tics during wakefulness, must be differentiated from SRRMD. If polysomnography is used, sequences of at least four movements with a frequency between 0.5 and 2 Hz should be looked for (American Academy of Sleep Medicine 2018).

TREATMENT

No double-blind, placebo-controlled treatment outcomes have been reported; only anecdotal reports with tricyclic antidepressants or benzodiazepine receptor agonists are available. One study from Israel showed a controlled restriction of sleep time that increases the sleep pressure and thus decreases sleep latency can be useful (Etzioni et al. 2005).

Propriospinal Myoclonus at Sleep Onset

DIAGNOSTIC CRITERIA

PSM is still a heavily debated entity. Diagnostic criteria include the following (American Academy of Sleep Medicine 2014b):

1. Patient complains of sudden jerks, mainly of the abdomen, trunk, and neck.
2. The jerks appear during relaxed wakefulness and drowsiness, as patient attempts to fall asleep.
3. The jerks disappear upon mental activation and with onset of stable sleep stage.
4. The jerks result in difficulty initiating sleep.
5. Disorder is not better explained by another sleep disorder, medical or neurological disorder, mental disorder, medication use, or substance use disorder.

PATHOPHYSIOLOGY

The pathophysiological mechanisms of PSM are unclear. A similar phenomenon, called *propriospinal myoclonus during wakefulness*, has demonstrated that most of the events apparently have a functional origin because the jerks are preceded by "Bereitschaftspotential" (readiness potential), which refutes an involuntary genesis of the movement (Erro et al. 2013; Esposito et al. 2014; van der Salm et al. 2014). It remains to be determined what percentage of suspected PSM in sleep-onset cases will also be shown to have a functional origin. On the other hand, it is not known if PSM at sleep onset might be symptomatic in some patients, because in other cases of symptomatic PSM (non–sleep related), lesions (myelopathy associated with antithyroid autoantibodies, low back trauma, lymphocytic myelomeningitis, thoracic disc hernia, cervical and thoracic lesions) and complications from progression of the underlying disease could be suspected (Manconi et al. 2005; Roze et al. 2009).

EPIDEMIOLOGY

The prevalence is unknown.

RISK FACTORS

Risk factors are unknown.

FAMILIAL PATTERN/GENETICS

Any familial patterns or genetic causes are unknown.

CLINICAL PRESENTATION, COURSE, AND COMPLICATIONS

PSM at sleep onset was described by Vetrugno and colleagues almost 20 years ago (Montagna et al. 2006). They observed sudden jerks of the trunk and the body, appearing in the transition from wakefulness to sleep, that ceased upon sleep onset. In multichannel electromyographic recording performed along with polysomnography, they were able to show that the jerks and electromyographic activation initiated from the midthoracic or abdominal muscles. It propagated from the initially involved muscles rostrally and caudally, with a propagation speed in line with propriospinal conduction (Montagna et al. 2006). PSM at sleep onset was only added to ICSD-3 in 2014 under the sleep-related movement disorders.

DIAGNOSTIC PROCEDURES, TESTS, AND QUESTIONNAIRES

In cases of suspected PSM at sleep onset, the following diagnostic procedures are required to confirm the diagnosis and rule out other diagnoses and a functional genesis:

1. Polysomnogram with multichannel electromyographic recording to demonstrate

   - Consistent onset of electromyographic activation in the midthoracic and midabdominal muscle segments
   - Typical propagation

2. Back averaging to exclude "Bereitschaftspotential"
3. Spinal MRI to exclude spinal cord lesions

DIFFERENTIAL DIAGNOSIS

The most important differential diagnosis is intensified periodic limb movements, which are sometimes seen in patients with dopaminergic-treated RLS or RLS augmentation as discussed in Chapter 17 (Mitterling et al. 2014). Also, hypnic jerks can be intensified and interfere with sleep onset (Calandra-Buonaura et al. 2014). Myoclonic events related to other extrapyramidal or epileptic disorders more rarely constitute a relevant differential diagnosis.

TREATMENT

In patients for whom the jerks interfere with sleep onset, a response to clonazepam has been reported (Antelmi and Provini 2015; Byun et al. 2017; Stefani and Högl 2019). However, due to the suspicion that many of these cases may be due to functional genesis, the diagnosis needs to be confirmed before clonazepam treatment is started.

Other Minor Movement Disorders of Sleep

Several other movement disorders of sleep are described in ICSD-3 for which the clinical relevance is unknown (American Academy of Sleep Medicine 2014b). Excessive fragmentary myoclonus, hypnagogic foot tremor, and alternating leg muscle activation are now listed in the ICSD-3 as a subcategory of "isolated symptoms and normal variants" within the sleep-related movement disorders section. Some movement disorders not yet described in ICSD-3 include high-frequency leg movements and REM-related head jerks (neck myoclonus).

EXCESSIVE FRAGMENTARY MYOCLONUS

EFM is often an accidental polysomnographic finding on the tibialis anterior muscle surface electromyogram observed in NREM sleep. According to the American Academy of Sleep Medicine scoring manual, the following define EFM (American Academy of Sleep Medicine 2018):

- Usual maximum electromyographic burst duration of 150 msec
- At least 20 minutes of EFM in NREM sleep
- At least five electromyographic potentials per minute

Nevertheless, it needs to be acknowledged that these diagnostic criteria are not based on large enough independent data sets but rather on an arbitrary definition of a historical convenience sample (Broughton et al. 1985; Raccagni et al. 2016). More recent studies have shown that EFM is almost ubiquitous in a large clinical cohort (Frauscher et al. 2011) and even in a healthy population, where 9% have been reported to meet these criteria for EFM (Frauscher et al. 2014). This suggests that although EFM might be a normal variant on the one hand, on the other the historical arbitrary cutoff is too low and will need to be revised in subsequent versions of the ICSD.

During differential diagnosis of EFM in the tibialis anterior muscle, the physician must remember that at least half of patients with EFM have peripheral neuropathy, L5 nerve root lesions, and benign fasciculations (Raccagni et al. 2016). Twitches that are reminiscent of EFM but only occur during REM sleep can be found in small amounts in normal REM sleep and in large amounts in REM sleep behavior disorder (see Chapter 15) (Högl et al. 2018; McCarter et al. 2014; Nepoticek et al. 2019).

HYPNAGOGIC FOOT TREMOR, ALTERNATING LEG MUSCLE ACTIVATION, AND HIGH-FREQUENCY LEG MOVEMENTS

Hypnagogic foot tremor, alternating leg muscle activation, and high-frequency leg movements all represent other "minor motor findings during polysomnogram" that are of unknown clinical significance and seem to belong to the same group of often ancillary findings, although some have been integrated into the ICSD.

Hypnagogic foot tremor was first described by Broughton in 1985 and defined as "grouped phasic tremor potentials at varying frequencies between 0.5 and 1.5 per second, recorded in general, independently from both anterior tibialis muscles, more so on the right" (Broughton et al. 1985). Alternating leg muscle activation was defined by Chervin et al. (2003) as an "alternating pattern of anterior tibialis activation." These two diagnoses have been added to the ICSD-3 (American Academy of Sleep Medicine 2014b). High-frequency leg movements, described by Yang and Winkelman (2010), have not yet been added.

A case report highlighted the similarities, more than the differences, of these three phenomena and suggested using the single and more generic term "high-frequency leg movements" for all of them (Bergmann et al. 2019). Discussion has also addressed whether the appearance of these minor repetitive movements on polysomnography during wakefulness or drowsiness should prompt questioning about undiagnosed RLS (Bergmann et al. 2019), because leg discomfort and the urge to move could produce such a pattern on a polysomnogram (as well as other movements, such as rhythmic tapping or scratching itchy skin).

HEAD JERKS: NECK MYOCLONUS DURING REM SLEEP

Neck myoclonus during REM sleep was defined in 2010 and is characterized by typical "stripe-shaped" movement-induced artifacts visible vertically over electroencephalographic leads in the polysomnogram, with a duration up to 2 seconds (Frauscher et al. 2010). In the original work describing neck myoclonus, this phenomenon was present in 54.6% of subjects (Frauscher et al. 2010). It was so frequent during REM sleep that in this sleep stage it was considered a physiological phenomenon. In a cohort of 100 healthy sleepers, neck myoclonus was present in 35% (Frauscher et al. 2014). It seems to be a physiological phenomenon that is part of the spectrum of physiological twitching during REM sleep.

Conclusion

Sleep-related movement disorders are a heterogeneous group of disorders and findings of unknown significance. Some are not currently listed in the ICSD-3; their clinical relevance, as well as their prevalence, needs to be further elucidated in future studies.

KEY CLINICAL POINTS

- Sleep-related movement disorders may be an incidental finding during polysomnography or may represent the reason for referral if they cause sleep disturbances.

- Sleep-related leg cramps are usually isolated. However, if 1) they occur very frequently, 2) are present during both daytime and nighttime, 3) occur not only in the legs but also in the upper extremities, or 4) other neurological symptoms, other neurological disorders (e.g., myopathies, myotonic dystrophy), or peripheral neuropathies are present, they need to be actively investigated and excluded.

- Sleep bruxism is a common sleep-related movement disorder. Protection of teeth against mechanical damage using a dental splint is recommended. Recently, understanding of genetic contributions has advanced with reports that the C allele carrier of serotonin 2A receptor (HTR2A) single nucleotide polymorphism rs6313 is associated with an increased risk of sleep bruxism.

- Propriospinal myoclonus during wakefulness seems to have a functional origin in most cases, as demonstrated by the presence of a "Bereitschaftspotential." It still has to be determined whether this is the case also for propriospinal myoclonus at sleep onset.

- The incidental finding of excessive fragmentary myoclonus during polysomnography may be associated with alterations in peripheral nerve function.

- Hypnagogic foot tremor, alternating leg muscle activation, and high-frequency leg movements are similar conditions with overlapping characteristics. They would likely be better classified as a single phenomenon.

- Neck myoclonus seems to be mostly a physiological condition during REM sleep. However, cutoffs have not yet been defined, and it is still not clear when it should be considered pathological (e.g., in cases of REM sleep behavior disorder presenting mainly with "excessive" neck myoclonus).

References

Abe Y, Suganuma T, Ishii M, et al: Association of genetic, psychological and behavioral factors with sleep bruxism in a Japanese population. J Sleep Res 21(3):289–296, 2012 22545912

American Academy of Sleep Medicine: AASM Manual for the Scoring of Sleep and Associated Events, Version 2.1. Darien, IL, American Academy of Sleep Medicine, 2014a

American Academy of Sleep Medicine: International Classification of Sleep Disorders, 3rd Edition. Darien, IL, American Academy of Sleep Medicine, 2014b

American Academy of Sleep Medicine: AASM Manual for the Scoring of Sleep and Associated Events, Version 2.5. Darien, IL, American Academy of Sleep Medicine, 2018

Antelmi E, Provini F: Propriospinal myoclonus: the spectrum of clinical and neurophysiological phenotypes. Sleep Med Rev 22:54–63, 2015 25500332

Attarian H, Ward N, Schuman C: A multigenerational family with persistent sleep related rhythmic movement disorder (RMD) and insomnia. J Clin Sleep Med 5(6):571–572, 2009 20465026

Bergmann M, Stefani A, Brandauer E, et al: Hypnagogic foot tremor, alternating leg muscle activation or high frequency leg movements: clinical and phenomenological considerations in two cousins. Sleep Med 54:177–180, 2019 30580191

Bertazzo-Silveira E, Kruger CM, Porto De Toledo I, et al: Association between sleep bruxism and alcohol, caffeine, tobacco, and drug abuse: a systematic review. J Am Dent Assoc 147(11):859–866, 2016

Blyton F, Chuter V, Walter KE, et al: Non-drug therapies for lower limb muscle cramps. Cochrane Database Syst Rev 1:CD008496, 2012 22258986

Borie L, Langbour N, Guehl D, et al: Bruxism in craniocervical dystonia: a prospective study. Cranio 34(5):291–295, 2016 26884222

Broughton R, Tolentino MA, Krelina M: Excessive fragmentary myoclonus in NREM sleep: a report of 38 cases. Electroencephalogr Clin Neurophysiol 61(2):123–133, 1985 2410221

Byun JI, Lee D, Rhee HY, et al: Treatment of propriospinal myoclonus at sleep onset. J Clin Neurol 13(3):293–295, 2017 28516739

Calandra-Buonaura G, Alessandria M, Liguori R, et al: Hypnic jerks: neurophysiological characterization of a new motor pattern. Sleep Med 15(6):725–727, 2014 24815789

Calic A, Peterlin B: Epigenetics and bruxism: possible role of epigenetics in the etiology of bruxism. Int J Prosthodont 28(6):594–599, 2015 26523718

Chervin RD, Consens FB, Kutluay E: Alternating leg muscle activation during sleep and arousals: a new sleep-related motor phenomenon? Mov Disord 18(5):551–559, 2003 12722169

Chiaro G, Maestri M, Riccardi S, et al: Sleep-related rhythmic movement disorder and obstructive sleep apnea in five adult patients. J Clin Sleep Med 13(10):1213–1217, 2017 28859719

Chirakalwasan N, Hassan F, Kaplish N, et al: Near resolution of sleep related rhythmic movement disorder after CPAP for OSA. Sleep Med 10(4):497–500, 2009 19324593

Cogen JD, Loghmanee DA: Sleep-related movement disorders, in Principles and Practice of Pediatric Sleep Medicine, 2nd Edition. Edited by Sheldon SH, Ferber R, Kryger MH, et al. Philadelphia, PA, Saunders, 2014, pp 333–336

Cruz-Fierro N, Martínez-Fierro M, Cerda-Flores RM, et al: The phenotype, psychotype and genotype of bruxism. Biomed Rep 8(3):264–268, 2018 29599979

De la Torre Canales G, Câmara-Souza MB, do Amaral CF, et al: Is there enough evidence to use botulinum toxin injections for bruxism management? A systematic literature review. Clin Oral Investig 21(3):727–734, 2017 28255752

El-Tawil S, Al Musa T, Valli H, et al: Quinine for muscle cramps. Cochrane Database Syst Rev (4):CD005044, 2015 25842375

Erro R, Bhatia KP, Edwards MJ, et al: Clinical diagnosis of propriospinal myoclonus is unreliable: an electrophysiologic study. Mov Disord 28(13):1868–1873, 2013 24105950

Esposito M, Erro R, Edwards MJ, et al: The pathophysiology of symptomatic propriospinal myoclonus. Mov Disord 29(9):1097–1099, 2014 24976412

Etzioni T, Katz N, Hering E, et al: Controlled sleep restriction for rhythmic movement disorder. J Pediatr 147(3):393–395, 2005 16182683

Ferreira NM, dos Santos JF, dos Santos MB, et al: Sleep bruxism associated with obstructive sleep apnea syndrome in children. Cranio 33(4):251–255, 2015 26715296

Flores-Mir C, Korayem M, Heo G, et al: Craniofacial morphological characteristics in children with obstructive sleep apnea syndrome: a systematic review and meta-analysis. J Am Dent Assoc 144(3):269–277, 2013 23449902

Frauscher B, Brandauer E, Gschliesser V, et al: A descriptive analysis of neck myoclonus during routine polysomnography. Sleep 33(8):1091–1096, 2010 20815192

Frauscher B, Kunz A, Brandauer E, et al: Fragmentary myoclonus in sleep revisited: a polysomnographic study in 62 patients. Sleep Med 12(4):410–415, 2011 21316297

Frauscher B, Mitterling T, Bode A, et al: A prospective questionnaire study in 100 healthy sleepers: non-bothersome forms of recognizable sleep disorders are still present. J Clin Sleep Med 10(6):623–629, 2014 24932141

Garrison SR, Dormuth CR, Morrow RL, et al: Seasonal effects on the occurrence of nocturnal leg cramps: a prospective cohort study. CMAJ 187(4):248–253, 2015 25623650

Gogo E, van Sluijs RM, Cheung T, et al: Objectively confirmed prevalence of sleep-related rhythmic movement disorder in pre-school children. Sleep Med 53:16–21, 2019 30384137

Grandner MA, Winkelman JW: Nocturnal leg cramps: prevalence and associations with demographics, sleep disturbance symptoms, medical conditions, and cardiometabolic risk factors. PLoS One 12(6):e0178465, 2017 28586374

Guaita M, Högl B: Current treatments of bruxism. Curr Treat Options Neurol 18(2):10, 2016 26897026

Hallegraeff JM, van der Schans CP, de Ruiter R, et al: Stretching before sleep reduces the frequency and severity of nocturnal leg cramps in older adults: a randomised trial. J Physiother 58(1):17–22, 2012 22341378

Hayward-Koennecke HK, Werth E, Valko PO, et al: Sleep-related rhythmic movement disorder in triplets: evidence for genetic predisposition? J Clin Sleep Med 15(1):157–158, 2019 30621834

Hoashi Y, Okamoto S, Abe Y, et al: Generation of neural cells using iPSCs from sleep bruxism patients with 5-HT2A polymorphism. J Prosthodont Res 61(3):242–250, 2017 27916472

Högl B, Stefani A, Videnovic A: Idiopathic REM sleep behaviour disorder and neurodegeneration: an update. Nat Rev Neurol 14(1):40–55, 2018 29170501

Khoury S, Carra MC, Huynh N, et al: Sleep bruxism-tooth grinding prevalence, characteristics and familial aggregation: a large cross-sectional survey and polysomnographic validation. Sleep (Basel) 39(11):2049–2056, 2016 27568807

Lobbezoo F, Visscher CM, Ahlberg J, et al: Bruxism and genetics: a review of the literature. J Oral Rehabil 41(9):709–714, 2014 24762185

Lombardi C, Provini F, Vetrugno R, et al: Pelvic movements as rhythmic motor manifestation associated with restless legs syndrome. Mov Disord 18(1):110–113, 2003 12518310

Maluly M, Andersen ML, Dal-Fabbro C, et al: Polysomnographic study of the prevalence of sleep bruxism in a population sample. J Dent Res 92(7 suppl):97S–103S, 2013 23690359

Manconi M, Sferrazza B, Iannaccone S, et al: Case of symptomatic propriospinal myoclonus evolving toward acute "myoclonic status." Mov Disord 20(12):1646–1650, 2005 16092107

Manni R, Terzaghi M: Rhythmic movements in idiopathic REM sleep behavior disorder. Mov Disord 22(12):1797–1800, 2007 17580329

Massignan C, de Alencar NA, Soares JP, et al: Poor sleep quality and prevalence of probable sleep bruxism in primary and mixed dentitions: a cross-sectional study. Sleep Breath 23(3):935–941, 2019 30569316

Mayer G, Wilde-Frenz J, Kurella B: Sleep related rhythmic movement disorder revisited. J Sleep Res 16(1):110–116, 2007

McCarter SJ, St Louis EK, Boeve BF, et al: Greatest rapid eye movement sleep atonia loss in men and older age. Ann Clin Transl Neurol 1(9):733–738, 2014 25493286

Mitterling T, Frauscher B, Falkenstetter T, et al: Is there a polysomnographic signature of augmentation in restless legs syndrome? Sleep Med 15(10):1231–1240, 2014 25129261

Montagna P, Provini F, Vetrugno R: Propriospinal myoclonus at sleep onset. Neurophysiol Clin 36(5–6):351–355, 2006 17336781

Mukherjee A, Dye BA, Clague J, et al: Methamphetamine use and oral health-related quality of life. Qual Life Res 27(12):3179–3190, 2018 30076578

Nepoticek J, Dostalova S, Kemlink D: Fragmentary myoclonus in idiopathic REM sleep behavior disorder. J Sleep Res 28(4):e12819, 2019 30676675

Ohmure H, Oikawa K, Kanematsu K, et al: Influence of experimental esopha-geal acidification on sleep bruxism: a randomized trial. J Dent Res 90(5):665–671, 2011 21248360

Ohmure H, Kanematsu-Hashimoto K, Nagayama K, et al: Evaluation of a proton pump inhibitor for sleep bruxism: a randomized clinical trial. J Dent Res 95(13):1479–1486, 2016 27474257

Ondo WG, Simmons JH, Shahid MH, et al: Onabotulinum toxin-A injections for sleep bruxism: a double-blind, placebo-controlled study. Neurology 90(7):e559–e564, 2018 29343468

Oporto GHV, Bornhardt T, Iturriaga V, et al: Single nucleotide polymorphisms in genes of dopaminergic pathways are associated with bruxism. Clin Oral Investig 22(1):331–337, 2018 28451935

Rabbitt L, Mulkerrin EC, O'Keeffe ST: A review of nocturnal leg cramps in older people. Age Ageing 45(6):776–782, 2016 27515677

Raccagni C, Löscher WN, Stefani A, et al: Peripheral nerve function in patients with excessive fragmentary myoclonus during sleep. Sleep Med 22:61–64, 2016 27544838

Roguin Maor N, Alperin M, Shturman E, et al: Effect of magnesium oxide sup-plementation on nocturnal leg cramps: a randomized clinical trial. JAMA Intern Med 177(5):617–623, 2017 28241153

Roze E, Bounolleau P, Ducreux D, et al: Propriospinal myoclonus revisited: clini-cal, neurophysiologic, and neuroradiologic findings. Neurology 72(15):1301–1309, 2009 19365051

Stefani A, Högl B: Diagnostic criteria, differential diagnosis, and treatment of minor motor activity and less well-known movement disorders of sleep. Curr Treat Options Neurol 21(1):1, 2019 30661130

van der Salm SM, Erro R, Cordivari C, et al: Propriospinal myoclonus: clinical re-appraisal and review of literature. Neurology 83(20):1862–1870, 2014 25305154

van Selms MKA, Marpaung C, Pogosian A, et al: Geographical variation of parental-reported sleep bruxism among children: comparison between the Netherlands, Armenia and Indonesia. Int Dent J 69(3):237–243, 2019 30411782

Walters AS, Hening WA, Chokroverty S: Frequent occurrence of myoclonus while awake and at rest, body rocking and marching in place in a subpopulation of patients with restless legs syndrome. Acta Neurol Scand 77(5):418–421, 1988 3414379

Walters AS, Silvestri R, Zucconi M, et al: Review of the possible relationship and hypothetical links between attention deficit hyperactivity disorder (ADHD) and the simple sleep related movement disorders, parasomnias, hypersomnias, and circadian rhythm disorders. J Clin Sleep Med 4(6):591–600, 2008 19110891

Yang C, Winkelman JW: Clinical and polysomnographic characteristics of high frequency leg movements. J Clin Sleep Med 6(5):431–438, 2010 20957842

Yeh SB, Schenck CH: Atypical headbanging presentation of idiopathic sleep related rhythmic movement disorder: three cases with video-polysomnographic doc-umentation. J Clin Sleep Med 8(4):403–411, 2012 22893771

Index

Page numbers printed in **boldface** type refer to tables or figures.